THE
PESCETARIAN
PLAN

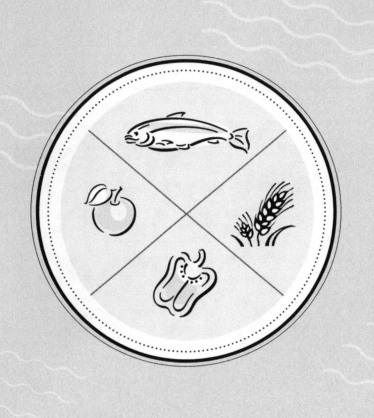

The
PESCETARIAN PLAN

The Vegetarian + Seafood Way to Lose Weight and Love Your Food

JANIS JIBRIN, M.S., R.D.

RECIPES BY **SIDRA FORMAN**

PHOTOGRAPHS BY **KATE HEADLEY**

WITHDRAWN

BALLANTINE BOOKS

NEW YORK

No book can replace the diagnostic expertise and medical advice
of a trusted physician. Please be certain to consult with your doctor
before making any decisions that affect your health,
particularly if you suffer from any medical condition or
have any symptom that may require treatment.

Copyright © 2014 by Janis Jibrin

Published in the United States by Ballantine Books,
an imprint of Random House, a division of Random House LLC,
a Penguin Random House Company, New York.

BALLANTINE and the HOUSE colophon are
registered trademarks of Random House LLC.

LIBRARY OF CONGRESS CATALOGING-IN-PUBLICATION DATA
Jibrin, Janis.
The pescetarian plan : the vegetarian + seafood way to
lose weight and love your food / Janis Jibrin, M.S., R.D.; recipes by
Sidra Forman; photographs by Kate Headley. — First edition.
pages cm
Includes bibliographical references and index.
ISBN 978-0-345-54716-3 (hardcover : alk. paper) — ISBN (invalid)
978-0-345-54717-0 (ebook)
1. Reducing diets—Recipes. 2. Weight loss. 3. Cooking (Fish)
4. Veganism. I. Title.
RM222.2.J523 2014
641.5'635—dc23   2013041935

Printed in the United States of America on acid-free paper

www.ballantinebooks.com

2 4 6 8 9 7 5 3 1

FIRST EDITION

Book design by Barbara M. Bachman

ACKNOWLEDGMENTS

If you've never equated "healthy" with "delicious," just wait until you get a load of Chef Sidra Forman's Shrimp Grilled with Barbecue Peach Chutney, Kale Soup, Chocolate Cupcake with Mint Glaze, and all her other delicious recipes. Thank you, thank you, Sidra, for translating *The Pescetarian Plan* so deliciously! (And simply—these recipes are a breeze to make.)

Another big thanks to photographer Kate Headley, who managed to capture the dishes' beauty and allure perfectly. I'm in good company: Kate's sophisticated-yet-relaxed images have appeared in *Martha Stewart Weddings* as well as *Brides, Southern Living,* and other national publications.

Registered dietitians Caroline Kaufman and Tracy Gensler provided invaluable research help, no easy task because nutrition science is something of a moving target. (Is saturated fat *really* so bad for you? See the state of the science on page 37.) Even my pescetarian agent Peter Steinberg sent cutting-edge research studies that made their way into this book. (I wish I could say I converted him, but he was already eating this way when we met.) And thanks to Gary R. Gensler, MS, for helping me do the math (literally) to confirm the great omega-6 to omega-3 ratios in the Pescetarian meals in this book.

Every writer needs an editor to trim and tighten text, but few are lucky enough to get two pros, as I did for this book. Donna Fennessy, whom I met when she was editing my articles for *SELF* magazine, gave invaluable feedback. Marnie Cochran at Ballantine helped me organize the book and coaxed me into cutting the excess (yes, this book could have been a lot longer).

—JANIS

CONTENTS

Acknowledgments   v

Introduction   ix

Part One   Your Body on Pescetarianism

Chapter 1:   Your Fabulous Pescetarian Figure   3

Chapter 2:   Age-Proofing Your Body   14

Chapter 3:   This Is Your Brain on Fish   25

Chapter 4:   Pescetarian Ultra-Nutrition   31

Part Two   Your Pescetarian Action Plan

Chapter 5:   The Seven Pescetarian Principles   53

Chapter 6:   Putting the Principles into Action   73

Chapter 7:   Upgrade Your Diet and Maintain Your Weight   81

Chapter 8:   Pescetarian Meal Basics   95

Chapter 9:   Exercise, Sleep, Love   103

Part Three   Pescetarian Cooking: Green, Clean, and Lean

Chapter 10:   Catches to Reel In, Catches to Toss Back   115

Chapter 11: Environmentally Friendly Pescetarianism 133

Chapter 12: Seafood Shopping and (Foolproof) Cooking 141

Chapter 13: Pescetarian Recipes 152

Appendix A: Pescetarian Tracker 279

Appendix B: Weight and Inches Log 283

Appendix C: Pescetarian Meals 285

Notes 317

Index 329

INTRODUCTION

~~~~~~~~

WHY BECOME A PESCETARIAN?

Eat fish and you'll protect your heart, plus you'll stay smarter and happier and—no joke—have a better sex life. Go vegetarian and you'll be thinner, dramatically reduce your risk of developing heart disease and cancer, and live longer. But why not have it all? You can! Just combine the two eating styles and become a *pescetarian;* it's a vegetarian diet with the addition of seafood (the word *pescetarian* comes from *pesce,* the Italian word for fish). It's a delicious, easy, and fun way of eating.

I realize that I just made a bunch of outrageous-sounding claims, like "thinner," "happier," "better sex life." And to be fair, I can't know *exactly* how your particular body will react to a pescetarian diet. But as a dietitian who has spent a career examining every imaginable type of diet, I can tell you that the case for pescetarianism is incredibly strong. The research *does* support my claims, as I'll show you later on in the book. In fact, it's so compelling that I can't find another type of diet that can touch it.

While *pescetarianism* isn't yet a household word, I predict it will be soon; it might be new to Americans, but it has a long track record. Just look around the world at people who live the longest and—more important—the healthiest. Their diets are pescetarian (or nearly so). For instance, pescetarianism is the backbone of two of the world's healthiest ways of eating: the traditional Mediterranean and Japanese diets. For *The Pescetarian Plan* I chose the Mediterranean approach, because that's the food I grew up on.

Scientists have picked apart these traditional diets and figured out what makes them tick: lots of vegetables, fruits, whole grains, healthy fats, not too much sugar, and seafood. And fish alone—especially fatty fish like salmon, trout, and sardines—is proving indispensable to our health. It provides the omega-3 fats our bodies need but that have nearly disappeared in the American diet. Starved of these important fats, we're more prone to heart disease, cancer, diabetes, depression, and Alzheimer's.

Meanwhile, red meat *promotes* those very diseases that fish helps protect us from. And poultry has its own issues such as salmonella and the unethical treatment of chickens. The Pescetarian Plan contains all the slimming, health-promoting elements of the traditional diets, without red meat and poultry. Your body will never have it so good!

Okay, you might be thinking, fish *used* to be healthy. But isn't it now full of mercury and other contaminants? Plus, what about the environmental issues? Overfishing has drastically diminished the world's supply of fish. And some fish farms leave too heavy an environmental footprint.

All true, but fortunately, if you choose carefully, you *can* put seafood that's clean, delicious, and "green" on your plate. And there's more good news: Governments, nonprofits, and industry are working on laws that protect the oceans, and there has already been some progress made. In chapters 10 and 11 I'll direct you to the best catches and inform you of ways that you can help save the oceans.

PESCETARIAN-MEDITERRANEAN

It's been called "The Island Where People Forget to Die," the small Greek island of Ikaria, and as you might imagine, it's a great place to live. Men here are four times as likely to hit the age of 90 as American men—and in good health to boot. Depression is virtually nonexistent among elderly men and women, and their brains stay sharp, with just a quarter the rate of Alzheimer's and other forms of dementia as in the United States.

What are they doing right? Well, their diet, for one. It's a diet very similar to the one you are holding in your hands! It's the traditional Mediterranean diet, the one that first piqued researchers' attention in the 1950s and 1960s, when they found that people on the Greek island of Crete were living longer, healthier lives.

But the Pescetarian Plan isn't just a Mediterranean diet—it's the healthiest interpretation of this diet. I say "interpretation" because there is not one Mediterranean diet. People in Spain, Greece, southern Italy, Lebanon, the South of France, and other countries along the Mediterranean serve up different cuisines. But what is the same: a core eating pattern that's mainly plant-based with fish as the primary animal protein and olive oil and nuts as the main fat sources, with wine accompanying the meals.

Put down that passport! You don't have to live in Greece or any other Mediterranean country to reap the benefits of this kind of diet. You simply have to adhere to the basic principles I've outlined in Chapter 5. In fact, researchers have developed a "Mediterranean Diet Score" to rate the "Mediterranean-ness" of their subjects' diets. What they found: The closer that people adhere to a traditional Mediterranean diet, the less likely they are to develop heart disease, cancer, type 2 diabetes, dementia, depression, and other chronic conditions.

Notice I keep saying "traditional Mediterranean diet"? If you've been to Greece, Spain, or other Mediterranean countries lately, you probably know that the diets of many of these people can no longer be described as "traditional." Instead, they're rife with fast food and junk food, (although still not as bad as the typical American's diet). And of course, these countries have increasing rates of overweight and obesity to show for it. That ultra-healthy Mediterranean diet that I'm referring to is the one of their parents, their grandparents, and generations further back.

The Pescetarian Plan has one-upped all other versions of the Mediterranean diet because it:

- Eliminates red meat and poultry (which, admittedly, were scarce to begin with on this diet);
- Uses the "cleanest" (low in contaminants) and most environmentally sustainable types of seafood;
- Includes a weight-loss component for those who need to lose weight, with clear portion guidance (chapters 5 and 6);
- Features true superfoods (ultra-nutrient-packed foods), whether they're traditionally eaten along the Mediterranean or not. For example, although sweet potatoes aren't traditional in Mediterranean countries, I've included them in this Pescetarian Plan because they're loaded with virtually every vitamin and mineral—not to mention phytonutrients. They're a serious superfood.

MY PESCETARIANISM

As an American kid growing up in Mediterranean countries (my father was in the Foreign Service), I ate lots of fish, fruits, and vegetables. My brother and I loved the food, but *boy,* did we play the martyrs. We whined about missing out on McDonald's, Twinkies, bologna sandwiches, and the like. But a funny thing happened when we spent those occasional summers back in the States: Junk food didn't taste very good.

Something else I noticed on those summers: Americans didn't seem as healthy as the Greeks, Lebanese, and Italians in our adopted countries. People in the United States were a lot heavier. My grandmother's friends were often homebound or in nursing homes. They weren't out farming, tending shops, running households, and walking from one village to the next like the elderly people I grew up with.

Now, as a nutritionist, I know why: The American diet was—and is even more so today—killing people. And the Mediterranean diet I grew up with has been proven to be extraordinarily healthy. In these pages, I've made it even healthier, by rooting out meat and poultry. It's the way I eat. Do I miss these foods? Truthfully—not at all. And on rare occasions I'll eat them (if I'm invited to someone's house for dinner and that's what's served, for instance). That's another thing you'll find about this diet—it's sane. You can adapt it to your budget and lifestyle, and you don't have to be rude at dinner parties!

You'll notice, in this book, that I stick with the science. That's always been my M.O. It's why my clients trust me—and get frustrated when I tell them to toss their wacky and dangerous weight loss supplements! It's why my editors trust me—I'm a contributing editor at *Self* magazine and have written hundreds of nutrition articles for many other popular publications. As the lead dietitian for TheBestLife.com—diet and fitness site of Bob Greene, Oprah's trainer—I make sure our hundreds of articles and blogs are firmly rooted in research. In books I've written with Bob and those I've done on my own, science rules. On Sharecare.com, a vetted search engine for health information headed by Dr. Mehmet Oz and Jeff Arnold (founder of WebMD), I not only answer questions but also serve on the board to help keep the nutrition information as accurate as possible.

So my pescetarianism springs from many sources: the diet I grew up on, the science I adhere to, and the way it makes me look and feel. It feels good to be healthy!

YOUR PESCETARIANISM

You can put any kind of culinary twist on this plan, as long as you're eating according to the healthy basics outlined below. For example, my uncle Sami Jibrin's diet is quintessentially Mediterranean (and mostly pescetarian) while incorporating cuisines from three countries: Syria (where he grew up), Brazil (where he's lived most of his adult life), and the United States (where he visits yearly).

I'm convinced that this way of eating has played a big hand in his extraordinary mental and physical health. Well into his eighties he's still in charge of his successful business and a prolific poet to boot! Here's a typical day for him (cooking courtesy of his wife, Najla, an inventive, health-oriented cook):

BREAKFAST
Oatmeal with tropical fruit

LUNCH
Fish broiled with lemon juice, garlic, and olive oil

Collard greens sautéed in olive oil, onions, and garlic

Bulgur wheat with pine nuts

Plain yogurt mixed with chopped cucumber, garlic, and mint

Cup of Arabic coffee

SNACK
Pistachios with herbal tea

DINNER
Lentil and rice pilaf topped with caramelized onions (an Arab dish called mujaddara)

Plain yogurt topped with green olives drizzled with olive oil

Green salad with tomatoes, chopped parsley and scallions, dressed in olive oil and lemon juice

A glass of wine

Grapes

YOUR CHEF

I didn't just want to hand you the world's healthiest diet; I wanted it to taste *really* good. As good as the Greek, Lebanese, and Italian food of my childhood. As good as it does when I go to my friend Sidra Forman's house.

So I was beyond thrilled when Sidra—a well-known chef here in Washington, D.C.—agreed to design the hundred-plus recipes in this book. What was also a thrill: Going to her kitchen and tasting every single one of them! As you'll find out, she manages the near impossible: healthy recipes that taste like food you really want to eat—not "diet food"—*and* are easy to make. (Most recipes take less than 25 minutes to make and average only eight ingredients including salt and pepper.) All this comes naturally to her because she's never been one to rely on cream, fatty meats, and loads of sodium. She knows how to let good ingredients do the talking.

PESCETARIAN Q & As

If burgers and fries are your mainstays, you might be wondering if you can handle giving up meat and eating more vegetables. Or maybe you're eating fairly healthfully, but cooking fish intimidates you. (Best-kept secret: Fish is a lot easier to cook than poultry or meat!) Here are some common questions I'm asked about the Pescetarian Plan. I'm hoping my answers will assure you that this way of eating is very doable.

- *Can I lose weight on this plan?* Absolutely—in fact, lots of it, if you need to. There is no magic diet that will melt pounds and keep them off. But I can tell you that this pescetarian way of eating is easier to sustain over the long run than a low-fat or low-carb diet. It has been successful with many of my clients, and there's some strong research backing this.
- *Can I have chicken, beef, pork, lamb, or other animal meats on this diet?* Sure. But try not to. I'm leaving them out, because my goal is to present the hands-down healthiest way of eating. If you want to eat these foods on occasion, go ahead. Burger lovers, you can still have your fun! Soy and pea-protein-based burgers (and other meat substitutes) have improved dramatically. They're so

good, they've fooled chefs, especially once they're in a bun with lettuce, tomato, and the fixins.

- *Why are chicken, turkey, beef, pork, duck, and lamb bad for you?* Red meat of any type is linked to higher rates of heart disease, cancer, and premature death (details in chapter 4). As for poultry, there are both nutritional and ethical issues. If you eat the skin, you're getting a mouthful of artery-clogging saturated fat. And low-fat turkey and chicken deli meats are loaded with sodium, and cancer-causing nitrites. True, cooking your own skinless poultry from scratch without salt makes for a nutritious protein (although not nearly as healthy as omega-3-rich fish). But personally, I have a hard time eating chicken because of the cruel, overcrowded conditions in which they're raised. Plus, when I used to cook with chicken, I was always worried about salmonella contamination.

- *Is sugar in or out on this plan?* It's in—but in moderation, as eaten in long-lived cultures like those along the Mediterranean Sea.

- *I have food allergies/intolerances—can I still follow this plan?* If you're allergic to all seafood, then I suggest you buy another book! If you can eat fish but are allergic to shellfish (or vice versa), hold on to this book—you can still follow the plan. If you can't eat gluten, soy, nuts, or dairy, you'll be fine here. There are plenty of recipes that exclude these foods, and for recipes that don't, you can easily make substitutions. Nuts are a core element of the plan, but if you're allergic to them, I'll give you a work-around.

- *How much time will I have to spend in the kitchen?* About two to five minutes for breakfast; somewhere between 5 and 30 minutes for most other meals. The recipes in the back of this book (which I hope you try—they're delicious) take, on average, 25 minutes to make from start to finish and contain an average of just eight ingredients—including salt and pepper!

- *Do I have to eat seafood every day?* Not at all! You can go vegetarian on Monday, have some shrimp on Tuesday, and go vegan on Wednesday. As long as your diet roughly follows the "Seven Pescetarian Principles"—basically how many fruits, vegetables, grains, proteins, and other foods to eat—you can be very flexible about what goes on your plate.

- **Isn't seafood expensive?** It can be, but I'll steer you to the less pricy picks. And the very inexpensive foods on this plan will balance out any extra dollars spent on seafood. For instance, you'll be eating vegetarian protein, like black beans, kidney beans, and tofu, all of which are cheap. And if you start preparing more meals at home—there are some really great choices in this book—you'll save a bundle over eating out. Many of these meals are cheaper than fast food! See "Pescetarianism on a Budget" in chapter 8 for meals as low as $1.27.

- **Will my family enjoy this plan?** Absolutely! Even picky eaters (small and grown-up) will find lots to love on this plan. Once your kids get a load of the Tilapia Fish Sticks (page 241), they might not ask for frozen fish sticks anymore. Potato and Celery Root Mashed with Basil make a wonderfully comforting side dish. Haddock Tacos (page 223) and Cornmeal Crusted Catfish with Cucumbers (page 215) are other familiar favorites, but with a healthier twist. And no one at the family dinner table is going to turn down Chocolate Cupcakes with Mint Glaze (page 260), Sesame Coconut Cookies (page 266), or any of the other desserts!

- **I don't live anywhere near water. Can I still do this diet?** Definitely—you just need a discerning eye (and nose) to ensure that the "fresh" seafood is actually just that. (See page 141 for tips.) If you live in a part of the country where seafood arrives from long distances or it's just not that popular (so there's slow turnover in the supermarket), quality is likely to suffer. Fortunately, frozen fish and shrimp can be delicious, especially if prepared with seasonings or as part of a pasta or vegetable dish (as opposed to simply grilling with a little salt and pepper). Tasty and easy-to-follow seafood recipes start on page 154.

HAVE FUN WITH THIS BOOK!

Becoming a pescetarian will be a fun ride, especially if you're a food lover like I am. I enjoy food too much to stand for restrictive fad diets, like a high-protein diet, a cookie diet (it might not sound so bad, but by day three you never want to look at another cookie), crazy juice fasts, and the like. I indulge in a glass of wine or a beer on occasion. (I'll tell you all about the pros and cons—mostly pros, fortunately—of alcohol in this book.) I like going out to eat, and I certainly don't want to worry that nothing on the menu fits my diet! A pescetarian diet works in real life while it's working its magic on your body. You'll see.

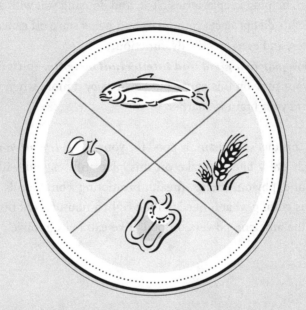

Your Body on Pescetarianism

Look around the world—wherever people eat a pescetarian-style diet, they live longer and healthier. It all goes back to the dramatic impact of lifestyle on health. About 80 percent of heart disease cases, 70 percent of cancer cases, and a whopping 90 percent of cases of type 2 diabetes are caused by poor diet and lack of exercise. On the flip side: Most people could avoid these diseases if they exercised and ate the type of pescetarian-Mediterranean diet I'm recommending in this book.

Here's how this diet can help you be your healthiest:

1. *It helps keep you at a healthy weight and shrinks your belly.* This puts you at a huge health advantage. Obesity alone is responsible for up to 30 percent of cancer cases, and having too much visceral fat—the deep "belly fat" that lodges in and around your organs—is a major cause of heart disease and type 2 diabetes.

2. *It fights aging in every single way.* By fending off chronic inflammation, helping keep arteries clear, and dousing you with antioxidants, this diet protects your heart and helps stave off cancer, type 2 diabetes, and even erectile dysfunction.

3. *It offers psychological and intellectual benefits.* You'll not only extend your time on this earth, but you'll *enjoy* it more when you're happier and your brain is sharper.

Why is this diet so amazingly good for your body? *It's ultra-nutritious;* pretty much every bite you take on this plan infuses you with vitamins, minerals, and phytonutrients (health-promoting compounds in plants). Your body is getting what it needs in the right amounts, so it thrives. I'll fill you in on the amazing powers of foods like extra-virgin olive oil, broccoli, and clams.

Chapter 1

YOUR FABULOUS PESCETARIAN FIGURE

In the beginning, I didn't plan on writing a weight-loss book.
When I initially started, my primary purpose was to guide you through a
way of eating that keeps your brain sharp and your heart healthy and also
reduces your risk for cancer, diabetes, and other conditions. But guess what?
The more I researched, the more it became crystal clear that this is the ideal
diet to help you lose weight—and lots of it, if you need to do so. The research simply confirmed my real-world experience: This is the diet I've
been giving my clients for decades, because it's the one that produces the
best long-term results.

What if you don't need to lose weight? Stay with me here, don't go anywhere! Being a pescetarian may very well be your best bet for preventing
unwanted pounds from creeping on.

THE PESCETARIAN WEIGHT-LOSS EDGE

I've found that it's easier to lose weight on a pescetarian diet than on a
vegan or vegetarian one. The reason: seafood. Seafood is a low-calorie
concentrated protein source, just what you need when you're trying to lose
weight. That's because protein, compared to carbohydrates and fat, is particularly appetite-quelling. Meaning, after a meal containing a high-protein
food, you last longer before getting hungry again.

Vegans and vegetarians do have tofu—also a healthy concentrated
source of protein—but how much tofu do you feel like eating? And vegetar-

ians also have eggs, but again, they're a little limiting. Legumes, which I recommend highly in this book as a healthy carb, aren't the best protein source if you're trying to lose weight. That's because you have to rack up a lot more beans—and calories—than seafood to get substantial protein levels. For instance, three ounces of cooked trout offers up 18 grams of protein for just 113 calories. To get that much protein from beans, you'd have to eat about one and a half cups of beans, for about 300 calories.

Loads of research from across the globe—the United States, Europe, northern Africa, or anywhere else—shows that people who eat along the lines of the Pescetarian Plan are slimmer. How much slimmer? Pescetarians are, on average, about 20 pounds lighter than regular eaters, according to a study tracking 89,000 Seventh-day Adventists in the United States and Canada. Adventists are an ideal group to study because their religion advocates a vegetarian diet (only about half are actually vegetarians, while another 10 percent are pescetarians; the rest are "regular eaters," eating meat, poultry, and everything else). Vegetarians and pescetarians also had about half the risk for diabetes and high blood pressure.

A Mediterranean diet is also slimming. As I've explained already, the Pescetarian Plan is basically a Mediterranean diet that takes a pass on poultry and red meat and embraces the form of animal protein favored in Mediterranean countries: seafood. A Spanish study tracking university students for five years after graduation found that men and women who closely followed a Mediterranean diet were only half as likely to gain 11 pounds or more compared to their classmates whose diets were furthest from a Mediterranean pattern.

How's this for a triple threat: The Pescetarian Plan rolls all three fat-fighting diets into one. It's Mediterranean and basically vegetarian with the addition of seafood.

You'd think that the words *diet* and *painless* would go together about as well as socks and sandals. But my clients tell me that the Pescetarian Plan is the most painless way they've ever lost weight. There are lots of biological and psychological ways this plan makes it easier to lose weight, including:

It tastes good. You're eating food you actually like, and the sky's the limit when it comes to recipes.

You won't walk around hungry. Personally, I can't last a day on a diet if I'm hungry. This diet is so filling that my clients often tell me they can't eat all the food! Not only are the meals large (thank you, fruits and vegetables) but the diet is designed to minimize spikes and dips in blood sugar. The brain reads blood sugar dips as "time to eat," while a nice even blood sugar suppresses appetite.

You'll have energy to exercise. What keeps energy high? Getting enough calories (but not too many); enough vitamins, minerals, and other nutrients; and the right kind of carbs (to stabilize blood sugar). Of course, sleep plays a role, too (sleep tips in chapter 9). With sleep and diet in place, you'll have more energy than ever to work out.

You can break your sugar or salty snack habit. Sugar begets more sugar—the same with chips and salty snacks. Even if your breakfasts, lunches, and dinners are reasonable, your treat habit can sabotage your effort to drop those pounds. For some people, these foods are as addictive as alcohol or drugs. The Pescetarian Plan acts as a junk food reset button, training your tastes away from high-sugar, high-salt foods such as cookies, candy, fries, and the like and allowing you to enjoy the tastes of real food like ripe fruit, grilled fish sprinkled with fresh herbs, and a grain-and-toasted-nut pilaf. (If you can handle a little treat daily, great! Those treat calories, for sweets, alcohol, or whatever you'd like, are built into the plan.)

Slimming Pescetarian Foods

The Pescetarian Plan is how trimmer people eat. Check out these results from the U.S. arm of INTERMAP—an international diet and blood pressure study. You'll note that those at a healthy weight ate a lot more fruit, seafood, and nuts: core Pescetarian Plan staples. And obese people ate a lot more of foods that are either off this plan (red meat and processed meat) or are recommended in moderation (alcohol).

Those at a healthy weight ate:

Three to five times more seafood as obese people

Twice as much fruit

Two to four times as many nuts

Obese people ate:

---

25 percent more red meat than those at normal weight

Twice as much processed meat (bacon, pepperoni, etc.)

Six times as much alcohol (only the men, no difference in women)

Three times as many sugary beverages, including soft drinks,

    fruit punch, and sweetened iced tea (only for women, not much

    difference in men)

THE DECK'S STACKED TO FAVOR MAINTENANCE

You can lose weight on any diet as long as you're cutting calories. But maintaining weight loss is still a gigantic challenge. The truth is, most people who lose weight don't keep it off. The reasons are both biological (for instance, metabolic rate—the rate at which you burn calories—slows) and behavioral (maybe you lost weight on a diet that was unsustainable or didn't instill good habits).

That's the bad news. But much more encouraging is the fact that enough people *do* maintain their weight loss to show clearly that it can be done. I know a number of them who have maintained large weight losses of 50 or 100 pounds, even more. The National Weight Control Registry, a study tracking the habits of more than ten thousand of these "successful losers," is documenting how they do it. They're exercising and eating a lot of fruit, vegetables, lean protein, and other mainstays of the Pescetarian Plan. Research shows that these foods can just about double your chance of successfully maintaining your weight loss.

It's not only the types of foods that make a difference—the percentages of each also play a role, according to research. The makeup—both types and amounts of foods—of the Pescetarian Plan promotes weight maintenance.

In other words, I've stacked the deck fully in favor of weight maintenance. Here's how:

- *Your metabolism will stay relatively high.* When you lose weight, your metabolic rate tends to drop. That's a major reason why it's so difficult to maintain weight loss. But research from the Boston Children's Hospital shows that eating along the lines of the Pescetarian Plan somewhat offsets that drop in the amount of calories burned.

- ***It's a diet you can live with.*** Unlike wacky, expensive, or restrictive fad diets, this one is easily adapted to your lifestyle. In some cases, it's just a healthier version of what you're already eating.

- ***You might be happier.*** My clients report feeling "good," "light," and "energized" on this plan. Sure, it feels great to shed pounds, but it's also the omega-3s that can perk up your mood, as explained in chapter 4. When your mood's up, so is your motivation to eat well and exercise. Which, in turn, puts you in a good mood. It's a happy cycle!

OUTSMARTING YOUR "FAT GENES"

You, your co-worker, and your friend could all go on *The Pescetarian Plan*, get the same amount of exercise, and lose very different amounts of weight. Why? Chalk it up to genetics.

If you've been heavy since childhood and seem to have a harder time than others keeping your weight down—despite valiant efforts—you probably have more than your fair share of "fat genes." Genetics are thought to account for 65 percent of the reason that one person has more body fat than another.

But don't despair! Genetics rarely fate you to be heavy. Fat genes need the right environment to thrive. That's why forty years ago, when the food environment was vastly different, the obesity rate in the United States was 13 percent compared to 35 percent today.

Our genes haven't changed—our environment has. We don't need to walk anywhere these days, most of our jobs involve sitting (plus all the time we spend in front of TVs and video games), and, of course, there are excessive amounts of food everywhere.

Fat genes devise sneaky ways to interact with the environment and pile on body fat. This was useful when we were hunter-gatherers and burned calories like mad all day and relied on our fat stores in times of food scarcity. But now, obviously, it's counterproductive.

The Pescetarian Plan is designed to outsmart your fat genes and our toxic food environment. How so?

How Your Genes Make You Fat: You have strong cravings for—or are even addicted to—fatty, salty, and sweet foods.

We're all wired to like these foods. They're the foods that kept our hunter-gatherer ancestors alive; it took a lot of berries, grubs, and lean antelope to rack up desperately needed calories. Salt was also hard to come by, and, believe it or not, you do need some to stay healthy.

It's even worse for some people—they have either a stronger genetic predilection for these high-calorie foods or a brain chemical imbalance that leaves them unsatisfied with a moderate amount (similar to the way a drug addict develops tolerance and needs higher doses).

How the Food Environment Makes It Worse: We live in a toxic food environment—28-ounce sodas, cookies the size of salad plates, and all the other ridiculous portions out there that are considered normal. Don't forget about the infestation of round-the-clock fast food joints with their super-sized, penny-pinching meals, and all the other ways we can easily satisfy our sweet, salty, and fatty cravings. In fact, food manufacturers design some foods to be addictive, a disaster for the people most wired for addiction.

The Pescetarian Solution: You'll get to enjoy fat, sugar, and salt, but you'll do it in a diet- and health-friendly way. For instance, you'll get your fair share of fat on this plan (35 percent of your calories from fat), but you'll get it from healthy sources like nuts and olive oil. As for salt, I'll show you how judicious use of the salt shaker at the table delivers a satisfying salt hit but keeps sodium levels reasonable.

Here's how we'll handle sweets on this plan: You'll get a certain amount of treat calories each day, and I'll point you toward lower-sugar options. Remember, the more sweets you eat and the sweeter the foods (think M&Ms vs. dark chocolate), the more you crave them. By limiting sweets and opting for lower sugar (but never artificially sweetened) choices, you could see your sugar cravings diminish dramatically in two weeks on this plan.

How Your Genes Make You Fat: Some people are genetically pro-grammed to deposit more fat deep in the abdomen. This "visceral fat" spurs on heart disease, cancer, and type 2 diabetes, so it's something you want to minimize. To find out whether you're carrying around too much visceral fat, check out the "Busting Belly Fat" section later in this chapter.

How the Environment Makes It Worse: Too much white flour and sugar tend to encourage fat deposition to your midsection more than to other areas of the body. So does being sedentary.

The Pescetarian Solution: You'll be eating foods associated with a smaller waistline: whole grains, fruits and vegetables, calcium- and fiber-rich foods, and lean protein. Added sugar like white sugar, honey, and other sweeteners stay under 6 percent of total calories, which is considered a healthy level. Throw exercise into the mix, and you've got the ultimate gut-shrinking plan.

How Your Genes Make You Fat: Your genes drive you to eat frequently. Again, that was adaptive for hunter-gatherers who were foraging all day, but not necessarily for most of us.

How the Environment Makes It Worse: You can't go anywhere—and I mean anywhere—without being faced with food. Think about it: There are candy bars at the counter of Home Depot and Staples and even a bowl of candy at my hair salon! The old "three squares" model has been thrown out the window—it's perfectly acceptable to eat anytime, anywhere.

The Pescetarian Solution: You don't have to work against your genes in this case—you can eat a number of mini-meals on this plan and keep your weight down as long as you stay within the guidelines for fruit, dairy, and the other food groupings. And for those (like myself) who prefer the "three squares plus snacks" approach, you can take that route on this plan as well.

How Your Genes Make You Fat: It takes a lot of food to feel full. It could be that your genes are stingy when it comes to making hormones like leptin, which quell appetite, or that you're somewhat resistant to their effects. Or you might be overproducing hormones that stimulate appetite.

How the Environment Makes It Worse: We're surrounded by calorie-dense foods, such as fried foods, doughnuts, Häagen-Dazs, french fries, and more. These foods contain extraordinary amounts of calories for a relatively small volume. You can scarf down a lot of these foods before your stomach really starts expanding.

The Pescetarian Solution: To fool you into feeling full on fewer calories, I've made these Pescetarian Plan meals large. Vegetables, fruit, and soup stretch the stomach on relatively few calories; nerves in a stretched stomach send a "full" signal to the brain. It's not the only signal, but it's a powerful one. Another appetite-quelling signal is a nice, stable blood sugar level, which you should experience on this plan thanks to its low glycemic index. (Such meals elicit a relatively small and slow rise in blood sugar; for details, see "The Glycemic Index," page 42.)

A Gut Instinct About Body Weight

I t's been called the "forgotten organ": the microbiota, or "intestinal flora," the hordes of bacteria—some harmful, most neutral or helpful—that populate our intestines. While the microbiota is not a true organ, it certainly behaves like one. The microbes in your gut, which outnumber the cells in your body (there are a hundred trillion of them), influence immunity, hormones, inflammatory compounds, and, as emerging research is starting to discover, your body weight.

Animal studies were one of the first tip-offs that your gut can, well . . . give you a gut! You can make a mouse fat simply by inoculating its gut with a small amount of intestinal flora from an obese mouse. And studies in humans are turning up microbiota differences between overweight and trim people.

Scientists are just beginning to figure out how those tiny single-celled organisms affect that number on your scale. For instance, they can wring more calories out of your food. Also, certain bacteria make it easier for your gut to absorb glucose (and its calories). Others put the brakes on metabolic rate, in other words make you burn calories more slowly and store more calories as fat. You might even be able to blame your microbiota when you reach for that third helping of mashed potatoes. Yes, the little bugs might also increase appetite!

Scientists are trying to develop probiotic supplements (consisting of friendly bacteria) that would shift the balance of bugs to help you lose weight. Also, changing your diet may help. Typical American fare seems to encourage the growth of intestinal bacteria that *promote* obesity. But a plant-based diet, like the one in this book, appears to favor a "skinny microbiota." Researchers at the University College in Cork, Ireland, have put 1,250 elderly people living in various European countries on either a Mediterranean diet (similar to the Pescetarian Plan) or their usual Western diets. Because diet changes take a while to influence the microbiota, the study will last a year. Stay tuned for those results—I'll be posting them on ThePescetarianPlan.com.

BUSTING BELLY FAT

I f you're overweight, you are perfectly justified in wondering whether it really matters to your health. You're certainly not getting any help from the media, where conflicting headlines either scare the heck out of you ("Obesity is killing you!") or make you wonder if you should let your gym membership lapse ("Being overweight makes you live longer!").

So which is it? It seems to boil down to this: *Where* you deposit your fat is much more important than how much fat you're carrying around. Too much visceral fat—also called "abdominal fat"—the deep belly fat that settles in and around your liver, pancreas, and other organs, is *very* risky. Being "apple-shaped" is a ticket to pre-diabetes, diabetes, and heart disease. It is also linked to cancer. This is in contrast to subcutaneous fat right under the skin, the more "pinch-able" fat, which appears to be medically neutral. Meanwhile, if you're "pear-shaped," packing more of your fat in your hips and thighs, you may actually be more *protected* from these diseases, according to new research.

Of course, you can be at a "healthy" weight but carry too much visceral fat. (Healthy, overweight, and obese are generally measured by the Body Mass Index or BMI, a number derived from a formula that includes a person's weight and height. For a link to a BMI calculator, go to ThePescetarian Plan.com.) While it's true that a BMI of 18.5 to 24.9 is considered "healthy weight" because it's generally linked to lower risk from chronic disease, all bets are off if your visceral fat levels are high. A National Institute on Aging study—a huge one, tracking approximately 250,000 men and women—showed that people with a "healthy" BMI but a large waistline were 20 percent more likely to die sooner than those with a healthy BMI and a smaller waistline.

How can you tell if you have too much visceral fat? In research labs, scientists use computed tomography (CT) scans or DEXA scans—X-ray images of cross-sections, or "slices," of the body, showing both visceral and subcutaneous fat. But you have a pretty good tool right in your sewing kit: a tape measure. In fact, waist measurement is used in a lot of research studies, and it has been found to correlate well with the fancier and pricier equipment!

So, summon up your courage and put that measuring tape around your waist. Here's how:

1. Stand up in front of a mirror.
2. Place the tape measure around your belly, just above your hipbones. Place the bottom edge of the tape measure at the top of your hipbones. This will probably correspond to the largest part of your belly, but not necessarily.
3. Check in the mirror—the tape should evenly circle your body (as opposed to riding up on one end and down on another).
4. Breathe out (but don't suck in your waist), make sure the tape is snug, but not pinching the skin, then measure.
5. Write down the number. Every few weeks, or at least once a month, remeasure to note your progress.

The risk for chronic diseases goes up with a waistline measurement greater than 35 inches for women or greater than 40 inches for men. (For Asians, disease risk increases at 31.5 inches for women and 35.5 for men.)

If you're over the cut-off points, don't panic! Instead, use this reality check to become extra-determined to stick to your chapter 5 portions and keep exercising: Exercise preferentially removes visceral fat. That's because visceral fat is the last fat to deposit, and it's the first your body removes.

Pescetarian Foods That Fight "Belly Fat"

Stock your cabinets and fridge with foods (or food components) that take aim at visceral fat. Note: If you're following the Pescetarian Plan, you'll be getting these in sufficient supply.

- Fiber. The Pescetarian Plan is high in fiber thanks to all the fruits, vegetables, whole grains, and legumes.
- Whole grains. The Pescetarian Plan recommends whole grains only and the healthiest form: the coarser type (like steel-cut oats) as opposed to the more pulverized flours (like what Cheerios are made from). That's important, as the bigger particles help reduce blood sugar and insulin, which, in turn, reduce visceral fat. Also, whole grains are rich in magnesium, which helps keep the body more sensitive to insulin.
- Calcium. Eating calcium-rich foods is linked to lower visceral fat levels.

The yogurt, nonfat and 1-percent milk, and calcium-enriched soy and other nondairy milks on this plan are chock-full of calcium.

- Fruits and vegetables. You're certainly getting plenty of these on this plan! The higher the intake, the lower the visceral fat, found a study tracking 22,570 Danish men and women for five years.

- Protein. That same Danish study has linked adequate protein levels with less visceral fat. (Other studies have confirmed the result.) The Pescetarian Plan provides not only adequate amounts of protein but also the healthiest forms: seafood, egg whites, and soy.

HIT THE SWEET SPOT:
SLIM DOWN AND STAY SATISFIED

For a minute, try to forget about all the negatives associated with cutting calories—you know, the panic that you'll never get to enjoy food again, the obsession with the scale, the hunger, the deprivation.

Instead, I want you to wipe the slate clean and take a different approach. I'm going to help you figure out how much food you really need—just enough to feel comfortable and satisfied. In other words, you're not walking around hungry (unless it's just before meal time). We're going to work on hitting the sweet spot where you get enough food to keep you happy but are still losing weight.

How much weight? Typically, about ½ to 1 pound per week, but if you have a lot to lose, it could be as much as two pounds a week, especially at the beginning. I can't—and wouldn't want to—promise you anything more than that because that's not only unrealistic but also unhealthy and unmanageable for the long term.

Let's make a pact: If you can live with gradual weight loss, I can deliver a way of eating that's satisfying and energizing. And, even better, it's one that you can maintain over the long term. Add exercise to the mix, and your chances of losing and maintaining skyrocket even further. Plus, as you'll read in the next few chapters, you'll get way more than a leaner body. This pescetarian plan also helps prevent and treat heart disease, reduces cancer risk, keeps your brain sharper, lifts your mood, and helps keep you young.

Chapter 2

AGE-PROOFING YOUR BODY

~~~~~

While it whittles your waistline, the Pescetarian Plan is also busy staving off pretty much every age-related condition, such as heart disease, cancer, diabetes, and erectile dysfunction. It can even give your skin a healthier glow!

But what if you already have heart disease, type 2 diabetes, or another ailment? This Pescetarian lifestyle can improve your condition—and possibly even reverse it. That's because it helps relieve inflammation, keeps you at a healthy weight, clears arteries, and is packed with the nutrients you need to thrive. While I don't want to oversell this plan as a miracle cure, it certainly works better than any drug at preventing and, in some cases, treating many of the diseases that debilitate or kill us.

DOUSING INFLAMMATION

Of all the ways the Pescetarian Plan fights aging, reducing chronic inflammation may be the most critical, as it affects every part of your body. *Inflammation* is one of the hottest buzzwords in health these days, and with good reason. It has been shown to trigger a host of killer conditions—heart disease, cancer, dementia, and others. And it shortens your telomeres—the little protective segments at the end of your chromosomes. Shorter telomeres can mean a shorter life span and are associated with all the diseases I just mentioned. Brand-new research led by Dr. Dean

Ornish (a giant in the disease prevention field) found, for the first time, that a healthy lifestyle can actually *increase* telomere length.

What exactly is inflammation? There are two types: There's *acute inflammation,* which is swelling and fluid buildup that happens when your immune system attacks invaders. You've seen it in action when your finger swells and reddens around a splinter. That's an indication that white blood cells and chemicals produced by your immune system have rushed to the area to destroy bacteria. As you can probably guess, this is the type of inflammation you want!

You don't want *chronic* inflammation, the second type. This type of inflammation can hang around for years, often at a level too low to cause obvious symptoms. This time, instead of targeting a foreign invader, the inflammatory compounds are directed at your arteries, your joints, and other tissues. It's a health double whammy: The inflammation *causes* or contributes to conditions like heart disease, diabetes, cancer, ulcerative colitis, and Alzheimer's, and these diseases, in turn, create more inflammation in the body.

Here's how you get chronic inflammation and how *The Pescetarian Plan* combats it:

INFLAMMATION TRIGGER	PESCETARIAN DEFENSE
Being overweight or obese. Especially damaging is the visceral fat (deep belly fat in and around the liver and other organs), which spews out inflammatory compounds.	***You're eating foods that quell appetite and aid your weight-control efforts.*** This way of eating sends the "I'm full" signal to the brain in so many ways. (1) Low glycemic-index carbs like steel-cut oats and whole-wheat pasta prevent blood sugar dips; (2) lean, high-quality protein like fish, shellfish, and tofu leave you feeling satisfied; (3) hearty portions of relatively low-calorie foods like vegetable and fruit fill you up; (4) foods like nuts contribute to satiety; (5) fruits, vegetables, whole grains, and other high-fiber foods promote "skinny" gut bacteria (see page 10 for details). Plus, by keeping sugar low and avoiding refined flour, you're helping prevent visceral fat in particular.

INFLAMMATION TRIGGER	PESCETARIAN DEFENSE
Not enough vitamins, minerals, and phytonutrients. Without enough of these anti-inflammatory foot soldiers, the pro-inflammatory forces win the battle in your body.	*This ultra-nutritious diet is rich in anti-inflammatory compounds.* Omega-3 fats in fish and walnuts and the vitamins, minerals, and phytonutrients found in tomatoes, basil, berries, and many other pescetarian staples wage war on inflammation. Some of these compounds fight it directly, while others trigger your body to produce more of its *own* anti-inflammatory compounds (and suppress the creation of pro-inflammatory elements). A recent study found that Italians adhering closely to a Mediterranean eating pattern had four times the levels of anti-inflammatory compounds in their blood and just a third of the pro-inflammatory compounds as those whose diets were closer to an American way of eating.
The wrong mix of fats in the diet. The typical American diet has too many of the types of fat that promote inflammation (omega-6 and saturated fats) and too few of the types that douse it (omega-3s and monounsaturated fat).	*The ratio of omega-6 to omega-3 fats is even in this plan, and the bulk of the fat is monounsaturated.* This is the most anti-inflammatory fat pattern. Monounsaturated fat is the main type in this diet thanks to your staple oil—olive oil. You're also getting the omega-3s you need from fatty fish, walnuts, chia, and flaxseed. Meanwhile, sources of omega-6 and saturated fats are at reasonable levels.
Too much sugar and white flour. In excess, these feed inflammation.	*Refined flour is eliminated, and added sugar hovers around a low 5 percent of your daily calories.* "Added sugars" are sweeteners that are added to your food either as an ingredient (like in cookies, candy, cereal, spaghetti sauce) or as a flavoring, like when you use white sugar or honey to sweeten your coffee or tea.

INFLAMMATION TRIGGER	PESCETARIAN DEFENSE
Having a chronic disease. Type 2 diabetes, certain allergies, heart disease, cancer, and other conditions create pro-inflammatory substances that not only worsen the disease but also cause other complications. For instance, type 2 diabetes can raise levels of inflammatory compounds called AGEs (advanced glycation end-products), which can damage the retina in the eye, worsening vision and even causing blindness. It's a vicious cycle, because inflammation is also a cause (or one of the triggers) for these diseases.	***The Pescetarian Plan will help prevent—and even treat—chronic diseases.*** How? Through every single recommendation in this book—diet, exercise, sleep, and emotional well-being.
Being sedentary. It's hard to fight inflammation when you just sit around. Lack of exercise sets you up for a wide variety of major diseases and disorders.	***Exercise helps remove visceral fat and prevent insulin resistance.*** It does much more, but just these two functions are the main ways it targets inflammation.

SKIP METABOLIC SYNDROME

There's a condition that ignites chronic inflammation, doubles or triples your heart disease risk, and bumps up your odds of getting type 2 diabetes anywhere from four- to tenfold. It strikes over a third of American adults, but it still isn't a household word. It's "metabolic syndrome," and it's characterized by *at least three* of the following symptoms:

- A waistline that's 35 inches or greater for women, 40 inches or greater for men (for tips on measuring your waistline, see page 12)
- Blood triglyceride (a type of fat in the blood) level of 150 milligrams per deciliter (mg/dL) or more
- HDL ("good" cholesterol) that's less than 40 mg/dL in men or less than 50 mg/dL in women
- High blood pressure
- Fasting blood sugar of 100 mg/dL or more
- Insulin resistance—a condition in which the body can't properly use insulin. It's usually measured in a lab by a glucose tolerance test (where blood sugar is measured after you drink a glucose solution).

The good news is that 90 percent of cases of metabolic syndrome can be prevented by diet and exercise. Simply losing weight can reverse this condition. But a University of Laval, Canada, study found that in people with this condition, dropping pounds on a Mediterranean diet lowered inflammation even further than on a typical American diet (26 percent lower by one marker called C-reactive protein).

ENJOY A STEAMIER SEX LIFE

Okay, maybe *The Pescetarian Plan* can't guarantee that things will be *steamier* in the bedroom, but it can certainly help ensure that all the necessary parts are *functioning* properly.

Erectile dysfunction (ED), the persistent inability to have or maintain an erection sufficient for satisfactory sex, affects at least 30 percent of men between the ages of 40 and 70. Its causes: psychological issues like stress or anxiety and often a physical problem, usually clogged arteries, the same way that plaque-filled coronary arteries cause heart disease. In fact, ED is considered a harbinger of heart disease because if the penile arteries are narrowing, the odds are high that the same thing's going on in the coronary arteries.

Studies show that a Mediterranean diet as well as exercise may reduce the likelihood of developing ED. For instance, a study from the University of Naples indicates that 52 percent of men with diabetes eating a more Western-style diet had moderate to severe ED compared to 39 percent of those with a more Mediterranean style of eating.

Women are often left out of this conversation, but they too suffer from sexual dysfunction. It's not as obvious as ED, but standardized questionnaires rating desire, arousal, lubrication, orgasm, satisfaction, and pain help diagnose the problem. While psychology and hormones are at play in women, so is artery narrowing, just as in men. Research is still sparse on this, but an Italian study suggests that women with type 2 diabetes whose diets most closely resembled a Mediterranean pattern were more apt to be sexually active (65 percent of women compared to 54 percent) and have less sexual dysfunction (47.5 percent versus 57.8 percent) than women whose diets were the least Mediterranean.

PROTECT YOUR TICKER

Take a moment to appreciate the amazing-ness of your heart. It'll beat about 100,000 times today, keeping you alive by sending out blood that oxygenates and nourishes every cell.

Now consider this: Nearly 40 percent of men and women aged 40 to 59 have heart disease, an umbrella term for a number of things that can go wrong with your heart: coronary heart disease, heart failure, congenital heart defects, and arrhythmia. That number jumps to 72 percent for people in their sixties and seventies and about 83 percent for those age 80 and up. But the vast majority of cases of heart disease can be prevented by eating right and moving more.

A diet like the Pescetarian Plan cuts your risk of developing heart disease (or dying from it) by 30 to 50 percent. Exercise can slash it by about 50 percent. And the combination of a good diet and exercise could reduce heart disease cases by a whopping 80 percent. How? By helping keep the arteries that supply blood to your heart muscle clear and flexible—that's what happens when inflammation is low and you're taking in nutrients (like those in nuts) that encourage blood vessels to relax, keeping blood pressure low. The Pescetarian Plan is also low in sodium—another boon to low blood pressure. (For ways to slash sodium, check out page 87.)

There are a jillion studies linking Pescetarian Plan components to heart disease prevention; here's just the tip of the iceberg:

- People who ate a diet highest in omega-3 were only *half as likely to die* from sudden cardiac death (due to arrhythmias) over a sixteen-year period compared to people who ate the least, shows a Harvard School of Public Health study. Even more impressive: The *omega-3 eaters lived 2.2 extra years on average!* The study, which excluded people taking fish oil supplements and looked at participants who were free *of heart disease at outset,* reflects the power of diet to prevent disease.
- People at risk for heart disease who went on a Mediterranean diet cut their chances of developing the condition by 30 percent compared to a group who followed a standard low-fat diet. The study, which was published in *The New England Journal of Medicine* in

2013, was cut short after four years because it was considered un-ethical to keep the control group off the Mediterranean diet.

- Eating fish just one to two times per week was associated with a 42 to 50 percent reduction in the risk of sudden cardiac death in healthy adults, according to a special report in the American Heart Association journal *Circulation*.

What if you already have heart disease? Then switching to this pescetarian way of eating could literally be a lifesaver. A diet like the one in this book can reduce the risk of a heart attack or dying from heart disease by up to 70 percent.

STAVE OFF (OR EVEN REVERSE) TYPE 2 DIABETES AND PRE-DIABETES

How's this for a shocker: More than a quarter of Americans have pre-diabetes, but only 11 percent know they have the condition. And of the 8.3 percent of the population that has diabetes, only 63 percent are aware they have it. You might *think* you're diabetes-free, but given how common these diseases are, it's absolutely worth getting tested. In fact, cases of type 2 diabetes are rising so fast that it's estimated that within forty years, one in three Americans will have it. About 90–95 percent of diabetes cases are type 2.

The reason for the twin epidemics of pre-diabetes and type 2? Another epidemic: being overweight or obese. Too much body fat is the cause of about 80 percent of the cases of type 2 diabetes, and it's roughly the same for pre-diabetes.

Type 2 diabetes occurs when your cells become resistant to insulin (the hormone that controls blood sugar) and/or you don't produce enough of it. Sometimes oral medication can control blood sugar, and in other cases, you must inject insulin. (Type 1 diabetes, in which you stop making insulin, is not on the rise because it's not related to diet or obesity but has an autoimmune origin.)

The encouraging research on prevention:

- If you're overweight, losing about 7 percent of your initial body weight (that's 14 pounds if you weigh 200 pounds) could be enough to reduce the incidence of developing type 2 diabetes by 58 percent. That's what the Diabetes Prevention Program Research Group showed. This landmark study proved that diet and exercise are even more effective than medication at staving off type 2 diabetes.

- In a study of men and women living in Spain who were at high risk for developing heart disease and type 2 diabetes, those who most closely followed a Mediterranean diet cut their risk for type 2 diabetes by 56 percent compared to those who didn't follow a Mediterranean diet.

If you have diabetes—either type 1 or type 2—*The Pescetarian Plan* can help stave off diseases triggered by your condition. For example, having diabetes makes it two to four times more likely that you'll develop heart disease. It can prompt painful neuropathy of the feet and other areas, dim your vision, and cause kidney disease.

To prevent all these complications, you want to keep blood sugar as close to normal as possible—that's what a good diet, enough exercise, losing weight (if you need to), and proper medication can do.

In some cases of type 2 diabetes—albeit a minority—you can reverse the condition, at least for a number of years.

- The Look AHEAD Trial found that 11.5 percent of people went into remission after changing their diets and exercising. Remission rates were even higher—15 to 21 percent—in the participants in the diet and exercise group who lost the most weight (more than 6.5 percent of starting weight) and made the biggest fitness gains.
- In an Italian study, only 44 percent of newly diagnosed diabetes patients (they were not yet on medication) who followed a Mediterranean-style diet required medication to control their blood sugar four years later. That's compared to 70 percent of those who ate a low-fat diet. Mediterranean dieters were essentially able to reverse their condition partly because they lost more weight than folks on the low-fat diet. Plus, they reaped other diet-related health benefits, including less inflammation, lower blood sugar and "bad" LDL cholesterol, and higher "good" HDL cholesterol compared to the low-fat dieters.

~~~~~~
GET THAT HEALTHY GLOW
~~~~~~

The saying "You are what you eat" is especially true when it comes to the skin. Most Americans are well nourished enough to avoid the all-out vitamin or mineral deficiencies that cause skin sores, spots, and cracking, but many have a borderline deficiency that can make skin more wrinkly and rough. Of course, wearing sunscreen and limiting sun exposure is your first line of defense, but a good diet can help offset the sun's damaging ultraviolet rays.

There are two basic skin-protecting compounds in the diet: antioxidants and healthy fats. The more antioxidants you have in your diet, the better equipped you are to fight off skin-damaging molecules called free radicals, which are formed in response to sunlight exposure. (Skin's number one enemy is the sun—it's the main culprit behind wrinkles and cancer.) Most of the fat in your skin is unsaturated—polys and monos—so you need adequate amounts of these fats in your diet.

Both a Mediterranean diet—and omega-3s in general—have been linked to skin health.

- People of various ethnicities (Greek, Australians, and Swedes) living in different areas (either their native country or abroad) who ate the most vegetables, olive oil, fish, yogurt, nuts, and legumes had the least amount of skin wrinkling. Meanwhile, high intake of butter, milk, meat, processed meat (like sausage), and sugar (from soft drinks and foods like cake and pastries) was linked to more wrinkles.
- People living along the Mediterranean Sea tend to have lower rates of melanoma, a potentially deadly skin cancer, despite the sunny climate. There are just 3 to 11 cases of melanoma per 100,000 inhabitants in Mediterranean countries, compared to 20 cases per 100,000 in the United States; 50 per 100,000 in Australia; and 9 to 22 per 100,000 in Scandinavia. While differences in skin pigment (darker skin is more protective), latitude (higher latitudes—further from the equator—are protective), altitude (the higher, the more risky), and how much people expose their bodies to the sun all come into play, so does diet.

CLOBBER CANCER

The stats still amaze me: Genetic defects are thought to be responsible for only 5 to 10 percent of cancer cases. That means that 90 to 95 percent of cancers are due to the way we live. This includes smoking, diet, alcohol, sun exposure, pollution, infections, stress, obesity, and a sedentary lifestyle.

Diet can prevent up to 35 percent of cancer cases (up to 75 percent for prostate cancer and colorectal cancer), exercise up to 40 percent. Pretty much everything about *The Pescetarian Plan* reduces cancer risk:

- Superfoods like broccoli and olive oil contain a wealth of antioxidants and other substances that disable carcinogens (cancer-causing substances) and slow cancer growth. The risk that avid extra-virgin olive oil eaters have of getting any type of cancer compared to infrequent users may be up to a third lower, according to a University of Athens review of the research. Extra-virgin olive oil appears to be particularly protective against breast cancer and cancers of the digestive system (colorectal, oral cavity, pharynx and esophagus, and pancreatic). Credit goes to the oil's monounsaturated fat and phytonutrients, both of which fight inflammation. The thirty-plus phenolic compounds in extra-virgin olive oil also disable cancer-causing substances before they can do harm. The diet quashes inflammation, which is a cancer trigger.
- The appetite-suppressing foods on this plan help you get down to—and maintain—a healthy weight, which can reduce cancer risk by 4 to 40 percent. (The higher numbers are for breast, colon, and endometrial cancers.)

While there are countless studies on how to prevent cancer, research into the best way to eat and exercise once you've had cancer (or are in treatment for it) is still paltry. The few studies that are out there indicate that the same things that help prevent the disease also help prevent a recurrence. I do want to point out results from the Harvard Nurses' Health Study: While close adherence to a Mediterranean diet didn't make it more or less likely that breast cancer survivors would die from the disease, it did appear to significantly lower their odds (by 60 percent) of dying of *other* causes, like heart disease and respiratory illnesses such as pneumonia. This is important to know, because cancer treatment can increase risk for these other illnesses.

Something else to keep in mind: There's a difference between getting a vitamin or other substance through food and through supplements. For instance, the beta carotene in carrots, cantaloupe, spinach, and many other fruits and vegetables protects against the development of cancer. But when smokers were given beta carotene supplements, their chances of developing lung cancer actually increased. So until the research makes a compelling case that taking supplements helps prevent cancer, I'm recommending that you stick with this healthy pescetarian approach. That means getting your nutrients through food and using supplements sparingly, if at all (more on supplements later in the book).

Chapter 3

THIS IS YOUR BRAIN ON FISH

Your brain consumes about a fifth of the oxygen in your body, and where there's oxygen, oxidants—molecules that can destroy cells—are formed. The antioxidants in all the fruits and vegetables and whole grains on the Pescetarian Plan fend off those oxidants. In conjunction with the program's anti-inflammatory and blood pressure–lowering agents, they also help clear the arteries, supplying blood to the brain and minimizing the risk of stroke. The Pescetarian Plan also keeps you well stocked with B vitamins, which are so crucial to cognition. And those are just a few of the protective elements!

The food that has attracted the most attention in the scientific community when it comes to brain health is fish. Its omega-3 fats are vital to proper brain function, helping you think more clearly and be happier. Omega-3s—especially the fish oil DHA—allow your brain cells (neurons) to do their job: talk to one another.

To picture what's going on in your brain, look at the image on the next page. The bottom neuron is "talking" to the top one. In order to get its message across, it has to "shout" over that little gap between them, called the synaptic cleft.

To do so, neurons send chemical messengers (little dots) over the cleft. These are called *neurotransmitters* or *brain chemicals*. They get picked up by receptors on the next neuron (the little wrenchlike structures at the end of the top neuron). Receptors are all shaped a little differently; they're tailored to accept specific types of neurotransmitters in the same way that a key fits into a lock.

There are scores of neurotransmitters that affect mood, reasoning, memory, desire, and other brain functions. For instance, serotonin can boost mood and make you think more clearly. Opiates relieve pain and stimulate pleasure. (Heroin, morphine, and other opioid drugs are shaped a lot like natural opiates and can also bind to their receptors, creating a drug high.)

For this neuron-to-neuron communication to run smoothly, the cells need a quality cell membrane or lining. (In the image below, it's the dark border on both the top and bottom neurons.) Here's where fish comes in. One of the omega-3 fish oils—DHA—plays a key role in keeping brain cell membranes healthy. This fat is actually part of the membrane, keeping it fluid, which eases communication across the synapses. It also helps repair injured brain cells and quash destructive inflammation in the brain. DHA even has a hand in creating brain chemicals. Every one of its functions in the brain ultimately affects mood and intellect.

But if your diet is low in DHA—like the typical American diet—other fats crowd into the membrane, which can impede neurotransmitter travel. And that can dampen mood, contributing to depression, anxiety, and possibly attention deficit hyperactivity disorder (ADHD). Americans' omega-6 to omega-3 ratio is about 16 to 1. The Pescetarian Plan has a 1-to-1 ratio—which our brain and bodies were designed for.

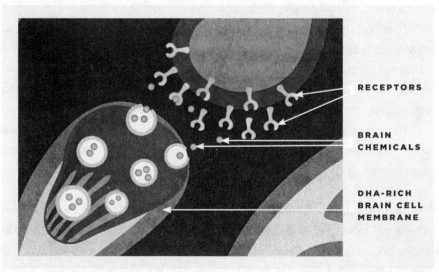

Image credit: National Institute of Mental Health, National Institutes of Health, Department of Health and Human Services.

It's not just omega-3s that give your brain a boost—it's also the blueberries, whole grains, nuts, and all the other ultra-healthy Pescetarian Plan foods that reduce inflammation and clear arteries (including those leading to the brain).

The result? Get a load of what this diet can do for your mood, memory, and cognition, as detailed below.

BOOSTS MOOD

"There's an epidemic of depression in the U.S. and in many other countries with low fish consumption. The bulk of the evidence shows that low levels of fish or omega-3s play a role," says Joseph Hibbeln, M.D., acting chief at the National Institute on Alcohol Abuse and Alcoholism. His pioneering research in the mid-1990s, based on his hunch that omega-3 intake was linked to mood, was the launching pad for thousands of subsequent studies.

- Depression rates are up to 65 times higher in countries where people don't eat much fish compared to those where fish is a regular menu item, according to Dr. Hibbeln's research.
- Young women who switched to a Mediterranean-style diet for just ten days had "significant improvements in self-rated vigour, alertness and contentment," conclude the authors of an Australian study, published in the journal *Appetite*.
- The healthy elderly of Ikaria (described in the introduction to this book) have varying levels of fish consumption. Those who ate the most fish—at least three fish meals *weekly*—were free of depression, while those who had fish three times a month or less were more likely to suffer from mild depression. (But keep in mind that overall, depression rates are very low in this population.)
- Eating fatty fish may lower the risk of depression by 25 percent; women seem to benefit even more than men in some studies. (Taking omega-3 supplements is also helpful; see chapter 7 for details.)
- Depressed people averaged 27 percent less DHA in their red blood cells than non-depressed people, reports a Dutch study.
- In countries where women eat more fish, the postpartum depres-

sion rates are lower, sometimes dramatically so. For instance, in Singapore, where moms eat twice as much seafood as in the United States, rates are less than 1 percent, compared to 12.5 percent for American women.

- During the final trimester of pregnancy, the fetal brain is rapidly expanding and loading up on DHA—one of the omega-3s in fish. To protect the developing brain, nature decided to give the fetus first dibs on DHA. So if mom's supply is low, the fetus gets it, leaving the mother deficient. That's a setup for depression, both during and after pregnancy.

IT'S SMART TO GET PHYSICAL

No matter how good your diet, if you just sit around, your brain will dull. Here's some motivation to go lace up your sneakers: Exercise triggers the formation of new brain cells—something you generally *lose* with age! It also preserves—and enhances—what you have by helping keep arteries leading to the brain clear, reducing inflammation, and triggering the release of feel-good brain chemicals. Exercise plays an enormous role in helping both prevent and treat depression. In research studies, about half the depressed people who take part in aerobic exercise programs go into remission.

MAKES US SMARTER

The Pescetarian Plan won't just sharpen your brain, it could give you smarter children. That's because the final trimester of pregnancy is a time of rapid brain development in the fetus. Supply enough critical omega-3s and you could influence IQ!

Do that by eating fatty fish three times a week during pregnancy *and* while breastfeeding. But what about the possible harm to your fetus by mercury in fish? You'll be fine if you choose the low-mercury fish recommended in chapter 10.

- The research linking omega-3 intake during pregnancy and offspring IQ is so compelling that the World Health Organization and the Food and Agriculture Organization (representing Europe) recommend that pregnant women take in an average of 200 mg of DHA daily through food. Three ounces of wild salmon, sardines, and most other fatty fish contain about 1,000 mg of DHA, so if you have a three-ounce serving of fatty fish three times a week, you're more than covered.

- Women who ate at least 12 ounces of fish per week during pregnancy were more likely to have children with higher IQs and who scored higher in tests of social, fine motor, and communication skills than kids whose moms ate fewer than 12 ounces, according to a study from researchers in Bristol, U.K. (Children were tested from six months old all the way to 8 years old.)
- Boys who regularly ate fish at age 15 scored higher in a battery of intelligence tests at age 18 than boys who ate little to no fish, in a Swedish study of nearly 5,000 young men. Specifically, those eating fish *more* than once a week scored 12 percent higher in tests of overall intelligence; 9 percent higher in verbal intelligence; and 11 percent higher in visual/spacial skill than those who ate fish less than once a week. Even eating fish just once a week sent scores up significantly. The brain boost held true even after accounting for other factors that impact intelligence, such as exercise and the parents' education level.

Adults also benefit:

- The more fatty fish people ate, the better they scored on a battery of cognitive tests measuring reaction time, memory, reasoning and problem-solving, and overall cognition, according to a Dutch study of 45- to 70-year-olds.
- Chicagoans aged 65 to 94 who had at least one fish meal per week had a 60 percent lower risk for developing Alzheimer's disease compared to those who rarely or never ate fish over the four-year period of the study by Chicago's Rush Institute for Healthy Aging.
- Elderly men who ate little to no fish had four times the rate of cognitive decline compared to men averaging about five ounces weekly, reports a five-year Dutch study. (Imagine what even more fish, as recommended on this pescetarian diet, could do!)

- Seniors with mild cognitive impairment, a precursor for Alzheimer's, whose diets closely followed a Mediterranean pattern were about half as likely to develop Alzheimer's over four years as those who didn't eat this way, according to a study from Columbia University Medical Center in New York City. The Alzheimer's Association recommends a Mediterranean diet.

Omega-3s and Beta-Amyloid

Omega-3 may be a weapon in the battle against Alzheimer's, suggests exciting new research from Columbia University in New York City. After examining the diets and blood of 1,219 men and women, ages 65 or older, who were free of dementia, the researchers made an important finding: The more omega-3s in the diet, the lower the blood levels of a marker for Alzheimer's. The marker is a type of beta-amyloid—the protein that causes destructive plaques in Alzheimer's disease. Other research has found that people who have higher levels of this beta-amyloid in their blood are more likely to develop Alzheimer's.

In this study, researchers looked only at food sources of omega-3s, not supplements. People who took in a gram of omega-3s from their diet daily—that's the amount in two ounces of salmon—had 20 to 30 percent lower beta amyloid levels than people who consumed half a gram. "We didn't hit a threshold amount after which it didn't matter how much omega-3 you consumed. The higher the levels, the lower the beta-amyloid count. The same thing has been found in animal research, and we're very excited to see the same in humans," says Nikolaos Scarmeas, M.D., a co-author of the study and associate professor of neurology at Columbia University's Taub Institute.

Chapter 4

PESCETARIAN ULTRA-NUTRITION

Adiet that can whittle your waistline, stave off killer
diseases, improve your skin, *and* boost mood and brain power? I wouldn't
blame you if you've become a little skeptical at this point in the book. But the
research doesn't lie; a Mediterranean-Pescetarian way of eating really works
because it meets your body's needs so beautifully. In this chapter, I'll show
you how.

Pescetarian Macronutrients

Strip a diet—any diet—to its core and you're left with four macronutrients:
protein, fat, carbohydrates, and, if you drink, alcohol. These are where your
calories come from. Choose your macronutrients wisely, and your diet will
be slimming, inflammation-quashing, and healthy in every other way.
Choose poorly (as in the typical American diet) and your macronutrients
can make you overweight and sick.

The protein (such as fish), fat (olive oil, nuts, seeds, and avocado), carbohydrates (whole grains, fruits, and vegetables), and even alcohol (red wine)
on the Pescetarian Plan conspire to put you in your best shape ever. How?
Keep reading. You're going to feel *great* about every bite you put in your
mouth on this diet!

PERFECT PROTEIN

Americans are big on protein; we average 41 ounces of beef, poultry, and pork a week (half of this is from beef). Meanwhile, we're eating only about five ounces of seafood weekly, about half of it shrimp. All that meat and so little fish has tragic health consequences.

Fatty Fish—a Pescetarian "Must-Have"

The stats are startling. Here's a CliffsNotes version of just a few studies: People who eat more fish live, on average, 2.2 years longer than those who eat little fish, according to a 2013 Harvard University study. A Norwegian study found that women who eat little to no fish were three times more likely to develop heart disease than women who eat fish once a week. Dutch men and women eating the most fish had just half the risk of suffering fatal heart attack than people eating very little fish. Fish eaters have a 12 percent lower risk for colon cancer, concluded an *American Journal of Medicine* review. These are just a few examples in a, um, sea of studies showing the extraordinary power of fish.

That's why fish—especially fatty fish—is a must on the Pescetarian Plan. What makes fatty fish so fabulous for you: omega-3 fats, which clobber inflammation, quiet heart arrhythmias (electrical disturbances of the heart rhythm that cause heart attack and stroke), lower triglycerides, and improve brain function. The omega-3s unique to seafood—EPA and DHA—are particularly potent anti-inflammatory agents, even more so than the omega-3s found in walnuts, flax, and other plant foods. With enough fish oils in your cells, you tend to produce fewer inflammatory compounds, such as eicosanoids and cytokines. Also, you make more molecules called "resolvins," which, as the name implies, help resolve inflammation, shutting down the process and preventing—or limiting—damage to tissues.

But omega-3s can't claim all the credit. Fish has a few other health tricks up its fins! It's rich in the organic acid taurine, which safeguards your arteries by reducing inflammation, blood pressure, LDL, and triglycerides. In the international Cardiovascular Disease and Alimentary Comparison (or CARDIAC) study, it was the most avid fish consumers—the Japanese—who had the highest levels of taurine in their bodies (measured by the amount excreted in their urine). And of course, the Japanese were at the lowest risk for heart disease than the other nationalities studied.

Fish is also notable for what it lacks, namely lots of calories and saturated fat (which, as explained earlier, may be a fat you want to eat less of). The numbers speak for themselves; I've provided some beef stats, too, in order to give you a comparison:

4 OUNCES OF RAW ...	Calories	Total fat (g)	Sat fat (g)	Omega-3 fat (g)
LEAN EXAMPLES				
Tilapia	109	2	0.7	0.2
Beef tenderloin, lean, trimmed of fat	174	7	2.7	0
FATTY EXAMPLES				
Atlantic salmon	161	7	1.1	2.2
Regular ground beef (typically used in burgers)	350	30	12.2	0.2

What's the Beef Against Red Meat?

Just as seafood is a Pescetarian "must," red meat is a "must-not." The news about red meat just keeps getting grimmer. How harmful is it? It can kill you. Sounds dramatic, but just look at what a quick sampling of many research studies shows:

- People who ate the most meat were 33 percent more likely to die over the course of a ten-year study than those who ate the least, according to a National Cancer Institute study of more than half a million people (an enormous amount for any study). The researchers found that the most avid meat-eaters were about 20 percent more likely to die from cancer. With heart disease deaths, it broke down differently by gender: Men who consumed the most meat were 27 percent more likely to develop the condition than men who ate little meat; the risk was higher—50 percent—for women who ate the most compared to the least.
- Every daily serving of red meat (3 ounces in this study) can raise your risk of dying by 13 percent. For processed meat, it's even worse: A serving of bacon (two slices) or a 1.5-ounce hot dog increased the risk of death by 20 percent. That's what Harvard University's ongo-

ing study of men (Health Professionals Follow-up Study) and women (Nurses' Health Study) found, looking at 121,340 people.

You read that right: Compared to a person who eats no meat, a person who averages one serving daily is 13 percent more likely to die over the course of twenty-two years (the length of time of the Harvard study). A person who averages two servings daily is 26 percent more likely to die. And a person who eats bacon and hot dogs is even more likely to meet an early end.

Keep in mind, these numbers are based on a three-ounce serving. We all know that restaurant portions are significantly bigger—they can be anywhere from four to ten ounces! At Outback Steakhouse, a *modest* order—the nine-ounce sirloin—racks up three meat servings. So you can see how easy it is to average one serving daily.

- Eating little to no meat for twenty years or more adds, on average, 3.6 more years of life, according to a review of the research by scientists at Loma Linda University in California.

Nutritionists have always thought that the saturated fat and cholesterol in red meat are to blame, especially when it comes to heart disease. But now that saturated fat/heart disease science is being questioned (as you'll see later in the chapter), other possible causes have surfaced. One prominent suspect: cancer-causing substances called "heterocyclic amines" that develop in meat when it's broiled, fried, or otherwise prepared using high cooking temperatures.

And in 2013, a completely different culprit emerged, a substance generated by our gut bacteria. It basically works like this: Meat is a rich source of L-carnitine, a substance that helps the body burn fat for energy. Sounds good so far, right? But in excess, microbes in our gut convert it to a compound called TMAO. TMAO is bad news—it prevents excess cholesterol from leaving the arteries so it hangs around and clogs them up. A study led by researchers at the Cleveland Clinic in Ohio found that people with high TMAO levels tended to have more coronary artery disease.

The takeaway: A meat-free diet that's rich in plant foods creates a healthier gut environment. And not just because there are fewer L-carnitine–chomping bacteria. Other studies show that a diet along the lines of the Pescetarian Plan can shift the balance of gut bacteria to help you lose weight and boost immunity.

TRULY HEALTHY FAT

The American diet is also seriously out of whack when it comes to fat. It's not that we're eating too *much* fat, believe it or not. There's nothing wrong with our 33 percent of total calories coming from fat. (Fat makes up about 35 percent of your diet on the Pescetarian Plan.) It's that we're eating too many bad fats and not enough of the good ones.

Fat 101

Before I explain how our fat imbalance is making us sick, I'm going to turn you into a fat expert, which is always useful when dinner conversation lags (just kidding!). You'll understand why you're using olive oil as your mainstay fat on this plan, why you're eating an omega-3 source daily, and why I'm even encouraging you to eat more almonds than pumpkin seeds. Here's what you need to know:

- There are three basic types of fat (also called "fatty acids") with different degrees of saturation. Saturation refers to the structure of fats—think of them as having a backbone of carbon with hydrogen molecules attached. (Still with me?) The degree of saturation makes a big difference to your body.
  - *Saturated fat* is fully loaded with hydrogen. Found in red meat, chicken skin, butter, whole milk, and coconut and palm oils, in excess, it raises cholesterol and promotes inflammation. But, as explained on page 37, new research suggests that the saturated fat–heart disease connection may not be as airtight as we thought.
  - *Monounsaturated fat* has middling levels of hydrogen. It's the main fat in olive oil, avocados, almonds, and certain other nuts and has been linked to lower risk of heart disease. It's the primary fat in the Pescetarian Plan.
  - *Polyunsaturated fat* (main types are omega-3 and omega-6) has the least amount of bonded hydrogen. While both are linked to lower risk of heart disease, in excess, omega-6s

may raise cancer risk. More on the difference between the two later in this chapter.

- Within each type are different fats. Just as there are two basic types of polyunsaturated fat—omega-6s and omega-3s—there are a number of different saturated fats and a few different monounsaturated fats. For instance, as luck would have it, stearic acid, the main type of saturated fat in chocolate, does not raise blood cholesterol, whereas most other saturated fats do.

- Individual foods contain a mix of fats. For instance, the fat in butter is 68 percent saturated, 28 percent monounsaturated, and 4 percent polyunsaturated fat. But it breaks down very differently in olive oil: 14 percent saturated, 75 percent monounsaturated, and 11 percent polyunsaturated.

- All fats have the same calorie count: 9 calories per gram (compared to 4 calories per gram for carbohydrates and protein, and 7 calories per gram for alcohol). That means, for instance, that olive oil, which is so rich in monounsaturated fat, has approximately the same number of calories per tablespoon as butter (high in saturated fat).

Plant vs. Fish Omega-3s

On the Pescetarian Plan you eat fatty fish three times a week. That's because these fish are the only source of the two most potent types of omega-3s: eicosapentaenoic acid (EPA) and docosahexaenoic acid (DHA). Countless scientific studies show that EPA and DHA tamp down inflammation, lower risk of heart disease, improve insulin sensitivity (which helps reduce the likelihood of pre-diabetes and type 2 diabetes), fight depression, raise infant IQ, and help ward off breast cancer and possibly other cancers. Another fish oil—docosapentaenoic acid (DPA)—is looking as though it's also protective, but scientists have only just begun to investigate it.

However, the omega-3 found in plants like flaxseeds, chia seeds, and walnuts—alpha linoleic acid (ALA)—doesn't appear to be as effective. It's healthy, don't get me wrong, because it does reduce inflammation and heart disease risk. But it's just not as potent as fish oils. And it's unclear whether it helps with any of the other conditions influenced by EPA and DHA. Our bodies do convert a little ALA to EPA and DHA, but probably less than 5 percent, so you can't depend on it.

HOW OUR FAT IMBALANCE IS MAKING US SICK

Compare the fat sources in a caveman's diet (nuts, seeds, wild animals, and fish) to the types of fatty foods on the typical American menu (corn-fed beef, fried chicken, potato chips, soybean oil-based salad dressing, ice cream, Oreos, pie crust, and countless others). It's clear that we're eating too much omega-6 fat and saturated fat and way too little omega-3.

OMEGA-6 AND OMEGA-3 IMBALANCE

We were designed for a 1-to-1 omega-6 to omega-3 ratio, but we're at 16 to 1 (if not higher). How did we wind up with so much omega-6 in the diet? Two main culprits: The first is our oils. We're eating a lot of soybean oil—it's the primary oil in processed food and what's sold as "vegetable oil" in our supermarkets—and it's heavy on omega-6s. And another oil in widespread use, corn oil, is predominantly omega-6.

Meanwhile, we're eating very, very little omega-3. Just look at the high omega-3 sources I recommend in this book—fatty fish, walnuts, chia seeds, and flaxseeds—who's eating those foods consistently? And, believe it or not, beef used to be a decent source of this fat, back when cattle grazed on grass, which contains omega-3. Corn, oats, and other grains now fed to cattle do not contain this healthy fat.

While omega-6s are healthy in moderation, in excess they may promote inflammation. (I say "may" because the research still isn't clear on this.) Making matters worse, they compete with omega-3s—which are anti-inflammatory—for entrance into cells. Given their numbers in the typical American diet, omega-6s win handily.

TOO MUCH SATURATED FAT . . . (PROBABLY)

I say "probably" because, once again, the science is in flux. For decades, the prevailing wisdom was that excessive saturated fat was one of the main contributors to heart disease. It seemed to make sense: People who have high levels of saturated fat in their fat cells and other cell membranes have more chronic inflammation, which causes a host of problems, as explained in chapter 2. Not to mention all the studies showing that when people switch to diets high in saturated fat, LDL cholesterol goes up. High LDL levels put people at greater risk for heart disease.

But there's a nagging dot that's not connecting: Populations that consume more saturated fat don't necessarily have higher levels of heart disease than those that consume less saturated fat. That's why researchers are rethinking the saturated-fat issue. Here's what I gleaned from a recent paper by Remko Kuipers, professor of molecular genetics of prokaryotes at the University of Groningen in the Netherlands:

- While it's true that too much saturated fat raises LDL, simply having a high LDL might not predispose you to heart disease. It's a particular type of LDL—oxidized small dense LDL—that is the real bad guy, and it is formed as a result of chronic inflammation. Interestingly, there's evidence that people with high LDL levels who eat a Mediterranean diet do not produce the dangerous small dense LDL.
- Populations that eat more saturated fat don't necessarily have a high risk of heart disease.
- Too much saturated fat *in your fat cells* can trigger inflammation. But the amount of saturated fat *in your diet* doesn't necessarily correspond to the amount in your fat cells. What *can* fill your cells with saturated fat: Eating a lot of refined flour and sugar—even if the rest of your diet is low in saturated fat. That's because your body breaks down those foods into glucose and then turns some of that sugar into saturated fat. In fact, replacing saturated fat with refined carbs actually *increases* heart disease risk.

So it's looking as though the true heart disease culprits might be white bread, white rice, cookies, candy, and all other foods made with refined flour and sugar. Your body is converting them not only to fat but to *saturated* fat. And that encourages inflammation, which, among other things, encourages benign LDL to become the dangerous oxidized small dense LDL.

On the other hand, carbs with a low glycemic index, like the whole grains, fruits, and vegetables on the Pescetarian Plan, which are rich in anti-inflammatory compounds, seem to help ward off inflammation and are linked with lower heart disease risk.

Even if the heart disease link doesn't pan out, too much saturated fat is associated with type 2 diabetes risk, and it may depress mood. So until the science is sorted out, I'm going with the "less than 10 percent of total calories" recommended by the U.S. Dietary Guidelines and other health organizations. That's right in line with the traditional Mediterranean diet.

TRANS FAT

Just a few years ago, trans fat would have been a major dietary concern. Some of the fat sources I described earlier on—Oreos, pie crust, and cookies—used to be rife with this ultra-unhealthy fat. That's because they were made with partially hydrogenated vegetable oil, which is loaded with trans fat. But this oil began disappearing from ingredient lists in 2006, when the Food and Drug Administration (FDA) required food manufacturers to include grams of trans fat on the nutrition label. As of press time the FDA is proposing a ban on partially hydrogenated oil.

But until that happens, it's still lurking in some processed and fast foods, usually in amounts small enough that the nutrition label reads "0 g trans." Don't be fooled! Thanks to an FDA ruling technicality, the product can still contain up to 0.49 grams per serving. Doesn't sound like much, but even 2 grams daily is considered harmful. So, theoretically, you could accumulate that much by having four servings of a food. There's a simple way to avoid trans fat: Simply read the ingredient list and avoid any product that contains partially hydrogenated oil.

There's also a little trans fat in fatty cuts of beef and lamb and in whole and 2-percent dairy products, but these foods aren't on the Pescetarian Plan, so you'll automatically avoid (or at least drastically limit) them.

RIGHTING YOUR FAT BALANCE

Stick with the Pescetarian Plan, and you'll achieve the optimal fat balance. (The specifics are in chapter 5.) No need to think about it much—just follow my guidelines, and your fats will fall into place. On this plan:

- *Your omega-6 to omega-3 ratio is 1 to 1.* That's considered an ideal range, a far cry from the 16-to-1 (or even higher) ratio in the American diet. Thanks to all the omega-3–rich foods on this plan, you'll average 3,000 mg of this healthy fat daily.

- *Monounsaturated fat is your primary fat.* That's thanks to all the olive oil, avocado, almonds, and other high-mono foods on this plan.

- *Saturated fat is less than 10 percent of total calories.* Until the science becomes clear, I'm sticking to this level, which is in line with the traditional Mediterranean diet. That translates to no more than 15 grams of saturated fat on a 1,500-calorie plan; less than 18 grams on a diet of 1,800 daily calories, and so forth. No need to memorize the numbers; you'll automatically stay within this saturated fat limit by following the food group plan in chapter 5. Keeping saturated fat in check isn't all that hard to do, because this plan eliminates a few of the big sources: red meat, chicken skin, and whole and 2-percent milk.

EXTRA-VIRGIN OLIVE OIL: A PESCETARIAN DIET "MUST"

Extra-virgin olive oil is considered one of the most effective health-promoters in the Mediterranean diet. It's made by simply pressing olives—pits and all—grinding them into a paste, decanting to separate oil and water from the solids, and then spinning to separate the oil from the water. This unrefined product is not only flavorful but imbued with phytonutrients.

You get a double health bonus in extra-virgin olive oil: monounsaturated fat *and* health-promoting compounds such as polyphenols. Some act as antioxidants, while others may actually put the brakes on tumor growth and kill cancer cells, according to new research at Catalan Institute of Oncology in Girona, Spain.

A number of studies comparing people in the same community show that those eating the most olive oil have a lower cancer risk. One analysis of the major research studies found that these high olive oil consumers cut their risk of any type of cancer by a third. Protection was even higher against breast cancer and cancers of the digestive system.

Monos Boost Mood?

Omega-3s are famous for their mood-boosting benefits, but monos may also perk you up. In a University of Vermont College of Medicine experiment, people reported being in a better mood after they switched out of their typical American diet to one high in monounsaturated fat (at levels similar to this Pescetarian Plan). Plus, they spontaneously became 12 to 15 percent more physically active.

GOOD CARBS

Whenever I'm asked (and I get this *a lot*): "Aren't carbs fattening?" I know, of course, the carb in question: starch. Yes, sure, starches can be fattening, but only if you eat too many—especially of the wrong type.

Before I explain why starch is not necessarily your enemy, and how much sugar, fruit, and milk (yes, it contains carbs) you can get away with, let's make sure we're on the same page. To understand carbs you have to know the three basic types and how they affect blood sugar (the glycemic index).

CARBS, THREE WAYS

What's a carb? Here are the three main types in your diet:

- Sugar, such as sucrose, which is table sugar; glucose and fructose, both of which are found in fruit and honey; and lactose, which is found in milk. (Close cousins of sugar are sugar alcohols, like xylitol and erythritol, which are used in sugarless gums and candies and have half the calories of sugar.)
- Starch, which is the main component of wheat, corn, other grains, legumes, potatoes, and other starchy vegetables. Starch is composed of hundreds of glucose molecules bound together; enzymes in our mouth and gut cleave off those glucose units so that we can absorb starch.

- Fiber is the outer coating of most grains (some, like oats and bar-ley, contain fiber all the way through), but it's also in fruits, vegeta-bles, and legumes. Like starch, fiber is made up of glucose units strung together, but in a form we can't break down, so it has no calories. However, it's fodder for the "good bacteria" in your gut, which do digest some of it (a good thing, as I explain on page 10).

THE GLYCEMIC INDEX

Ever notice that after eating a bowl of oatmeal, you're able to last a little longer in the morning before the hunger pangs begin than if you'd had corn flakes? That's the glycemic index at work.

The glycemic index (GI) is a measure of how fast and steep blood sugar rises after eating a set amount of a carbohydrate-containing food. It's a 1–100 ranking of carbohydrate-containing foods based on their effect on blood sugar. High glycemic index foods (rated 70 and higher) send blood sugar soaring quickly, medium-GI foods (56 to 69) take a little longer to turn into blood sugar, and low-GI foods (55 or lower) take the longest time to convert to blood sugar.

WHAT AFFECTS GI?

Before your body can transform grains, sugar, vegetables, fruit, milk, or yogurt (dairy foods contain "milk sugar," or lactose), these foods have to be digested and absorbed. You do this in a jiffy for high-GI foods like sugar, white bread, and other foods made with refined flour. But it takes your digestive tract a lot longer to break down fruit, vegetables, and coarsely cut or intact whole grains (low-GI foods). That means a slower rise in blood sugar.

Notice I said "coarsely cut or intact whole grains"? They're the ones with a low glycemic index. Foods made with whole-grain flour, especially finely pulverized flour, can actually have high GIs, the same as refined flour. For instance, whole-wheat bread made from fine whole-wheat flour has a GI similar to white bread—about 75. But bulgur wheat (cracked wheat) has a GI of 46. Cheerios, made from pulverized oat flour, has a high GI of 74, but plain oatmeal, which is a much coarser cut, has a low GI of 42. So the more intact and coarsely cut, the lower the GI.

What you eat with your high-carb food also affects GI. Protein and fat in a meal tend to lower GI. Vinegar does as well. Refrigerating potatoes, rice, and other starches overnight produces a fiber-like substance called "resistant starch," which also reduces glycemic index.

PESCETARIAN CARBS

By incorporating low-GI foods and controlling the total number of carbs eaten, the Pescetarian Plan is a low-GI diet. Numerous studies show that people are able to lose weight and maintain weight better on these types of diets. Why?

- Sticking to low-GI carbs helps keep blood sugar on an even keel, minimizing spikes and dips. Those dips signal "hunger" to the brain, so avoiding them helps keep appetite in check.
- Insulin, the hormone responsible for normalizing blood sugar and promoting fat storage, tends to be lower on a low-GI diet. Lower insulin levels mean that fat is less likely to be stored and more likely to be burned for energy. Always helpful when weight loss is your goal!

SMART STARCHES

Legumes and whole grains, mainstays of the traditional Mediterranean diet, are what I call "smart starches"; people who regularly eat these (and few refined grains) tend to be thinner and healthier. Also traditional in Mediterranean cultures is physical activity; most people were out farming, walking, and burning calories in other ways to afford a fair amount of starch.

Because most of us are sitting at a desk all day, we have to watch *all* our portions, including healthy starches. Here's how you do so on this plan, and why pescetarian starches are so "smart":

1. *You don't eat too many of them.* Stick with the number recommended in the Seven Pescetarian Principles (and study up on just what a portion looks like), and you can enjoy potatoes, pasta, and other starches guilt-free.

2. ***They're easy on the blood sugar.*** Intact whole grains (think steel-cut oats vs. Cheerios or cracked wheat vs. whole-wheat flour) and legumes are the mainstay starches on this plan. As explained in "The Glycemic Index" earlier in this chapter, they elicit a slower and smaller rise in blood sugar, which, among other benefits, helps control body weight.

3. ***They're loaded with nutrients.*** When grains like wheat get refined into white flour, they lose their two most nutritious parts: the bran and the germ. But whole grains are rich in phytonutrients, B vitamins, iron, magnesium, and other minerals.

YOUR FIVE PERCENT SUGAR PLAN

How bad is sugar? Consider this: Soft drinks and sugary beverages alone are blamed for 180,000 deaths worldwide each year, 25,000 of them in the United States. Type 2 diabetes, heart disease, and cancer triggered by excessive consumption of these drinks are behind the deaths, according to a Harvard University study.

Intuitively, you know that sugar's not good for you; it's the classic "empty calories" ingredient (a can of soda is basically water, sugar, and chemicals with zero nutrition). Plus, of course, sugary foods tend to be loaded with calories.

But new research is indicating an even more sinister side to sugar—inflammation. Here's how sugar—and to some extent, white bread and other foods made with refined flour—goes on the attack. Keep in mind that a little sugar (and white flour) won't hurt you; it's the excess that does you in.

- Sugar, especially fructose, directs your body to lay down more visceral fat, the toxic deep belly fat in and around your organs that is especially pro-inflammatory.
- In your gut, sugar encourages the growth of bacteria that (a) cause you to extract more calories from your food and (b) promote inflammation.
- Your body converts excess sugar into saturated fat, the most inflammatory type (more on this on page 38).
- If your blood sugar is high from pre-diabetes or diabetes, you're forming high levels of "advanced glycation end-products," or

AGEs. These sugar-based compounds trigger inflammation and have been linked to heart disease, cancer, vision loss, and more. While we all form them, they can wreak havoc when we produce too many. A high-sugar (and refined flour) diet, coupled with high blood sugar, is the perfect breeding ground for AGEs.

- If sugary foods have crowded out vegetables and other inflammation fighters, you're in even more trouble!

Frightening stuff, but keep it in perspective: A little sugar won't hurt you. Personally, I wouldn't want a diet devoid of chocolate, the occasional cookie, or other treat. On the Pescetarian Plan, added sugar is no more than 5 percent of total daily calories. I recommend that you stick to that level if possible, by staying within your daily treat level spelled out in part 2 of this book. Your absolute max should be the 10 percent of total calorie mark recommended by the World Health Organization. What's "added sugar"? It's any sweetener (other than artificial) stirred into a cup of coffee, baked into cookies, or added to store-bought salad dressings, cereal, and so many other foods. Examples: white table sugar, high fructose corn syrup, honey, and maple syrup. Most sweeteners are a 50–50 split of glucose and fructose. (Despite the bad rap high fructose corn syrup has gotten over the years, research shows there isn't anything particularly evil about the sweetener, which is 55 percent fructose. The one I avoid is agave syrup, which is about 85 percent fructose.)

Flipping through the recipes, you'll see some sugar in the nutrition analyses. Most of that sugar is naturally occurring. It's the sugar found in fruit, milk, and plain yogurt as well as the little bits in vegetables and grains. Because nature packaged this sugar in foods that are so high in vitamins, minerals, and/or phytonutrients, you don't have to limit naturally occurring sugar except in one circumstance: fruit juice. Unlike whole fruit, fruit juice is a very concentrated source of sugar and calories. For example, you'd have to eat two oranges to get the sugar grams (and calories) in one cup of orange juice. If you love juice, make it one of your daily treats (details in chapter 5).

BRING ON THE FRUITS AND VEGETABLES

Other than being careful about your juice intake, one of the glorious things about the Pescetarian Plan is that you *don't* have to worry about portions of fruits and vegetables. These are the ultimate "good carbs"—nutrient-rich and calorie-poor (in a good way)! The only reason I even bothered suggesting a certain number of servings in chapter 5 is so that you get *enough*.

While all fruits and vegetables are healthy, some, like arugula, broccoli, Brussels sprouts, grapes, kiwi, and oranges, are outstandingly so. That's because they are particularly rich in vitamins and/or phytonutrients. The latter are plant compounds—there are thousands of them—that promote our health in a variety of ways. For instance, anthocyanins, plant pigments that give blueberries, blackberries, beets, and other fruits and vegetables their purplish or deep reddish hues, produce substances in the body that kill stomach cancer cells while protecting normal cells. Another phytonutrient that targets cancer cells: sulforaphane, found in broccoli, Brussels sprouts, and other cruciferous vegetables. Find these and other superfoods in the Pescetarian Standout Superfoods chart (see chapter 7).

DAIRY: THUMBS UP OR DOWN?

Why am I putting dairy in the "Carb" section? Because a cup of milk has nearly as many grams of carbohydrates as a slice of bread. Milk and yogurt are a mix of carbohydrates, protein, and fat (unless you use fat-free).

Dairy is controversial—it's been blamed for a lot of nasty things, from increasing mucus to raising cancer risk. But my review of the research shows that dairy's plusses far outweigh any minuses. (And no, I'm not an undercover agent for the dairy industry!) The accusations—and my findings:

- It's unnatural for adults to have dairy—that's why so many people are lactose intolerant. While it's true that some people lose the ability to digest lactose (milk sugar), many others have no problem with it. So if you're lactose intolerant, you can avoid dairy, drink soy milk or other nondairy milks, or try Lactaid or another brand of milk that cleaves the lactose molecule into its component sugars, glucose and galactose. Most people do well on this type of milk.
- Dairy causes allergies. A small number of people are allergic to proteins in dairy. Like allergies to nuts, eggs, and other foods, your body mistakenly reads that protein as a harmful allergen. If you're allergic, you need to avoid dairy.

- Dairy makes you produce more mucus. Again, if you're having a true allergic reaction to dairy, mucus could be one of the symptoms. But otherwise, studies don't prove a link.

- Dairy makes you fat. While it's true that cheese, ice cream, cream, whole and 2-percent milk, and sugary yogurts are high in calories, the bulk of the research shows that dairy eaters are either slimmer or no different in body weight than people who consume little to no dairy. It could be all the calcium in dairy—calcium tends to signal the body to burn fat instead of store it. Also, calcium may shave off a few calories from your meal by binding with some of the fat you just ate and whisking it out of the body.

- Dairy clogs up your arteries. Cheese, whole and 2-percent milk, and yogurt are high in saturated fat, and saturated fat raises LDL ("bad" cholesterol), which in turn is linked to clogged arteries and heart disease. But research indicates that dairy eaters—even if they're eating higher-fat stuff—are less likely to suffer from heart disease and stroke. It could be that the types of saturated fat in dairy aren't so artery-clogging (and, as I've mentioned, the saturated fat/heart disease connection is being questioned these days). Also, it's probably the calcium at work once again—it lowers blood pressure. Low-fat dairy (nonfat and 1-percent milk and yogurt)—the type recommended on this plan—sends blood pressure even lower than high fat dairy, according to the Harvard Nurses' Health Study.

- Dairy increases cancer risk. Some studies show that men who eat the most dairy have a higher risk for prostate cancer, but others show no link. Of all the lobs fired at dairy, this one may have the most weight behind it, but even so, the association is considered weak at best. The link between dairy and ovarian cancer is even weaker. One study showed an increased risk in women who had three or more servings of dairy a day (the Pescetarian Plan recommends just two servings), but then other studies showed that dairy *reduces* the risk of this cancer. Meanwhile, people consuming more milk and other dairy foods appear to have a *lower* risk of colorectal, bladder, breast, and colon cancers.

A reason to say yes to yogurt (and to kefir, a drinkable fermented milk product made with different types of bacteria than yogurt): Their "friendly bacteria" may confer a health advantage over other dairy products. Commonly used strains such as *Lactobacillus acidophilus, Bifidobacteria,* and *Lactobacillus casei* can lower cholesterol production, reduce inflammation, and boost immunity. Studies indicate that yogurt fans, especially among the elderly, have stronger immune systems. And a study in Australia linked yogurt (not milk or cheese) consumption to lower levels of plaque in the carotid artery, the one leading to the brain that you want to keep nice and clear to prevent strokes.

The bottom line on dairy: You can have a perfectly healthy diet with or without it. If you like milk, yogurt, and cheese and are not lactose intolerant or allergic to dairy, you should benefit from the two daily servings (preferably from nonfat or 1-percent milk, plain yogurt, or plain Greek yogurt) that I recommend in chapter 5. That's the amount eaten, usually in the form of cheese or yogurt, on Mediterranean diets. (And even if you are lactose intolerant, you might do well on lactose-free milk or small quantities of yogurt, milk, or cheese.)

And if you prefer to do without dairy, you can substitute in soy milk, almond milk, or other nondairy milks.

BETTER BOOZE

You've got to love a diet that actually *encourages* drinking wine. And let's raise a glass to the scientists who've made Merlot, Cabernet, and your other favorite reds even more enjoyable by showing that yes, they truly are one of the reasons the Mediterranean diet is so good for you.

When it comes to heart health, the studies are nearly unanimous: Wine is protective. And not just wine—you may be surprised to discover that *all* alcohol has heart benefits. Gin, vodka, beer, and the like help prevent heart disease, heart attack, and stroke because they make blood less inclined to form clots while raising HDL (good cholesterol). Plus, alcohol helps tame chronic inflammation, a trigger not only for heart disease but also for cancer and diabetes.

However, wine, especially red wine, appears to be most protective. Its potent antioxidants like anthocyanins and resveratrol offer benefits beyond those of plain old alcohol. They protect LDL (bad cholesterol) from oxidation, which is the first step to artery-clogging plaque. They also reduce the risk of blood clots to a greater degree than other alcohols. Red wine has about ten times as many health-promoting compounds as white. That's because unlike white wine, red wine is fermented along with nutrient-rich grape skins.

So red appears to take first place. It's a close race for second between white wine and beer. Yes, beer! Beer contains a number of antioxidants and other agents derived from hops and has been shown to lower LDL.

But while wine and beer may be good for your heart, they may not be so good when it comes to cancer risk. The alcohol-cancer link isn't clear. Some studies show that *any* alcohol, even red wine, promotes the risk of breast and other cancers. Then there's research showing that wine may actually *lower* the risk of basal cell carcinoma (a type of skin cancer) as well as cancers of the lung, colon, and prostate.

Whether alcohol is or isn't a cancer trigger appears to come down to genetics. For example, a National Cancer Institute–funded study found that for women with a certain variation in a gene responsible for metabolizing alcohol, drinking was linked to a 34 percent increase in breast cancer risk compared to women who did not have that genetic variation. The risk was particularly high for women drinking more than three drinks daily.

The bottom line, starting with a few "ifs":

(a) If you don't abuse alcohol (alcoholism and binge drinking are terrible for your health);

(b) If drinking doesn't weaken your determination to stick to reasonable portions of food; and

(c) If your healthcare provider gives the go-ahead after you discuss cancer risk and other downsides associated with drinking.

Then enjoy in moderation!

By moderation, I mean no more than one drink per day for women, two for men. This is crucial—any more than this is linked to an *increase* in risky visceral fat. And keep in mind, a drink is 5 ounces of wine; 12 ounces beer, or 1½ ounces of gin, vodka, whiskey, or other hard liquor. Those are the *upper* limits on the Pescetarian Plan. The healthiest sips: red wine, followed by amber or dark beer, then white wine.

If, for any reason, you just don't like to drink, there's no compelling reason to take it up. You're getting doused with enough health-promoting foods on this plan that you really don't need alcohol.

PART

2

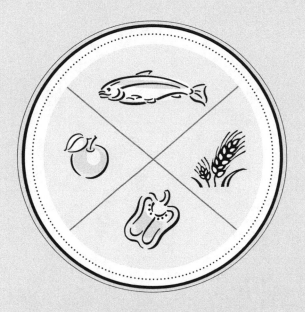

Your Pescetarian
Action Plan

Chapter 5

THE SEVEN PESCETARIAN PRINCIPLES

You're about to take control over your diet and health—maybe for the first time ever. You're in the driver's seat here. Instead of simply handing you a diet, I'm turning *you* into an expert. How? By teaching you the "Seven Pescetarian Principles." Nail these, and you'll soon be enjoying your own version of pescetarianism—one that keeps calories in check (without having to count calories), is wholesome and health-promoting, and suits your taste buds and lifestyle. Most important, this way of eating works over the long run.

Perfect these principles, and you'll sail through any food situation: restaurant menus, dinner parties, theme parks, and even buffet tables! It's going to be *such* a relief when you:

- *Can confidently fill your plate with the right type—and amount—of food.* That's because you'll have mastered the Pescetarian food groups, knowing by sight *just what a portion of grains, fat, and other foods looks like.* You'll also know *how many servings* of each you need to eat to either shed pounds or maintain a healthy weight.
- *Stop counting calories.* You'll simply track Pescetarian food groups instead. This is a *lot* easier. In no time, it'll become automatic—you'll barely need to think about how many grain or

protein servings you've accumulated. The only calories you have to track are for treats like ice cream, cookies, and alcohol.

- *Go at your own pace.*
- *Really enjoy your food.* And you will—I mean it!
- *See inches and pounds disappear* (even more quickly if you also exercise).
- *Feel a lot better.*

Think "Process," Not "Diet"

All you have to do is make this critical shift in vocabulary and mind-set, and boy, is this going to get easier! That's because being on a diet invokes all sorts of guilt, a sense of deprivation, and those crazy impossible standards that you're bound to break.

But accept that becoming a nutritious eater or a regular exerciser is a process instead of an all-or-nothing, I'm-on-or-off-my-diet affair, and everything changes. And it's a process that you own and are actively engaged in—not something you're doing for your doctor or anyone else.

But isn't *The Pescetarian Plan*, well . . . a diet? Yes, it is, in that it's a way of eating. But you're not following a strict set of rules, nor are you walking around hungry all day from consuming too few calories. (At least, you'd better not be—that's why you have a range of calorie levels to choose from. It may take a little trial and error, but you'll hit a daily calorie level that helps you shed pounds, if that's what you need, or helps you maintain your weight.)

Here's how I suggest you tackle the principles:

- Simply read through them first.
- Don't worry about the daily calorie levels mentioned in each of the seven principles. You might be thinking, "Wait a sec! Didn't she just say I won't have to count calories?" Aside from tallying treat calories, you won't. But you do have to choose an overall *daily* calorie level so you know how many servings of grains, seafood, and other foods to have every day. Not yet, though—I'll help you figure that out in the following chapter.

- After you've read through all the principles, turn to the next chapter for your "action plan." Here's where you'll pick up the tools that will bring the seven principles to life . . . as soon as your next meal!

Pescetarian Principle No. 1:
Dump Meat and Poultry, and Eat
Recommended Amounts of Protein

As I mentioned earlier, the Italian word for fish is *pesce,* and therein lies the fundamental, distinguishing feature of pescetarianism: You cut out meat and poultry and get your protein from fish, other seafood, and vegetable protein.

If you're a little shaky on your seafood cooking skills, the step-by-step instructions in chapter 12 are very easy to follow. And there are some terrific recipes in chapter 13 and seafood meals in the meal plan starting on page 285.

PROTEIN SERVINGS PER DAILY CALORIE LEVEL:

1,500 daily calories: 6 daily
1,800 daily calories: 7 daily
2,100 daily calories: 7 daily
2,500 daily calories: 8 daily

A PESCETARIAN PROTEIN SERVING (55 CALORIES) IS:

- Fish, fatty (see list on page 56): 1 ounce
- Fish, white-fleshed (cod, flounder, perch, tilapia, rockfish, etc.): 2 ounces
- Cheese, reduced-fat: ¾ ounce
- Cheese, regular: ½ ounce
- Edamame (young, green, soybeans): ⅓ cup
- Egg, medium: 1
- Egg whites: 3 (from a large egg) or ½ cup liquid egg white in a carton
- Shellfish, shell removed: 1½ ounces (3 medium clams, 3 medium mussels, 5 Eastern [smaller] oysters, 2 Pacific oysters, 3 large or 7 small scallops, 7 or 8 medium shrimp)
- Tofu: 2–4 ounces, about a third of a cup (check label for how much you get for 55 calories, as products vary)

PROTEIN POINTERS:

1. *You'll typically have more than one serving in a meal.* Although a protein serving is just an ounce or two, remember, you get six or more servings daily. So it's fine to have three to six ounces in one meal.

2. *Start out by having fatty fish twice a week, then work up to having it three times a week.* The following species are low in mercury, so they should be your mainstays:

   - Arctic char
   - Mackerel (but not king mackerel, which is high in mercury)
   - Salmon (canned or fresh)
   - Sardines (canned or fresh)
   - Trout
   - Tuna* (fresh or "chunk light" canned)

   * Limit to no more than six ounces six times a month, due to tuna's mercury content. See "Catches to Reel In, Catches to Toss Back" chart on page 121 for servings per month of canned albacore and many other types of fish.

3. *Limit the following high-cholesterol proteins to twice weekly.* Have 4 ounces of shrimp, 4 ounces of squid, or 2 eggs no more than twice weekly. For example, if you have 2 eggs on Monday and 4 ounces of shrimp on Friday, you've eaten all your high-cholesterol foods for the week and should choose only low-cholesterol proteins for the remainder of the week.

4. *Have no more than 2 ounces of either regular or reduced-fat cheese per day.* Cheese is high in saturated fat, and while this fat doesn't appear to be as harmful as once thought, it's better to be safe than sorry until the research is clear!

Using Legumes as Your Protein

Although black beans, kidney beans, lentils, and other legumes contain protein, they're so carbohydrate-rich that they're nutritionally closer to grains than they are to fish, tofu, and other high-protein foods on this list. That's why I put them in the "Grain/Starchy Vegetable" list on page 62.

That said, you can still use them as your protein source. If you are trying to lose weight, do this at no more than one meal a day. That's because you don't get nearly as much protein for the calories as you do with seafood, egg whites, or tofu. And as I've mentioned, protein is particularly appetite-quelling, so it's a key weight-loss tool. So if you're trying to lose weight and closely following the number of servings in each food group on this plan, you would consider three-quarters of a cup of beans *both* a grain/starchy vegetable *and* a protein serving. For instance, if you had three-quarters of a cup of chickpeas in your salad, you've used up one grain/starchy vegetable serving and one protein serving.

If you don't need to lose weight, sub them in as you like.

Pescetarian Principle No. 2:
Eat Your Fruits and Vegetables!

One nice perk to this principle is that, unless you're already a produce fiend, you get to *add* food—fruits and vegetables—to your diet. Even if you think you're eating the right number of fruits and vegetables recommended for your calorie level, it's best to take some time to measure and make sure. Most people aren't quite there yet—in fact, a third of Americans eat *less than one serving* of fruits and vegetables daily. If you've been skimping, then this one dietary change can be a significant turning point in your health.

To help you ramp up your produce servings:

- Keep washed and sliced carrots, celery, cucumbers, radishes, and peppers in the fridge. Ditto for fruits (sliced apples and pears keep pretty well).
- Aim to have vegetables or fruits in at least two meals daily. Or have one big salad—that'll more than cover all your vegetables for the day.
- Throw a handful or two of spinach or other greens into soup.
- Lean on frozen fruits and vegetables if fresh ones aren't looking so fresh (or don't taste that good). Interestingly, thawing causes frozen produce to leach out vitamins, so don't thaw before cooking or adding to a smoothie. Buy plain, unsweetened fruit and plain, unseasoned vegetables to spare yourself the sodium, and use your own herbs and a light touch with the salt shaker, if needed.

- Keep dried fruit around to have when you run out of fresh. Just watch the portions, as calories can add up fast. (As mentioned below, a portion is 2 tablespoons.)
- Don't worry about what type of fruit or vegetable you're eating— we'll work on making the highest-nutrition choices later on, when you're comfortable with the basics.

FRUIT SERVINGS PER DAILY CALORIE LEVEL:

1,500 daily calories: 2 daily
1,800 daily calories: 2 daily
2,100 daily calories: 3 daily
2,500 daily calories: 4 daily

Want to enjoy even more fruit? If you're not watching your weight, you can have as much fruit as you like. Even if you need to shed pounds, another daily serving won't hurt. In fact, you may be able to get away with even more—if you love fruit, go ahead and try. The reason I limited fruit at all is to keep to my promise that I'm delivering a specific daily calorie level.

Have any type of fruit you like. Later on, you can work on getting a greater variety and making sure you're eating the nutritional superstars.

A PESCETARIAN FRUIT SERVING (60 CALORIES) IS:

- a small fruit (like a kiwi or small apple)
- ½ a large fruit (like a banana, grapefruit, or mango)
- ½ cup of cut-up fruit or berries, fresh or frozen
- 2 tablespoons dried fruit (like raisins) or 1½ dried figs
- ½ cup 100% juice (It's better to eat whole fruit because it's more filling and lower in sugar for the volume and contains fiber, but if you love juice, you can count it as *just one* of your daily fruit servings, then use your daily treat calories to cover any more juice you have.)

VEGETABLE SERVINGS PER DAILY CALORIE LEVEL:

1,500 daily calories: 4 or more daily
1,800 daily calories: 5 or more daily
2,100 daily calories: 6 or more daily
2,500 daily calories: 7 or more daily

A PESCETARIAN VEGETABLE SERVING (25 CALORIES) IS:

- 1 cup salad greens or chopped herbs
- ½ cup raw vegetables (other than salad greens)
- ½ cup frozen vegetables
- ½ cup cooked vegetables (fresh or frozen)
- ½ cup canned vegetables (such as canned tomatoes)
- ½ cup vegetable juice (Make this only one of your daily vegetable servings because it lacks fiber; if you have any more, you'll have to use your treat calories.)

If you want even more vegetables, go for it! These are really minimums. Vegetable calories are negligible (many of these portions are actually less than 25 calories); I've never heard of anyone gaining weight by eating too many vegetables!

In the next chapter, I'll point you to the most nutritious vegetable choices. For now, just focus on eating enough vegetables—period!

Food Face-off: Organic vs. Conventional?

You're definitely doing the environment a favor when you buy organically grown produce, but does it matter to the body? It depends. Some studies show organic produce can have a slight nutrition edge over conventional, but a review of the research published in the *Annals of Internal Medicine* in 2012 found no difference. As for safety, if you wash conventionally grown produce well, you can remove all—or nearly all—the pesticides. The produce in the "Highest in Pesticides" column (on the next page) requires more scrubbing—if you want to splurge on organic, these would be the ones to buy. (These lists are courtesy of the Environmental Working Group.)

What's more important than organic or conventional is freshness: The closer you eat a fruit or vegetable to the time it was picked, the more nutrients you get.

Lowest in Pesticides	*Highest in Pesticides*
Asparagus	Apples
Avocado	Bell peppers
Cabbage	Blueberries (domestic)
Cantaloupe (domestic)	Celery
Corn (sweet)	Cucumbers
Eggplant	Grapes (imported)
Grapefruit	Green beans
Kiwi	Kale/collard greens
Mango	Lettuce
Mushrooms	Nectarines (imported)
Onions	Peaches
Peas (sweet)	Potatoes
Pineapple	Spinach
Sweet potatoes	Strawberries
Watermelon	

Pescetarian Principle No. 3:
Tame Treats (Including Alcohol)

How would you describe your relationship with chips and other salty snacks, or sweets like ice cream, cookies, cake, and candy? To alcohol? If you're in control—in other words, you can easily stop at a reasonable portion—then you should do well with the amount offered on this plan.

If you feel out of control, as in, you tend eat the entire box of cookies instead of just a few, then for a few weeks, try avoiding your "trigger" foods. You might be able to reintroduce trigger foods later on, or you might find you're better off crossing them off your list for good. Meanwhile, use your treat calories on other favorite foods that *aren't* addictive.

Aim to stay within your daily treat calories at least five days this week with the goal of eventually doing this every day. (If you drink, stay within your alcohol guidelines *every day* this week because if you overdo it, you might lose you resolve and overeat as well.)

TREATS PER DAILY CALORIE LEVEL
(CANDY, COOKIES, CHIPS, FLAVORED YOGURT, ALCOHOL, OR ANY OTHER INDULGENCE)

Because portions for treats are all over the map, this is the one food group that you will have to measure in calories rather than portion sizes. But you'll find plenty of treat examples, at all four calorie levels, in the meal plans starting on page 285.

DAILY TREAT CALORIES:

1,500 daily calories: 100 calories every other day
   (or 50 calories daily)
1,800 daily calories: 150 calories daily
2,100 daily calories: 200 calories daily
2,500 daily calories: 225 calories daily

If you're on the 1,500-calorie plan, you're probably not thrilled about the stingy treat allotment. I don't blame you! But squeezing in all the nutrition you need on just 1,500 calories is nearly impossible, and that's why there's so little room left for treats. Remember, this plan is flexible—if you find you can get away with a little more (like 100 calories daily), then please do! And you can save up for bigger splurges by forgoing a treat on one or more days.

ALCOHOL ADVICE:

1. *Stick to the safe limits.* That means, if you drink, have no more than one drink per day if you're a woman; no more than two drinks daily if you're a man. Even if there are still treat calories left after this alcohol limit, don't spend them on extra alcohol; have a cookie, dark chocolate, or another treat instead. A drink is 5 ounces of wine (a little over ½ cup), 12 ounces of beer (1½ cups), 1½ fluid ounces (3 tablespoons) of 80 proof spirits, or 1 fluid ounce (2 tablespoons) of 100 proof spirits. ("Spirits" are gin, vodka, whiskey, or any other "hard" liquor.)

2. *Drink with your meal.* That's the way it's done in Mediterranean countries, where red wine is linked with health and longevity. You don't get as tipsy this way, and you have more control. (Believe me, though—you'll still enjoy that glass of wine!)

3. *If it triggers appetite, skip it.* If you notice that you tend to overeat

after having even one drink, consider abstaining from alcohol until you reach a healthy weight (and even then, still be careful).

Pescetarian Principle No. 4:
Get a Handle on Starches

There's a wide range of starchy foods from the least healthful (think french fries and croissants) to super-healthful (steel-cut oats, sweet potatoes, and wheat berries). The healthy starches can, in moderation, actually help you lose weight by quelling appetite and promoting satiety—that full, satisfied feeling following a meal. Many studies show that whole-grain eaters are thinner than people who eat refined grains. But, of course, even these healthy carbs contain calories—so you have to keep servings in check.

When you start on my Pescetarian Plan, you'll want to measure *every* grain product or starchy vegetable, at least at the beginning. You might be surprised to find that your regular portions are bigger than you imagined. If you eat cold cereal, you'll have to check the label for calories, because these vary so widely. Remember, a Pescetarian serving is 80 calories of cereal (it's perfectly fine to have two servings at once).

GRAIN/STARCHY VEGETABLE SERVINGS PER DAILY CALORIE LEVEL:

1,500 daily calories: 5 daily
1,800 daily calories: 5 daily
2,100 daily calories: 6 daily
2,500 daily calories: 7 daily

A PESCETARIAN GRAIN/STARCHY VEGETABLE SERVING (80 CALORIES) IS:

- Bagel: ¼ of a large one or ½ of a small one (100 percent whole-grain)
- Bread: 1 slice (100 percent whole-grain; check label for calories)
- Cold cereal: Amount varies—check label to see how much you get for 80 calories. For instance, 80 calories is a half-cup of shredded wheat, and not even a full ¼ cup of Ezekiel 4:9 Almond. They're both terrific cereals—you just can't put the same amount of each in your bowl. I mix Ezekiel (low volume for the calories) with shredded wheat or flaky cereals (more volume for the calories). Cereals should be 100 percent whole-grain.

- Corn: ¾ cup (kernels)
- Corn meal or polenta: ⅓ cup cooked (stone ground whole)
- English muffin: ½ muffin (100 percent whole-grain)
- Flour, whole-wheat, or other whole-grain: 3 tablespoons
- Grains, whole, including barley, bulgur wheat (cracked wheat), couscous, rice, wheat berries: 2 tablespoons uncooked; ½ cup cooked
- Hot cereal: ¼ cup dry, ½ cup cooked (100 percent whole-grain, such as oatmeal, mixed whole-grain)
- Legumes, including black beans, chickpeas (garbanzo beans), kidney beans, white beans, lentils, etc.: ⅓ cup cooked or canned; 2 tablespoons dried
- Pasta: ¾ ounces uncooked; ½ cup cooked or canned (100 percent whole-wheat, quinoa, or other whole-grain)
- Steel-cut oats: ⅛ cup dry or ⅜ cup cooked
- Sweet potatoes, potatoes, or green peas: ½ cup cooked

STARCH SUGGESTIONS

1. *Distribute your grain/starchy vegetable servings however you like.* If you're at five daily servings, I often recommend having:

    - 2 at breakfast (a nice bowl of cold or hot cereal)
    - 2 at lunch (so you can have a sandwich if you want one)
    - 1 at dinner

2. *Make at least half of your grain servings whole grains.* When you feel ready, switch over entirely to whole grains.

3. *Eat legumes at least four times a week.*

4. *If you have to avoid gluten, don't forgo whole grains.* Some of the gluten-free offerings in stores are made with refined corn flour or other refined gluten-free flours. Avoid these and instead use buckwheat, whole-grain corn grits, oats (gluten-certified), quinoa, and whole-grain rice. And, of course, you can sub in the healthy starchy vegetables listed above.

5. *"Stretch" starch dishes with fruits and vegetables.* Starches are a lot more caloric than fruits and vegetables. A half-cup of cooked grains, potatoes, or legumes comes to 80 to 90 calories. Contrast that to about 40 calories for the same amount of fruit and about 10 calo-

ries for a half-cup of raw vegetables. By pumping up starch dishes with fruits or vegetables, you get a bigger, more satisfying portion for fewer calories. Case in point: the Quinoa with Lemon, Olive Oil, and Pomegranate recipe on page 190, contains as much herbs and pomegranate as quinoa. I usually use more vegetables than pasta in my dinners. Likewise, my cereal bowl is about 50–50 fruit and grain.

For examples of meals that use whole grains and legumes, turn to Appendix C. And to figure out what a whole grain is, check out the box below.

Is It a Whole Grain?

A whole grain contains the outer bran layer, the middle starch section, and the inner germ (as in wheat germ). Refined grains, such as white flour, are pure starch; the bran and germ have been removed (as well as all the nutrients).

Misleading food labels can make it difficult to know if you're getting a whole-grain product. For instance, "made with whole grain" may still mean that there's more refined flour than whole grain. "Multigrain" simply means a variety of grains were used—it could be that they are all refined.

But the ingredient list doesn't lie. To help you decipher it, here's your guide:

Whole Grains	*Not Whole Grains*
Amaranth	All-purpose flour
Barley*	De-germed cornmeal
Buckwheat	Enriched flour
Bulgur	Rice, rice flour
Brown, red, black rice	Rye flour
Groats	Semolina**
Millet	Unbleached flour
Oat flour	Wheat flour
Oats, oatmeal, steel-cut oats	White rice
Popcorn	
Rye berries	
Sorghum	

Triticale

Wheat berries

Whole corn

Whole rye

Whole semolina

Whole spelt (often just "spelt")**

Whole-wheat, whole-wheat flour

Wild rice

* Pearled barley has some of the bran removed, but that's all right because it's still high in fiber and nutrients.

** Even without the word *whole*, this grain is often whole. You can't be sure unless the product is billed as "100% whole-grain" on the label.

Pescetarian Principle No. 5:
Switch to Low-Fat/Nonfat Dairy (or Nondairy Milk)

If you're a whole or 2-percent milk drinker, I strongly recommend switching to 1-percent or nonfat. You'll lower the saturated fat and calorie content of your diet, and you can spend those extra calories elsewhere. And if you prefer a nondairy milk, such as soy or almond milk, that will work just fine on this plan. (Read about the pros and cons of dairy in chapter 4.)

If you just can't stand milk, yogurt, or nondairy alternatives, then you can skip this Pescetarian food group. Instead, make up your two dairy servings by having two extra protein servings and one more grain/starchy vegetable serving each day (for instance, 2 ounces of fish and 1 slice of whole-grain bread). And you'll have to make up the 600 milligrams of calcium provided by two dairy servings by taking calcium supplements. However, as explained in chapter 7, this isn't ideal.

You'll notice that I didn't include cheese here; instead, I've placed it with high-protein foods. That's because cheese is mainly protein and fat—it contains very little of the lactose (milk sugar) contained in milk and yogurt.

DAIRY/NONDAIRY SERVINGS PER CALORIE LEVEL:

1,500 daily calories: 2 daily

1,800 daily calories: 2 daily

2,100 daily calories: 2 daily

2,500 daily calories: 2 daily

A PESCETARIAN DAIRY SERVING (90 TO 100 CALORIES) IS:

- Nonfat or 1-percent milk: 1 cup
- Nonfat or low-fat (usually around 1.5%) plain yogurt: ¾ cup
- Calcium- and vitamin D–enriched almond, coconut, hemp, rice, or soy milk: 1 cup
- Soy yogurt, plain: ½ cup

DAIRY TIPS

1. *If you're used to whole or 2-percent milk, ease down to 1-percent gradually, so your milk doesn't feel too "thin."* If you're drinking whole milk, mix it with 2-percent and have that until it runs out. Then, use 2-percent alone for about a week. Follow that with a mix of 2-percent and 1-percent. You can stop at 1-percent or keep going until you're used to nonfat. *I promise* that once you get used to the lighter milks, you'll prefer them, and fattier milks won't taste right.

2. *Buy plain yogurt.* Vanilla and fruit yogurt are fine as desserts or treats, but they are too high in sugar to be part of your meals and snacks. Plain yogurt is not only lower in sugar, but it also has more calcium (because the sugar and fruit in sweetened yogurt displace the actual, calcium-containing yogurt). If you like your yogurt a little sweet, start by adding a teaspoon of honey (6 g sugar) or maple syrup (4 g sugar) per cup. That's just a fraction of the 13 extra grams of sugar found in just 6 ounces of sweetened yogurt.

3. *If using almond, coconut, hemp, or rice milk, consider adding protein to your meal.* Cow's milk and soy milk have about 8 grams of protein per cup; these other milks have just 1 or 2 grams. That's not a problem if your meals have other sources of protein, but if it's just cereal, milk, fruit, and nuts for breakfast, then your meal will be lacking in protein. That's okay on occasion, but, especially if you're trying to lose weight or maintain a weight loss, those 8 grams of high-quality protein from cow or soy milk go a long way to help quell appetite.

Add protein to breakfast by scrambling up an egg white, buying a breakfast cereal that includes soy (like Kashi GoLean), or having an ounce of cheese or fish (smoked salmon or even leftover fish from the night before), or two ounces of tofu. If making a smoothie, add 2 tablespoons of soy or whey protein powder.

And whatever nondairy milk you choose, make sure it's enriched with calcium and, ideally, vitamin D as well. (On the nutrition label, you should see at least 25 percent of the Daily Value for calcium and about the same for vitamin D.)

Pescetarian Principle No. 6: Enjoy Healthy Fat

One reason this Pescetarian diet tastes so good is that it's *not* a low-fat diet. In keeping with the Mediterranean diet, about 35 percent of total calories in this plan come from fat. But it *is* a "healthy-fat diet" averaging 3,000 mg of omega-3s daily. Because even healthy fat is high in calories, *portions matter,* so stick closely to my daily portion recommendations in this section.

You'll notice that olive oil and nuts and seeds are a "must" on this plan. If you have an allergy to a particular nut or seed mentioned in the recipes or meal plans, just substitute with a nut or seed that you are *not* allergic to. (For instance, if you have a peanut allergy but do fine with sunflower seeds, swap in sunflower seeds for peanuts.) If you cannot eat any nuts or seeds, then replace them with olive oil, avocado, or another healthy fat from the lists on page 68.

Olive oil ensures that you get the right balance of fat. Nuts and seeds do the same, and because they are "high-satiety" foods, they keep you feeling fuller longer for the calories. A number of studies show that people who eat nuts tend to be trimmer than those who don't. Nuts also help lower cholesterol and are linked to a lower risk for heart disease. That said, you still have to watch portions, because the little kernels are quite high in calories.

FAT SERVINGS PER DAILY CALORIE LEVEL:
  1,500 daily calories: 7 daily; at least 1 should be extra-virgin olive oil, and at least 3 should be nuts or seeds.
  1,800 daily calories: 8 daily; at least 2 should be extra-virgin olive oil, and at least 3 should be nuts or seeds.
  2,100 daily calories: 10 daily; at least 3 should be extra-virgin olive oil, and at least 4 should be nuts or seeds.
  2,500 daily calories: 13 daily; at least 3 should be extra-virgin olive oil, and at least 6 should be nuts or seeds.

A PESCETARIAN FAT SERVING (45 CALORIES) IS:

- Avocado: 3 tablespoons chopped (⅕ Hass avocado)
- Coconut flakes, unsweetened: 2 tablespoons
- Oils (canola, peanut, olive, walnut, etc.): 1 teaspoon
- Mayonnaise, regular: 1½ teaspoons (½ tablespoon)
- Mayonnaise, light: 1 tablespoon
- Nuts: 1 tablespoon (about 7 almonds, 5 cashews, 6 hazelnuts, 5 pecans, 8 peanuts, 13 pistachios)
- Olives: 5 medium (because these are high in sodium, eat them only occasionally)
- Seeds (such as chia, flaxseeds, pumpkin, sesame, and sunflower): 1 tablespoon
- Nut or seed butter (such as peanut butter, almond butter, or tahini): 1½ teaspoons (½ tablespoon)

HEALTHY FAT BALANCE STRATEGY:

In order to get the most healthful fat balance, follow these guidelines:

Eat Daily: Fats High in Monos and Omega-3s

Most of the fat in your diet should come from the following sources, which are high in monounsaturated fat and/or omega-3s. You'll definitely be eating nuts daily, as they are built into your Seven Pescetarian Principles.

HIGH MONO:	HIGH OMEGA-3:
Almonds and almond butter	Chia seeds
Avocados	Flaxseed oil
Canola oil (it's also omega-3–rich)	Flaxseeds
Cashews and cashew butter	Walnuts
Olive oil (this is your principal oil)	
Peanut oil	
Macadamia nuts	
Peanuts and peanut butter	
Pistachios	
Pecans	

Note: You're also going to be eating three omega-3–rich fatty fish a week, such as salmon, sardines, and trout. The list of high-omega fish are on page 121.

Eat Daily: Fats High in Omega-6 (Ideally, no more than 2 servings)

One or two daily fat servings can come from these sources, which are high in omega-6, a polyunsaturated fat.

> Brazil nuts
>
> Corn oil
>
> Grapeseed oil
>
> Pumpkin seeds
>
> Safflower oil (except "high-oleic," which is high in
>   monounsaturated fat)
>
> Sesame oil
>
> Sesame seeds and sesame seed butter (tahini)
>
> Soybean oil
>
> Sunflower seeds and sunflower seed butter
>
> Margarine made without partially hydrogenated oil

Limit: Fats High in Saturated Fat

Limit the following fats to no more than once per day—less often if you have heart disease. These foods are all high in saturated fat. If you're currently eating a lot of foods in this column, replace them with foods that are high in polyunsaturated and monounsaturated fats. Do *not* replace those calories with refined carbs—that could cause your triglyceride levels (a dangerous blood fat) to rise.

> Butter
>
> Coconut oil
>
> Cream
>
> Cream cheese
>
> Sour cream

Avoid: Fats Containing Trans Fat

Avoid foods made with partially hydrogenated oil. This oil is the main source of the über-unhealthy trans fat in the diet.

SAT FAT SUBSTITUTES

The left side of this chart is a who's who of popular American foods, many of which are not only high in saturated fat (which can raise cholesterol) but are also rife with sodium or sugar and low in nutrients. The processed, or "cured" meats—hot dogs, sausage, pepperoni, and bacon—are even more noxious to your health than plain old red meat, as explained in chapter 4.

Fortunately, for every unhealthy food, there's a much healthier alternative, listed in the right-hand column.

SATURATED FAT-LADEN FOOD	G SAT FAT	PESCETARIAN ALTERNATIVE	G SAT FAT
Buffalo wings (10) with blue cheese dressing	24	Grilled shrimp (12 large)	1
Regular ground beef patty (4 oz. cooked)	9	Wild salmon burger (4 oz. cooked)	1.4
Hot dog/sausage (4 oz. cooked)	10–18	Vegetarian hot dog or sausage (4 oz. cooked)	3
Pepperoni/bacon (2 oz. cooked)	8	Smoked salmon (2 oz.)	0.5
Fried chicken (4 oz. cooked)	4	Breaded and baked white fish (4 oz. cooked)	1–2
2-percent or whole milk (1 cup)	3–4.5	1-percent or nonfat milk or soy milk (1 cup)	0–1.5
Danish, donut, or croissant (3 oz.)	5–7	Carrot Muffin (page 156)	2
Butter (1 tablespoon)	8	Olive oil (1 tablespoon)	2
Premium ice cream, like Ben & Jerry's or Häagen-Dazs (½ cup)	10	Regular ice cream, like Breyers Original (½ cup)	2–4

Pescetarian Principle No. 7:
Become a Smart Sipper

On the Pescetarian Plan, water is your main beverage. You'll also be drinking milk (or nondairy milk) and, if you like, coffee, tea, and wine. But other drinks—even fruit juice—are a waste of calories, in my opinion. They don't leave you feeling as full as eating fruit or other solid foods. In fact, soda, very sweet iced tea, fruit punch, fruit drinks, sweet coffee concoctions, and other sugary drinks are considered culprits in the obesity crisis.

Need a nudge to drink more water? It perks up energy, endurance, and brain power (even slight dehydration makes for muddier thinking). And drinking enough water can make you slimmer. Here's why:

- You take in fewer calories. Water drinkers average 9 percent fewer calories—about 194 fewer—than non–water drinkers. Shaving off that many calories could mean a 20-pound weight loss in a year.
- It makes weight loss easier. People who drank two cups of water before a meal lost 44 percent more weight on a 12-week weight loss program, in research led by Virginia Tech University in Blacksburg, Virginia.
- It raises your metabolic rate, the rate at which you burn calories. This has been shown in both adults and children.
- Drinking water before and during a meal increases satiety (you feel fuller on fewer calories).
- It boosts exercise endurance and keeps motivation up while exercising.
- It displaces all the calorie-loaded sugary beverages that Americans are drinking way too much of.

WATER SERVINGS AT ANY DAILY CALORIE LEVEL:
A minimum of 6 cups (a cup is 8 fluid ounces) per day.

HYDRATION HINTS:

1. ***Drink plain water.*** Most tap water in the United States is safe to drink. But if yours isn't—or if you don't like the taste—drink filtered (Brita, Pur, etc.) or bottled water. If you're a sparkling water fan, as I am, it's probably best to limit it to two of your six daily servings. Too much carbonation can lead to acid reflux in susceptible people. And taking in too much of the stuff *may* cause tooth enamel erosion, although there aren't enough studies out to confirm or refute this.

2. ***Six cups is the daily minimum***—more might be necessary if you're exercising hard or sweating a lot or when the temperature gets hot. Remember, water isn't your only source of hydration—fruit and vege-

tables are mostly composed of water, and you get plenty of them on the Pescetarian Plan.

3. *Stay hydrated—let your urine be your guide.* You know you're properly hydrated when urine is straw-colored or the color of light lemonade. If it's darker, that's often a sign you need more water. If it's virtually colorless, you might be drinking *too much* water.

4. *Coffee and tea count toward your total beverage intake.* Ideally, you'd drink 6 cups of water *and* coffee and tea on top of that. But if you don't get in the full 6 cups, you can count coffee and tea toward your total. If you drink caffeinated coffee and tea, have your last cup by about noon so that it doesn't interfere with sleep. (Personally, I prefer decaf—I find I have more energy when I go off caffeine.)

5. *Minimize—or completely avoid—sugary beverages.* There are just too many studies linking colas and other soft drinks, fruit juice drinks, punch, sweetened iced tea, and sweet coffee drinks to obesity. If that's how you want to spend your daily treat calories *on occasion* (no more than two sodas or other beverages with added sugar a week), it probably won't hurt you. And I'd avoid diet beverages unless they're a temporary fix to help you wean off regular ones. The safety of the artificial sweeteners used in these drinks is still unclear.

6. *If you drink alcohol, do so in moderation.* See what "moderation" means and other alcohol tips in the "Treats" step on page 61.

EXERCISE: THE HONORARY 8TH PESCETARIAN PRINCIPLE

The seven principles on the preceding pages will help you take in the right amount of food either to drop pounds or to maintain a healthy weight. But calories *expended* are just as important. So carve out time to exercise. Chapter 9 spells out how many exercise minutes you need for general health and how much is needed for weight loss. Studies show that people do best when they exercise *and* change their diet at the same time, rather than starting with one and then adding on the other.

Chapter 6

PUTTING THE PRINCIPLES INTO ACTION

Say hello to reasonable portions and good-bye to supersized madness! As you tackle portions food group by food group, you'll do the following with every step:

1. Make good use of measuring cups and spoons. Yes, it's low-tech, but it's the most effective way! You don't have to measure forever, just long enough to get a good feel for what a portion looks like.
2. Use everyday items to gauge portions:

    - ½ cup is about the size of a tennis ball.
    - 1 cup is the size of a baseball or a woman's fist.
    - 1 ounce of a thin cut of fish is about the size of your forefinger and middle finger held together.
    - A thin 3-ounce serving of fish is about the size of a checkbook; a thicker cut is about the size of your palm or a deck of cards.
    - ½ ounce of cheese is the size of four dice.
    - 1 tablespoon of nuts, peanut butter, or mayonnaise is a little smaller than a ping-pong ball.

3. Log portions in the Pescetarian Tracker on page 279. The research is clear: This simple act can mean the difference between losing or not

losing weight. Why? It keeps you accountable. You can't be in denial when your food log says you had two beers and a bag of chips!

In addition to food, you should also record hours of sleep, hunger level, and emotions or situations occurring before you eat. This is a gold mine of information, helping you identify those all-important triggers to overeating (that candy bar that materializes right after your boss dropped a pile of work on your desk). You'll also figure out factors that keep you on track (like getting enough sleep).

Either track just the food group you're working on (for instance, fruits and vegetables, as laid out in Principle no. 2), or log your entire diet. You don't have to track it forever, but track as many days of the week as you can as you adopt the seven principles in chapter 5.

NOTE: Ideally, you should fill out the tracker for four days before even beginning this eating plan. This gives you a valuable baseline reading, identifying trouble spots ("Wow, I rack up 500 calories of sweets daily?") and where you're right on track ("I tend to have a least two fruit servings daily"). You'll also start getting clued in to triggers for overeating (such as when you're stressed at work or didn't get enough sleep). While going through the seven principles, you can also work on solutions to the triggers.

4. Weigh yourself and measure your waistline weekly. You can use the Weight and Inches Log in Appendix B to track your progress.

TRACK PESCETARIAN PORTIONS—NOT CALORIES

I'm a dietitian, and I rarely count calories. I figure there are better uses for my brain than keeping a running tally all day. A more intuitive way to eat: Keep track of the number of servings of starchy foods, fruit, dairy, and a few other food types.

The result: You'll be firmly in control of your portions—and of your body weight.

To do this, you need to learn what a serving looks like. That's what the seven principles are all about. For instance, a cup of nonfat or 1-percent milk or soy milk is a milk/yogurt serving. An example of a fat serving is a teaspoon of oil (of any type).

So yes, I'm putting you to work—it takes a little concentration to learn serving sizes. Your efforts will be rewarded on the scale. And I think life's more fun when you're no longer chasing down calorie counts for everything you put in your mouth.

Life's also more fun when you can be flexible. That's another major perk of the Pescetarian Plan. For instance, you can splurge at one meal and scale back at another. Looking forward to a big plate of pasta this evening or a large piece of fish? Enjoy! Just "save" for the bigger portions by having fewer protein servings or fewer grain servings at breakfast and lunch. When you know how many servings you get of various foods, you can play around with them and have them when you most want them.

There's another huge plus to letting Pescetarian portions be your guide: health. By ensuring that you get *enough* of the healthy stuff (fruits, vegetables, and healthy fats), you're also slowing down the clock and helping prevent age-related killers.

WHEN CALORIES *DO* COUNT

All that said, there *are* a few instances where calories *do* matter on the Pescetarian Plan. But very few! Here's when you have to pay attention to calories:

1. You'll pick a *daily* calorie level. Your total daily calorie level—1,500, 1,800, or more—determines how many servings of grains, fish, and other foods you can squeeze in.

2. You'll tally up the number of "treat" calories you can have daily. On this plan, I encourage you to have a daily indulgence, whether it's alcohol, cookies, chips, ice cream, candy, or other treats. (See Principle no. 3.) But unfortunately, there's no easy way to set a portion size for treats because calories can vary dramatically for the exact same amount of food. For instance, a half-cup of Häagen-Dazs is generally *twice* the calories as the same amount of Breyers ice cream.

3. Occasionally, you'll need to check calories on packaged foods. For instance, the first time you try a new cereal, you'll have to see how many cups you get for a grain serving, which is 80 calories. Or if you're buying a microwave meal, you can check its calories, keeping in mind that you should be getting somewhere between a fourth and a third of your daily calories per meal. So if you chose the 1,500-calorie plan, you can confidently buy a frozen meal that's 400 to 500 calories.

~~~~~~
PICK YOUR DAILY CALORIE LEVEL
~~~~~~

Your seven principles hinge on your daily calorie level, which will be the basis for determining the number of fruits, vegetables, and other foods on this plan. I'll help you pick a calorie level, and if it winds up being too high or too low, it's simple to adjust.

Whether you need to lose weight or merely maintain it, there's a calorie level for you. From past experience, you might know that level. If not, here's a rough guide—tweak your calories up or down as needed.

WOMEN WHO WANT TO LOSE WEIGHT:

- If you work out hard at least three times a week, try 1,800 calories.
- If you're not working out at least three times a week, start with 1,500 calories.

WOMEN WHO ARE MAINTAINING THEIR WEIGHT:

- If you lost weight and are maintaining that loss and you work out hard at least three times a week, try 1,800 calories. If you're hungry the first or second day, jump to 2,100 calories. (If you fall somewhere in between, the "Pad Your Plan" section later in this chapter will show you how to add 100 calories at a time to an 1,800-calorie plan.)
- If you lost weight and are maintaining that loss, but you're *not* getting in at least three workouts weekly, try 1,500 calories.
- If you are maintaining your "natural" weight (you didn't have to lose more than five pounds to reach this healthy weight) and working out hard at least three times a week, you probably fall between 1,800 and 2,100 calories. Start with 1,800—if it's too little, then try 2,100 calories. If somewhere in between seems best, go to "Pad Your Plan" to add 100 calories or so to the 1,800 plan.
- If you are maintaining your "natural" weight (you didn't have to lose more than five pounds to reach this healthy weight) and you're not working out at least three times a week, try 1,800 calories.

MEN WHO WANT TO LOSE WEIGHT:

- If you work out hard at least three times a week, try 2,100 calories.
- If you're not working out at least three times weekly, try 1,800 calories.

MEN WHO ARE MAINTAINING THEIR WEIGHT:

- If you lost weight and are maintaining that loss and work out hard at least three times a week, try 2,100 calories daily and move up to 2,500 if that's too little. Or land somewhere in between by adding on 100 or so calories to the 2,100-calorie plan with "Pad Your Plan."
- If you lost weight and are maintaining that loss and you are not exercising at least three times weekly, try 2,100 calories.
- If you're maintaining your "natural" weight (you didn't have to lose more than five pounds to reach this healthy weight) and working out hard at least three times a week, try 2,500 calories. (If you need more, see "Pad Your Plan.")
- If you're maintaining your "natural" weight (you didn't have to lose more than five pounds to reach this healthy weight), and you're not working out at least three times a week, try 2,100 calories. If you fall somewhere between 2,100 and 2,500, the "Pad Your Plan" section will show you how to tack on calories in a healthy way.

You know you've hit on the right calorie level when you're maintaining a healthy weight or losing weight (if you need to) and you aren't hungry, except before meal and snack times. If you're losing weight but feel hungry too often, jump up to the next calorie level or tack on 100 calories or so by following the advice in "Pad Your Plan." (This advice also applies if you need more than 2,500 calories.)

If you need to lose weight and it's not happening, drop down a calorie level or exercise more.

If you're an emotional eater or an addictive eater, you probably can't rely on hunger as your guide to the right daily calorie count. That's because (as you well know) you're often eating when you're not hungry. Or you never let yourself get hungry. Still, I recommend that you pick a calorie level and follow the plan as best you can. Meanwhile, start tackling your emotional or addictive eating (see suggestions in chapter 9).

PESCETARIAN CHEAT SHEETS

The charts on the following pages lay out the entire diet. Keep in mind that you don't have to tackle it all at once. You can work on one food group (that is, one of the seven principles from chapter 5) at a time.

Think of these charts as your Pescetarian cheat sheets that you can refer to when you need a reminder of number of servings and serving size. You can print them out from ThePescetarianPlan.com; you might even carry them around with you while you're still memorizing Pescetarian portion sizes.

HOW MUCH TO EAT?

NUMBER OF SERVINGS AT YOUR DAILY CALORIE LEVEL

Type of Food	1,500	1,800	2,100	2,500
Fruit	2	2	3	4
Vegetables	4 or more	5 or more	6 or more	7 or more
Grains/starchy vegetables	5	5	6	7
Milk/yogurt/non-dairy milk	2	2	2	2
High protein	6	7	7	8
Healthy fat (include at least this many nut/seed servings*)	7 (3)	8 (3)	10 (4)	13 (6)
Treat/alcohol calories	100**	150	200	225
Water †	6	6	6	6

* The number in the parentheses indicates the number of servings that should consist of nuts. If you're allergic to nuts but not to seeds, then eat seeds instead. If you're allergic to all nuts and seeds, then skip them and eat the other healthy fats listed in chapter 5.

** On the 1,500-calorie plan, have a 100-calorie treat every other day.

† You can drink other beverages on this plan; see the "Smart Sipper" section in chapter 5.

WHAT DOES A SERVING LOOK LIKE?

Here's a rough guide. You'll find serving sizes for more foods and specific information on those serving sizes, such as how many fatty fish servings to eat per week, in chapter 5. I included treats on this chart just to remind you that you do get them! But because treat portion sizes vary so much, you must track calories for just this one food group.

TYPE OF FOOD	A SERVING LOOKS LIKE ...
Fruit (60 cal.)	½ cup fruit or berries, 1 small fruit (kiwi), 2 tablespoons dried fruit (raisins)
Vegetables (25 cal.)	1 cup salad greens, ½ cup chopped, raw or cooked
Grains/starchy vegetables (80 cal.)	½ cup cooked grains, sweet potatoes, potatoes, or ¾ cup cooked or frozen corn. Cereals vary, so check labels and figure out how many cups equal 80 calories. ⅓ cup cooked or canned legumes (black beans, kidney beans, chickpeas, lentils, etc.), 3 tablespoons flour, 2 tablespoons uncooked grains (like quinoa and steel-cut oats)
Milk/yogurt/non-dairy milk (100 cal.)	1 cup nonfat or 1-percent milk, or calcium- & vitamin D–enriched soy milk or other non-dairy milk, ¾ cup plain nonfat or low-fat yogurt
High protein (55 cal.)	1 ounce fatty fish, 2 ounces white fish; 1½ ounces shrimp or other shellfish (without shell), ⅓ cup tofu or edamame, ½ cup egg white, ½ ounce regular cheese, ¾ ounce reduced-fat cheese
Healthy fat (45 cal.)	1 teaspoon olive, canola, or other liquid vegetable oil, ⅕ Hass avocado (or 3 tablespoons) Nuts and seeds: 1 tablespoon (⅓ ounce) almonds, hazelnuts, peanuts, walnuts, or any other nut of your choice; or seeds, such as chia, pumpkin, or sunflower seeds or ground flaxseeds; ½ tablespoon peanut butter or other nut or seed butter
Water (0 cal.)	1 cup
Treats (calories vary)	Portion sizes vary—see page 75

PAD YOUR PLAN

If none of the four calorie levels are exactly right for you, then you may need an in-between level. Here's how to create one:

1. Start with the calorie level that's a little too low as your base. For instance, say you're a little hungry on 1,800 calories but find that a 2,100-calorie plan is too high—then start with 1,800 calories.

2. Add 100 calories. Try that for a few days; if that's not enough, add another 100 calories, and so on. Because we're thinking in terms of food groups, not calories, here are some food-group combos that equal 100 calories (and keep the Pescetarian Plan in balance):

Choose any one of the following—they all equal approximately 100 calories:

- 1 fruit serving + 1 fat serving. For example, have an extra piece of fruit for breakfast and an extra teaspoon of olive oil in your dinner salad.
- 1 high protein serving + 2 vegetable servings. For example, have an extra ounce of salmon and an extra ½ cup of green peppers in your stir-fry, an extra ½ cup of tomatoes in your salad.
- 2 fat servings. For example, have an extra 2 tablespoons of nuts.
- 1 grain/starchy vegetable serving + 1 fat serving.* For example, have an extra third of a cup of beans and an extra 6 tablespoons (about a third of a cup) of avocado.

* Use this combo as *just one* of your "pads," otherwise the diet will become too high in carbohydrates. In other words, if you need to pad your diet with more than 100 calories, use this combo just once, and for the next 100 calories, use one of the other suggestions on this list. Exception: If you work out daily or near daily and take in more than 2,500 calories per day, you can get away with a higher-carb diet, so go ahead and use this combo more than once.

Chapter 7

UPGRADE YOUR DIET AND MAINTAIN YOUR WEIGHT

Iff you've started adopting the *Seven Pescetarian Principles*, you're enjoying a great diet and, if you need to, losing pounds and subtracting inches off your waistline. Now what?

Your next steps:

1. An even more nutritious diet. Believe it or not, there's still room for improvement over the Seven Pescetarian Principles! Stick with your portions but bring in more superfoods or make a few other tweaks.
2. Maintain your weight loss. This is the holy grail of weight loss and your biggest challenge on this plan. For all the many reasons I explained in chapter 1, *The Pescetarian Plan* is an ideal program to maintain on. I'll give you a maintenance roadmap in this chapter.

Upgrade Your Diet with Superfoods

While the Seven Pescetarian Principles steered you to a nutritious diet, its main focus was on *quantity* of food. Once you've nailed that down, you can shift to refining your diet *quality*. There's only so much a brain can take at once—even a sharp omega-3-improved pescetarian brain!

Your first diet upgrade is to eat mainly superfoods. Superfoods—and the legions of disease-fighting nutrients they contain—are making headlines weekly. Foods that bear this label have extra doses of vitamins, minerals, or phytonutrients. Phytonutrients—there may be ten thousand of them—are beneficial compounds in plants *other* than vitamins and minerals. Plants use them to defend themselves against insects (since escape is not an option), molds, and even harsh sunlight. Happily, those same phytonutrients help defend us against cancer and other chronic diseases. Labs the world over are demonstrating the powers of phytonutrients, and there's living proof in the health and longevity of people eating along the lines of *The Pescetarian Plan.*

Over the next weeks and months, start replacing your white rice with brown rice (or quinoa, bulgur, or other whole grains), iceberg and romaine lettuce with arugula, kale, and other dark greens, eat more berries than bananas, and find other ways to eat more foods from the Pescetarian Standout Superfood chart in this chapter.

Truth be told, nearly every ingredient in the meal plans (Appendix C) and recipes (chapter 13) are superfoods. Apples, peaches, high-fiber cereal, haddock, celery, and so many others are both nutritious and slimming. And then there are the *extraordinary* nutrition standouts; those I'm calling "Pescetarian standout superfoods," listed on the chart on the next page. You'll get plenty of ideas on how to work these foods into your diet from the meal plans and recipes in this book.

Be prepared! You'll never look at broccoli, trout, kiwi, or any of the other Pescetarian standout superfoods as just "food" again. Instead, these picks are edible health miracles!

Note: Looking at the foods on this chart, you'll notice that some are very seasonal, like strawberries and blueberries. Eating seasonally is fine. If you get a hankering for an out-of-season fruit or vegetable and find imports too pricy, try frozen. Frozen food retains much of its nutrition, even if its texture sometimes leaves something to be desired. I find the best place for frozen fruit is the blender (see the smoothie recipes, pages 160, 251, and 252) and frozen vegetables in spaghetti sauces, soups, or casseroles.

You'll also see that some of these foods are so vital to your health that I recommend having them daily or at least several times a week.

PESCETARIAN STANDOUT SUPERFOOD:	WHAT MAKES IT SO SUPER:
SUPER FRUITS	
Berries (blackberries, blueberries, strawberries, raspberries)	These four berry types are packed with phytonutrients, including anthocyanins—which give the berries their purple and red hues—and are linked to heart disease protection and possibly enhanced memory.
Citrus fruit (oranges, grapefruit, tangerines, lemon, lime)	Each of these fruits has its own set of citrus flavonoids, which battle cancer and heart disease. Be sure to use the rind as well, as it contains powerful cancer-protectors. (Grated rind makes a delicious addition to grain dishes, fruit salads, salad dressings, and marinades.)
Grapes	Red wine put the heart-healthy compound resveratrol on the map, but you can also get it from red and purple grapes. Scientists keep finding new benefits for this compound—it fights cancer and may even improve balance, which declines with age.
Kiwi	Just two kiwi offer twice your daily vitamin C requirement. It's the combination of vitamin C and other phytonutrients that gives kiwi a high antioxidant ranking.
Mangos	These delicious fruits contain polyphenols that have potential cancer-fighting powers.
Papaya	This fruit is rich in beta-carotene and vitamin C. The red type also contains lycopene, the powerful antioxidant responsible for the red pigment in tomatoes.
Plums and prunes (dried plums)	Plums and prunes offer a trifecta of heart-helping benefits: fiber to control spikes in blood sugar, phenolic compounds to lower LDL cholesterol, and potassium to tame high blood pressure.
Pomegranate	They contain a wealth of phytonutrients, and emerging research is showing they have promise in fighting cardiovascular disease, diabetes, and prostate cancer.
SUPER VEGETABLES	
Cruciferous vegetables (arugula, bok choy, broccoli, broccoli sprouts, Brussels sprouts, cabbage, cauliflower, collard greens, kale, kohlrabi, mustard greens, radish, rutabaga, turnips, turnip greens, watercress) *Eat at least five times weekly.*	Cruciferous vegetables contain compounds called glycosinolates, which convert to powerful cancer-fighters—for instance, isothiocyanates—in the body. They protect against cancer by acting as an antioxidant to destroy cancer-causing molecules (carcinogens), blocking carcinogens from landing on DNA and causing mutations that lead to cancer, and helping halt the spread of cancer.

PESCETARIAN STANDOUT SUPERFOOD:	WHAT MAKES IT SO SUPER:
SUPER VEGETABLES	
Dark greens (any of the greens listed under "cruciferous," plus others such as chard, dandelion greens, oak leaf lettuce, spinach, sweet potato leaves) *Eat at least five times weekly.*	Rich in lutein, which is also found in our eyes, this compound helps prevent macular degeneration, a leading cause of blindness. Most dark greens are also rich in beta-carotene, which is linked to reduced cancer risk and reduced skin wrinkles.
Red tomatoes *Eat at least five times weekly (in the winter, canned, no-salt-added is fine).*	Tomatoes get their red color from lycopene, which not only is an antioxidant but also lowers blood cholesterol, fights inflammation, and "thins" the blood. All of these factors protect your heart. Some studies suggest that tomatoes also protect against cancer.
SUPER GRAINS AND STARCHY VEGETABLES	
Black rice	Also called "forbidden rice" because at one time it was reserved for Chinese emperors, it is especially tasty and contains the same types of powerful antioxidant—anthocyanins—found in blueberries.
Legumes (all beans and lentils) *Eat at least four times weekly.*	They're rich in fiber and resistant starch (explained in "The Glycemic Index" in chapter 4), loaded with B vitamins, and contain iron, magnesium, and a variety of antioxidants. This all adds up to protection from heart disease, diabetes, high blood pressure, and inflammation.
Oats and barley	Both grains are rich in a type of fiber called "beta-glucan," which traps some of the cholesterol and fat from the foods you eat and escorts them out of your body before they can be absorbed.
Quinoa	While it gets lumped in with grains because it is high in carbohydrates, quinoa is technically a seed that is related to other superfoods like spinach and Swiss chard. While not necessarily all that high in protein compared to other grains, it has a stellar amino acid profile. Amino acids are the building blocks of protein; quinoa contains a good supply of the ones your body can't make (or make quickly enough).
Sweet potatoes	They contain a laundry list of virtually every vitamin and mineral, with vitamin A (from beta-carotene) a particular standout—a mere half a cup covers 5 times your daily needs.

PESCETARIAN STANDOUT SUPERFOOD:	WHAT MAKES IT SO SUPER:
SUPER GRAINS AND STARCHY VEGETABLES	
Wheat berries and cracked wheat (bulgur)	These more roughly cut, larger particles of whole wheat (as opposed to whole-wheat flour) give them a low glycemic index (see chapter 4). Bulgur wheat can be found in health food stores and Middle Eastern markets where it comes in at least two different "grades": one is more finely cut for use in tabouli (a Middle Eastern salad that also includes tomatoes, onions, and parsley). The coarser cut is perfect for a grain side dish and cooks up in about 20 minutes, just like rice. A delicious variation is "freekeh," which is made from younger, green wheat and grilled for a wonderful smoky taste.
SUPER NUTS AND SEEDS	

All of them
Eat daily (check chapter 5 for amounts). In particular, aim for about 1 tablespoon daily of chia seeds or ground flaxseed.
	They're all brimming with good fats, and many are rich in magnesium and other heart-healthy compounds that lower cholesterol, "relax" blood vessels (which lowers blood pressure), and reduce inflammation. Plus, they can help you lose weight: Calorie for calorie, they are one of the most satiating foods—meaning they make you feel fuller, longer, than many other foods.
	    Almonds and walnuts are particularly well-researched, proving helpful at lowering heart disease risk. Almonds are a staple of the Portfolio Diet, developed by University of Toronto researchers, which reduces cholesterol as effectively as statin drugs.
	    Chia seeds and flaxseeds also deserve special mention because of their extraordinary levels of omega-3, the healthy fat that we need more of. For suggestions on how to incorporate them into your meals, see page 158 and page 285 in Appendix C.

SUPER HERBS AND SPICES	
Basil, cilantro, mint, oregano, parsley, rosemary, thyme *Eat at least four days a week.*	It's a little unfair to lump these together, because while some share common nutrients and phytonutrients, they're each unique. I could spend many pages on them, but the bottom line is that you should use them often and abundantly because they're so rich in health-promoting nutrients. A few highlights: Rosemary can suppress cancer tumor development in animal and test-tube studies; basil may help keep blood pressure down; oregano is a powerful antioxidant; mint may lower blood pressure; thyme helps prevent inflammatory AGEs (see pages 44 and 149); cilantro is rich in beta carotene and other antioxidant carotenes.

PESCETARIAN STANDOUT SUPERFOOD:	WHAT MAKES IT SO SUPER:
SUPER HERBS AND SPICES	
Cinnamon, coriander, cumin, ginger, turmeric (found in curry powder)	Like the herbs on the previous page, these spices have too many health benefits to fit in this chart. The highlights: A daily teaspoon of cinnamon may lower blood sugar; a powerful inflammation-fighter in turmeric called curcumin kills cancer cells and may help fight insulin resistance (which causes type 2 diabetes); coriander also offers protection against type 2 diabetes; ginger not only reduces the risk for heart disease and diabetes, it also can help quell nausea; and cumin may suppress some of the destructive inflammation that occurs with type 2 diabetes.
Chives, garlic, leeks, onions, scallions	These members of the "allium family" (*allium* is Latin for garlic) are as important to your body as they are to your broth. They have antitumor powers, especially when it comes to the gastrointestinal tract. In a study of 238 men in Shanghai, those who ate more than 10 grams of allium vegetables a day had a 51 percent lower risk for developing prostate cancer than those who had less than 2 grams per day. One garlic clove weighs about 3 grams, and ¼ cup of chopped onions is 40 grams. Garlic has also been associated with a reduced risk for cancers like stomach, colon, esophageal, pancreatic, and breast. And although the results are mixed, it appears to have heart benefits because it lowers LDL and blood pressure. The World Health Organization recommends that adults have one garlic clove a day for general health benefits. There's no need to go overboard on one specific type of allium vegetable because they all contribute to disease protection.
SUPER SEAFOOD	
Arctic char, wild salmon, sardines, trout *Eat three times weekly.*	Four ounces of any of these fish provide 1 to 2 grams of omega-3 fats—a gold mine! As "musts" on the Pescetarian Plan, I give them a special shout-out on page 56.
Clams, mussels, and oysters	Beef is touted as high in minerals, but it can't hold a candle to any of these shellfish. Oysters must be the most zinc-rich food on the planet; 4 ounces contains an impressive *twelve times* your daily requirement of this immune-boosting mineral. With 4 ounces of clams, you hit 85 percent of your daily iron needs; that same amount of mussels covers a day's worth of selenium, essential to your body's antioxidant defense system. These shellfish douse you with anywhere between *5 and 22 times* your daily B12 needs (important for healthy blood and brain cells). Take that, beef!

PESCETARIAN STANDOUT SUPERFOOD:	WHAT MAKES IT SO SUPER:
SUPER FATS	
Avocado	You'll see a lot of avocados in the meal plans and recipes in this book—their high monounsaturated fat content helps keep that fat supreme in this diet. Avocados are also rich in vitamin K, folate, potassium, vitamin E, lutein, magnesium, vitamin C, fiber, and vitamin B6. Tip: Avocados tend to be less expensive in Latin and Asian markets than in supermarkets or natural foods stores. A 2013 study of nearly 18,000 American adults discovered that those who ate half an avocado a day had a better overall diet quality and were half as likely to have metabolic syndrome compared to non-avocado eaters—*even though* their overall diet was higher in total fat (mostly the healthy monounsaturated kind). Their diets were also higher in vitamin E, fiber, magnesium, potassium, and vitamin K, all of which play a role in health from blood pressure to cancer prevention to immunity. Bonus: They tended to be thinner with a lower BMI and a smaller waist circumference, too!
Extra-virgin olive oil *Eat daily or almost daily.*	This oil is rich in healthy monounsaturated fat plus other health-promoting compounds. It's so integral to the Pescetarian Plan that I've given it more play on page 40.
SUPER BEVERAGES	
Cocoa, coffee (regular and decaf), and tea (regular and decaf; green, oolong or black)	Each has its own distinct phytonutrient profile, but I'm lumping them together because they're all hot beverages that help protect your heart.
Red wine and beer *No more than 1 drink per day for women; 2 for men.*	Although white wine also has heart benefits, red is the superior sip. Its anthocyanins and resveratrol reduce heart disease risk by fighting inflammation and making your LDL cholesterol less likely to oxidize and form plaque on the arteries. Beer has been shown to lower LDL and contains a number of antioxidants and other agents derived from hops that may play a role in cancer prevention. More is not better—if you overdo it, all benefits are lost! Stick to the recommended amounts to stay healthy (see the specifics on pages 49 and 61).

SLASHING SODIUM

Your second diet upgrade: Reduce sodium. Weirdly, you can have a diet that's perfectly healthy in every way but still take in too much sodium, which can raise blood pressure. Unless you make everything from scratch (which you do *not* have to do on this plan) and never go to a restaurant, it's hard to keep sodium levels within the 2,300 mg/day upper limit. That's because even "healthy" foods like whole-grain English muffins, bean burritos, and salad dressings can have sky-high sodium levels.

But with a little vigilance, you can rein in sodium. Here's how:

- *Eat mostly "whole" natural foods.* That means fresh vegetables, fruit, and from-scratch grains. (Don't let that scare you—you can make whole-wheat couscous in about 7 minutes; bulgur wheat in 20.)

- *Use no more than an eighth of a teaspoon of salt per every four portions when cooking or preparing foods.* (In other words, if you're making a dish that serves four, use an eighth of a teaspoon for the entire thing.)

- *Use the salt shaker.* Yes, you read that right! Just 5 percent of sodium in the American diet comes from the salt shaker (the rest is from processed and restaurant foods). Studies show that if you cook with little or no sodium and add just a light sprinkle at the table, you have a good chance of meeting your sodium limits.

- *Whether it's a recipe from this book or one of your own, when you sit down to eat, taste the food.* If it can use some salt, then add just a few crystals, no more than ¹⁄₁₆ of a teaspoon total, to the portion on your plate. (That's 150 mg sodium.) The impact of an undissolved or semi-dissolved salt crystal hitting your tongue is more powerful than if you'd cooked with much more salt.

- *Buy "no salt added" products.* For example, canned beans, canned tomatoes, canned tuna, salmon or sardines, crackers, grain mixes, and the like. If you can't find no-salt-added, go for reduced sodium.

- *Always compare labels for sodium.* You might be surprised—an organic spaghetti sauce can have twice the sodium of the mainstream brand, one type of whole-wheat bread can be a lot higher in sodium than another. Scanning for sodium is truly eye-opening.

- *Quiz your waiter.* When ordering at a restaurant, explain to the waiter that you want flavor, just not a lot of salt. He may direct you to lower-sodium options (if he's aware of them). And request that dishes be made without salt, but be clear that you do want all the other herbs, spices, and sodium-free flavors. This trick may not work every time, but it should save you a little sodium.

If you wind up at a fast food or other chain restaurant, check out sodium levels online (thank goodness for smartphones), or ask if they're available onsite. It's a sodium jungle out there, but you may be able to skirt the worst of it.

DO YOU NEED TO SUPPLEMENT?

If you eat enough nutritious food and get enough sunshine, you probably don't need vitamin and mineral tablets. If you have a cupboard full of vitamins (and I've seen plenty of those), I know this sounds like sacrilege. But hear me out: The Ikarian Greeks I told you about in the introduction don't owe their long lives and vitality to vitamin pills. In fact, they take no supplements at all. Instead, they eat a diet like the one in this book, which is positively brimming with vitamins, minerals, phytonutrients, fiber, and good fats. And there's something else that's crucial: They get a lot of sunshine. That means they're up to snuff on vitamin D, a nutrient many Americans are short on.

But here's the rub: You *should* limit sun exposure to protect your skin from cancer and wrinkles, so that means a vitamin D supplement is probably in order. Then, depending on your age, diet, and health issues, you might benefit from an omega-3 supplement, a multivitamin/mineral tablet, and possibly vitamin B12.

Unless you have a deficiency—say, you have iron-deficiency anemia—you probably don't need anything more. In fact, overloading on certain vitamins and minerals can be harmful. Someday, when genetic testing becomes more sophisticated, a blood test will determine what supplements you need. But for now, we have to go with the existing "recommended dietary allowances," or RDAs, set by the Institute of Medicine.

You might be wondering why calcium isn't on the chart on the next page. It was always assumed that you need a lot of calcium to prevent osteoporosis—the bone-thinning disease responsible for bone fractures and disability. For this reason, calcium RDAs were set high (1,000 mg daily; 1,200 mg for older adults) to prevent the disease. Most health organizations recommend getting your calcium through a mix of dairy foods and supplements.

But new evidence suggests that calcium supplements may not be all that protective to bones—and might even be bad for your heart! So, until the science sorts itself out, I'm recommending that you get your calcium from your two daily dairy/nondairy milk servings (see page 65) and from the 300 to 400 mg of calcium sprinkled throughout the rest of the Pescetarian Plan. But, of course, if your health care provider prescribes calcium supplements, then take them!

Here's a guide to whether supplementation is in order, and if so, what to take:

SUPPLEMENT	YOU NEED IT IF . . .	TYPE AND AMOUNT

Vitamin D	• You don't get much sun exposure or you slather on the sunscreen (as you should).
	
	• A blood test shows that you're under the proper level.
		• You can take the RDA, which is:
		
		   • 600 IU daily for men and women age 70 and younger
		
		   • 800 IU daily for men and women age 71 and up
		
		• But experts generally agree that 1,000 IU daily is safe for adults.

Multivitamin/mineral	• You're pregnant.	• If pregnant, take a prenatal supplement.
	• You're cutting calories. Even on the ultra-nutritious Pescetarian diet, it's hard to get RDA levels of every vitamin and mineral when calories dip below 1,800.	• If cutting back on calories, take a standard multi (see ThePescetarianPlan.com for details) either every day or every other day.
B12	• You're age 55 or older; that's when, for some people, levels of stomach acid decline. The acid is necessary for proper absorption of B12.	• Take 417 percent (25 mcg) to 833 percent of the daily value, which is 50 mcg (micrograms). • You can get this amount through an "adult" (a euphemism for "over-50") multi or a single B12 tablet.

SUPPLEMENT	YOU NEED IT IF . . .	TYPE AND AMOUNT
Fish oil (EPA and DHA)	• You have coronary heart disease (CHD). • You have high blood triglyceride levels. • You have heart failure. • You have rheumatoid arthritis or osteoarthritis. • You have mild, beginning-stage Alzheimer's (research doesn't show improvement for more advanced). • You're depressed. • You have bipolar disorder. • You are healthy and are betting that the research proves there's a benefit.	• Take 1,000 mg daily for CHD, heart failure, mild Alzheimer's, depression, bipolar disorder, osteoarthritis, and if you're healthy but want to give it try. • Take 2,000 to 3,000 mg daily to lower triglycerides. • Take 2,600 mg daily if you have rheumatoid arthritis. • Buy oil derived from small species of fish, such as sardines and menhaden. These fish have a lot less mercury and PCBs—manmade compounds that can cause cancer—than bigger fish. (More on this in chapter 10.) Krill oil, derived from tiny shrimp-like creatures, is also low in contaminants, although some environmental groups fear that overharvesting krill could upset the oceans' ecosystems. (Krill is the dietary staple of some whales, seals, and other sea life.)

MAINTAINING YOUR WEIGHT LOSS

The Pescetarian Plan is both a weight loss and a weight maintenance diet. My clients lose weight on it, they maintain a weight loss on it, and those who never needed to lose weight eat this way to stay healthy.

If you're maintaining a weight loss, try not to be discouraged by the grim stats showing that most people don't maintain their weight loss. Instead, remain vigilant, and take a page from the 20 percent or more who *are* successful at weight maintenance. Terrific studies on these "successful losers" offer invaluable tips on the factors that predict success. I'll list the biggies here; for much more guidance, I recommend *The Life You Want: Get Motivated, Lose Weight, Be Happy*, which I co-wrote with Bob Greene and Ann Kearney-Cooke.

Your weight maintenance road map:

1. ***Increase calories.*** Once you've lost the weight, go to the "How Much to Eat?" chart on page 78 and bump up calories to the next level. For instance, if you lost the weight on 1,500, try maintaining on 1,800. If that's too high (meaning you're gaining weight), find an in-between daily calorie level by following the "Pad Your Plan" instructions in chapter 6.

2. ***Stick with the Seven Pescetarian Principles.*** Even when you can afford more calories, it's still critical to eat in this high-satiety, hunger-suppressing manner. That's because after a weight loss, your body may try to pile those pounds back on by ratcheting up hunger. That's one of the things that makes weight maintenance so tricky.

3. ***Keep up the exercise!*** As you'll see in chapter 9, it usually takes more than 150 minutes of aerobic exercise per week to maintain a weight loss. The research is incredibly clear: You have to exercise to maintain a weight loss.

4. ***Weigh yourself once a week.*** If you're maintaining a weight loss, you may want to do this for life. It's a lot easier to nip a two-pound gain in the bud than a five- or ten-pound gain. Stepping on the scale weekly catches any upward creep before it's too late.

5. ***Starting to gain weight? Whip out your Pescetarian Tracker and log.*** Record food, exercise, sleep, as well as the rest of the columns. Do this for a week, and analyze it carefully to pinpoint where you're going astray. It could be too many treat calories, not enough exercise or sleep, or an emotional eating issue. Tracking can help you reset back to weight stabilization mode.

   Another tactic: Follow the Pescetarian Meals starting on page 285 for a few days. They come in handy when you're feeling out of control—they're something concrete to follow.

6. ***Find your motivators.*** Your doctor may be telling you to lose weight to bring down your blood pressure, cholesterol, and future risk of heart disease—but that might not resonate with you. That's okay, just search for what does. It might be a semi-long-term goal, like keeping up with your family on the vacation you plan to take nine months from now. Or the prospect of enjoying your retirement, even if it's decades from now.

   And to keep you motivated day to day, eat foods you like, and do physical activity that you enjoy (or at least don't dislike). Take ownership of the process, as I explained on page 54.

7. *Periodically review the "Practices That Predict Maintenance Success" below.* Take advantage of the good science on the habits that predict successful weight maintenance.

8. *Enjoy yourself.* Enjoy your new weight, the new health, and the increased energy!

Practices That Predict Maintenance Success

How come some people are able to keep their weight off, when so many others gain it right back? Now we have good studies that reveal habits that spell success. For instance, a Penn State University study of 1,165 men and women found that pretty much everything recommended in *The Pescetarian Plan* raises your odds of maintaining a weight loss, such as eating plenty of fruits and vegetables, sticking with lower-fat protein sources, controlling portions, consistent exercise, and reminding yourself why it's important to control your weight.

In addition, here are tips from the National Weight Control Registry (NWCR), a long-running national study tracking the habits of more than ten thousand men and women who have lost, on average, 66 pounds and *kept* it off for an average of five and a half years:

- Eat breakfast daily.
- Weigh yourself every week.
- Watch no more than ten hours of TV weekly (compared to thirty-five hours for the average American).
- Exercise daily (they average one hour daily).
- Do both aerobic exercise and weight training.
- Get a handle on emotional eating.
- Don't be a perfectionist or a black-and-white thinker (as in you're either "on" or "off" your diet). Accept setbacks as part of the process and just continue your healthy habits.

Take heart from the fact that maintenance gets easier over time. The NWCR participants who clear the two-year mark are only half as likely to gain back even five pounds as those who have maintained for less time. If they stick it out for five years, that five-pound creep is only 30 percent as likely to happen.

What's also heartening—everyone will tell you it's worth it. Among the Registry participants, 95 percent report an improved quality of life, including higher levels of self-confidence, mood, energy, and improved relationships. What more could you ask for?

Chapter 8

PESCETARIAN MEAL BASICS

Who says *"diet food" can't be delicious? The Pescetarian* Plan is a plan that embraces delicious food! It encourages you to drizzle on the olive oil, have a little chocolate and wine, and experiment with recipes so tasty no one would ever suspect that they're "diet food."

You'll find dozens and dozens of meals in Appendix C that exemplify the Pescetarian way of eating. They translate the Seven Pescetarian Principles outlined in chapter 5 into real, live breakfasts, lunches, dinners, snacks, and treats that you can combine however you'd like. Some meals are based on chef Sidra Forman's terrific recipes (chapter 13). Others are more basic—like a peanut butter sandwich, carrot sticks, and a glass of milk.

In this chapter, I'll show you how to make the best use of the meal plan in Appendix C, and also, how to create your own meals.

APPENDIX C MEAL PLAN HOW-TO

Instead of a rigid meal plan dictating what to eat for breakfast, lunch, dinner, and snack on Monday, then what to eat on Tuesday and the rest of the week, *you* do the choosing. Here's how it works:

1. Know your daily calorie level. (If you haven't picked a calorie level yet, go back to page 76 in chapter 6 for pointers.)
2. Choose any breakfast, any lunch, any dinner, any snack, and any treat at your calorie level from the lists in Appendix C.

3. Tailor them to your tastes by swapping one fruit for another, changing up the grains, or making other substitutions (more on this below).

4. Enjoy! It's really that simple.

STICKING TO—AND STRAYING FROM— THE MEAL PLAN

- I recommend eating these meals fairly faithfully for at least a week. That's enough time to familiarize yourself with portions and to get in the swing of a pescetarian way of eating.

- If you need to lose weight, consider eating these meals for about a month. That way, you can be sure you're sticking to a calorie level, which will help you drop some pounds. A month of prescribed meals sounds constricting, but it doesn't have to be. As you'll see from the FAQs on the next page, there's *loads* of flexibility on this plan. You can substitute any food for another, as long as they're roughly nutritionally equivalent (for example, tomatoes for green pepper, rice for bread, and so on).

- If you prefer to make your own meals from the get-go, that's fine. Just make sure that by the end of the day, you've racked up the right amount of servings of fruit, protein, and the other Pescetarian Portions at your particular daily calorie level (all of this is laid out for you in chapters 5 and 6).

At the very least, I encourage you to *glance* at the meals. Why? Because they show you what a balanced meal looks like. The type of fats used puts you at a healthy 1-to-1 omega-6 to omega-3 fat ratio, which in the United States is an extraordinary accomplishment (more on this in chapter 4). They demonstrate the broad range of this plan—from vegan to vegetarian to pescetarian meals. They'll spark ideas. And you might even try a few, tweaking them to suit your tastes and your timetable. For example, maybe you don't have time to make the complete Black Rice with Arugula Shrimp Salad (page 297), but you might have the five or so minutes it takes to make the arugula shrimp salad and eat it with a slice of whole-grain bread instead.

PESCETARIAN MEAL FAQs

- *Can I substitute one food for another?* Please do! To keep calories—and nutrition—in check, sub in foods of similar nutritional value. For instance, swap white beans for garbanzo beans or another type of bean; red pepper for tomatoes or another vegetable; strawberries for blueberries or any other fruit; parsley for cilantro or another herb; trout for salmon or another fatty fish; scallops for shrimp or another lean fish, and so forth.

- *I'm allergic to a food (or foods) recommended on the plan—how should I handle it?* Follow the same advice as above—just make sure you're substituting foods of comparable nutritional value. So, if you have to avoid gluten, sub in a slice of gluten-free whole-grain bread or a third of a cup of cooked brown or black rice or half a cup of corn kernels for a slice of regular bread (or other gluten-containing starch).

  If you're allergic to tree nuts but not peanuts, then swap in peanuts or soy nuts for the other nuts. If you're allergic to both nuts and soy, then simply eat more olive oil and avocados in place of nuts. Remember, a tablespoon of nuts is one Pescetarian fat portion, equivalent to a teaspoon of olive oil or 3 tablespoons of avocado. (More details on fat portions in chapter 5.)

  If you have a dairy allergy or just don't want to consume dairy, then soy milk is the closest substitute for regular milk because it's comparable in protein. Almond, coconut, hemp, and rice milks have little to no protein—not a problem if there's already protein in the meal, but if not, then add a little extra protein to that meal or the next one.

- *You didn't include beverages—how should I fit them in?* Any beverage that doesn't have calories or artificial sweeteners is fine. That means you can have coffee, tea, and water as you'd like. Have at least a cup of water at every meal and a few more cups over the course of the day.

- *Do I have to eat the snacks in the order presented in this chapter?* Not at all. My general rule for snack time: Have a snack whenever you're hungry and a meal is still at least an hour away (or when you're hungry a few hours after dinner).

- *What if I want to eat meals from this plan as well as my own dishes?* That's exactly what I'm hoping you'll do! The whole idea behind these meals is to start you off so that you can more easily compose your own.
- *Do I have to eat certain Pescetarian food groups at each meal?* No, but to help quell appetite, it's best to include a protein source (seafood or dairy), a grain/starchy vegetable (sweet potato or cereal), a fat (olive oil or nuts) and a fruit or vegetable at each meal.

DESIGNING YOUR OWN MEALS

One of the beauties of the Pescetarian Plan is flexibility—you can create your own meals. You're in the driver's seat; you might decide to have all your daily fruit servings in one meal or have one for breakfast and one for a snack. The same goes for the other food groups.

However, as I mentioned in the FAQs, for weight-control purposes, it's a good idea to have some protein, fat, and carbohydrate at each meal. This balance tends to keep you feeling fuller longer, which helps control appetite.

Here's a very loose sample meal pattern that offers a nice balance of carbs, protein, and fat. There's no need to follow these examples to a T—in other words, you don't have to have a fruit serving at breakfast, or two to three fats at lunch, or follow any of the other suggestions below. However, seeing it laid out this way might help you get started. And for loads more examples, go to Appendix C. (And remember, you may need more or fewer serving sizes than shown in this example depending on your total daily calorie level.)

PESCETARIAN PORTIONS	EXAMPLES		
BREAKFASTS:	Cereal-based	or	Toast and nut butter–based
2 grain/starchy vegetables	About a cup of whole-grain cereal		2 slices whole-grain toast
1 fruit	½ cup berries on top of cereal		1 apple, sliced (place some slices on toast instead of jam)
1 dairy	1 cup milk with cereal		Glass of milk
1–2 fats	1–2 tablespoons walnuts topping cereal		½ to 1 tablespoon nut butter on toast
1 water	Glass of water		Glass of water
HIGH CALCIUM SNACKS:	Latte-based	or	Yogurt-based
1 dairy	12-ounce latte		6 ounces plain yogurt with a little honey
1–2 fats	1–2 tablespoons roasted almonds		1–2 tablespoons sunflower seeds
LUNCHES:	Salmon salad sandwich	or	Salad with tuna and chickpeas
2 grains/starchy vegetables	2 slices whole-grain bread		⅔ cup chickpeas (garbanzos)
2–3 proteins	2–3 ounces canned wild salmon		2–3 ounces chunk light tuna
2–4 vegetables	Chopped celery and carrots for salmon salad + 1–1 ½ cups celery and carrot strips on the side		1 cup arugula, 1 cup chopped tomatoes
2–3 fats	½ –1 tablespoon mayonnaise for the salmon salad		2–3 teaspoons olive oil for the salad dressing
1 water	Glass of water		Glass of water
DINNERS:	Vegetarian chili and rice	or	Salmon and sweet potato
1 grain/starchy vegetables	½ cup side of herb brown rice		½ sweet potato
3–5 proteins	1–1 ½ cups tofu and bean chili		3–5 ounces salmon
2–4 vegetables	2–3 cups salad greens and 1 cup chopped vegetables		1 cup sautéed spinach

PESCETARIAN PORTIONS	EXAMPLES	
2–3 fats	2–3 teaspoons olive oil to dress the salad (plus vinegar)	2–3 teaspoons olive oil to sauté the spinach
1 fruit	An orange for dessert	½ cup berries for dessert
1 water	Glass of water	Glass of water
TREATS:	Dark chocolate or	Cookie
100–250 calories (depends on your plan)	¾–1 ¾ ounces dark chocolate	1–2 oatmeal cookies
1 water	Glass of water	Glass of water
FRUIT OR VEGETABLE SNACKS**	3 fruit or	Fruit and nuts
	1 banana (considered 2 fruit) and an orange	1 apple and 2 tablespoons nuts

* If you're following the 2,500-calorie plan you should have two of these snacks, or have one and another snack made up of 1 grain/starchy vegetable and 2 nut servings (i.e. 80 calories of whole-grain crackers spread with 4 teaspoons nut butter), or 1 fruit and 2 nut servings (i.e. a cup of strawberries with 2 tablespoons walnuts). Or create your own snack that uses up your remaining food groups for the day. On the meal plans in Appendix C, this extra snack is 150 calories; helpful information if you're considering a fruit and nut bar or other packaged goods.

** For those on the 2,100- and 2,500-calorie plans only.

How to Size Up Any Plate

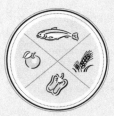

When in doubt, here's how to ensure your plate is not only well-balanced, but moderate in calories: Just imagine the Pescetarian Plan logo (left). As you can see, half the plate is filled with fruits and vegetables (on your plate it could be just fruit, or just vegetables), a quarter contains whole grain (or it could be legumes, sweet potatoes, and other healthy starches), and the final quarter should be fish or another Pescetarian protein.

Pescetarianism on a Budget

Think that healthy meals have to slim your wallet while also slimming your waistline? Sure, it's true that you can pay $17 per pound for fresh wild salmon and $5 per pound for red bell peppers. But there are loads of healthy foods that are real deals.

For instance, at 6 to 12 cents per ounce, dried lentils and beans are dirt cheap. That ounce—about 2 tablespoons—turns into a heaping third of a cup of cooked lentils or beans, a perfect Pescetarian grain/starchy vegetable portion. Even *canned* beans, at about $1.30 per 15-ounce can, are a steal, making that third cup cost just 25 cents. Canned tuna and canned salmon vary in cost but can be about half the price of fresh farm-raised. For examples of Pescetarian Plan meals starting at 52 cents, go to ThePescetarian Plan.com.

My shopping strategy is to buy what's on sale that week in both the produce section and at the seafood counter. As much as possible, I buy in-season fruits and vegetables, which are not only less expensive but also taste better.

PESCETARIAN MEAL PLAN
CALORIE BREAKDOWN

Although this is *not* a calorie-counting plan, in order to make the Appendix C meal plans mix-and-match, I had to pick a calorie level for all the breakfasts, ditto for the lunches, dinners, snacks, and treats. I'm sharing this with you in the chart on the next page, because you might be curious, and also, because it will help you incorporate convenience meals and restaurant meals into the meal plan. For example, when you're buying a frozen dinner or looking at the calorie count of restaurant menu items, you cannot only size them up by food groups, but see how their calories compare to the meal plan.

And just to cover myself: Calories in the Pescetarian Meals starting on page 285 may be slightly higher or slightly lower than those in the chart—but they're close!

	..............DAILY CALORIES..............			
	1,500-cal.	1,800-cal.	2,100-cal.	2,500-cal.
APPENDIX C MEAL	CALORIES PER MEAL, SNACK, OR TREAT			
BREAKFAST	390	390	440	440
High-calcium snack	150	150	150	150
LUNCH	425	500	500	600
Fruit/ vegetable snack	not on plan	not on plan	200	200
DINNER	500	600	600	700
Extra snack	not on plan	not on plan	not on plan	150
TREAT	100 calories every other day	150	200	250

Bon Appétit!

Now turn to the meal plans, which start on page 285, and give them a whirl. Mix and match as you like, combining any breakfast with any lunch, dinner, snack, or treat.

Chapter 9

EXERCISE, SLEEP, LOVE

As slimming and healthy as this Pescetarian eating plan is, it's not enough to put you in the ranks of the long-term weight loss maintainers. It alone can't catapult you to a level of health where you're buzzing energetically and enthusiastically through your day (and through the many days and years to come).

To get a firm grip on your weight and achieve that high-energy, feel-good health, you need three more things: exercise, sleep, and emotional nourishment.

In fact, without these three things, it's difficult to *sustain* this Pescetarian way of eating. Here's why:

- If you forgo exercise, you lose that "calorie cushion" and you'll have to eat ridiculously little to keep your weight down. Who wants to stay at 1,200 calories or even 1,500 to lose weight or to keep it off? No one! That's one reason most diets fail. And exercise is one of the main reasons people *do* maintain their weight loss, according to a great many studies.
- When you skimp on sleep, you'll have a much harder time controlling your appetite.
- When you feel lonely, stressed, or overwhelmed, healthy eating and exercise go out the window. Even worse, food can become your coping mechanism.

EXERCISE

I'm no athlete, but what I can say is that I'm faithful to fitness: I'm at the gym three times a week, pretty much every week. And on non-gym days, I walk. What's the key to my consistency? I've made exercise a priority, and I set achievable goals.

Sure I'd like to try a bunch of cool new exercise classes and do more strength training. But if I shoot for those things, I'm setting myself up for failure, given the other demands on my life. Instead, I make sure to get 150 minutes of aerobic exercise weekly—often more. I periodically increase the resistance at the elliptical and the slope on the treadmill. When my strength routine starts feeling too easy, I move up to the next heaviest weight. If things calm down someday and I have more time, I'll probably do more. But for now, I've hit upon a plan that works for me.

My approach gets the nod from exercise physiologist Bob Greene. "It's better to consistently exercise at a middle level of fitness than reach a higher level but go on-and-off again," says Bob, who has written a number of best-selling diet and fitness books, such as *The Best Life Diet* and *Total Body Makeover* (the latter of which I strongly recommend as your how-to-exercise book).

Working with Bob for a number of years, I've watched him inspire totally sedentary people to get moving. How? He meets them at their own exercise level—and doesn't make them feel bad about it. Then he helps them gradually move up. Plus, his unmistakable passion for exercise mixed with a gentle "no excuses" vibe is hard to resist! Through his books and television appearances (he counts Oprah among his clients), he has motivated millions to start moving.

You're next! If you're not hitting your 150 minutes of exercise per week (or working up to it), what's holding you back? "There are lots of reasons not to exercise, but I've never heard a good one," says Bob. The top three excuses he hears:

1. *"I don't have time."* When something is a priority, you drop something else (like a few hours of TV) or reconfigure your schedule to *find* the time. And Bob notes, "Flexibility is key. When you can't do your regular workout—maybe you're traveling, or it's snowing, or things got extra busy at home or work—always have a Plan B. If the

most time-pressed people can do it, so can you! Even new moms (who could be more time-pressed?) can invest in a jogging stroller or work out to exercise videos." (Bob has been spotted running up and down the stairwells of hotels for exercise as his Plan B.)

2. ***"I have an injury."*** This is a tough one—I've seen regular exercisers stop moving after being injured in an accident or fall. "First, ask yourself (and your doctor) what you *can* do, and start there," says Bob. In fact, he says, exercise is usually prescribed to *treat* injuries. "While you're on the mend, work on building strength elsewhere. For instance, if you've injured your leg, work out your upper body with weights, stretches, and if you have access to one, an upper-body ergometer (it's like an exercise bike for your arms). You might even be able to swim. Your goal is to keep up as much endurance and strength as you can so you can go back to your prior workout level, or close to it, once you've recovered."

If your injury is chronic—say, back problems that preclude running or jumping—you can usually find an exercise that keeps you fit. "Try a stationary bike or even a recumbent bike. You might not be able to *run* on a treadmill, but if you can gradually increase the slope, you can have just as challenging a workout that way," he advises.

3. ***"I don't enjoy it."*** "People who hate exercise have often had traumatic experiences, sometimes going back to their school days. Maybe they were last to be picked for a team or were ridiculed by their gym teacher. Or later on in life, they may have tried a brutal workout class or got into some other over-your-head exercise situation," Bob says. If this sounds familiar, Bob has two tips for you: "This time, start with an activity you like, such as walking on a beautiful trail with a friend, dancing, or swimming. You can turn virtually any form of exercise into a calorie-burning workout."

Second, he recommends recasting exercise as "non-negotiable," the same way you take medication if needed or brush your teeth every night, even when you're tired.

Why You Can't Live Without It

A fifteen-minute walk around your office building at lunch every day could grant you three extra years of life, according to a study of 416,175 Taiwanese men and women. That's just one example in a litany of studies demonstrating the dramatic impact of exercise on disease prevention and treatment and longevity.

One look at the list of exercise benefits below, and it becomes clear that our bodies were designed to be active. Physical activity:

- Enhances weight loss, especially fat loss (belly fat, in particular)
- Makes it a lot easier to maintain your weight loss over the long term
- Lowers risk of heart disease, cancer, type 2 diabetes, and pretty much every other disease
- Enhances your sex life
- Gives you a tighter and more toned look
- Allows you to eat more
- Boosts energy
- Improves mood
- Sharpens the brain
- Reduces the risk for dementia later in life
- Suppresses inflammation
- Lowers blood pressure
- Raises "good" cholesterol
- Regulates blood sugar
- Enhances immunity

EXERCISE RX

How much exercise is "enough"? Here are the latest recommendations from the American College of Sports Medicine (adopted by most of the major health authorities). For a sample exercise program, take a look at "Adding Physical Activity to Your Life" on the Centers for Disease Control's website or the "Get Moving" plan on ThePescetarianPlan.com. A solid, basic book that'll get you started on both an aerobic and strength-training program is *The American College of Sports Medicine Complete Guide to Fitness and Health.*

Aerobic (Cardio) Exercise

This type of exercise includes walking, jogging, biking, working out on an elliptical machine, or any exercise that gets your heart pumping and lungs working a little harder for a sustained period of time. How much do you need? Here's what the American College of Sports Medicine and other major health organizations recommend.

- To help prevent weight gain, heart disease, and other chronic conditions, aim for *at least* 150 minutes of moderate-intensity exercise per week, preferably spread out over five days (for instance, five sessions of 30 minutes each per week).

  Or log *at least* 75 minutes of vigorous-intensity exercise per week, done on at least three days of the week. (On the next page is a section on exercise intensity.)

- If you need to lose weight or maintain a weight loss, do *at least* 250 minutes of moderate-intensity exercise weekly.

  Or rack up *at least* 125 minutes of vigorous-intensity activity weekly. Less than this—150 to 250 minutes of moderate-intensity exercise weekly—is associated with just modest weight loss. It appears that you need to break 250 minutes for significant pound shedding.

The big caveat: These guidelines apply to *healthy* adults. If you're not a regular exerciser, even if you're pretty sure you're healthy, check with your doctor or other health care provider before increasing your exercise levels.

If you're thinking that 60 minutes a week is a challenge, much less 150 minutes, just remember: You can work up to these goals at your own pace, continually challenging yourself to add more minutes.

MEASURING INTENSITY

You'll notice that the guidelines require working out twice as long at "moderate" intensity than at "vigorous" intensity. Intensity, or how hard your body works during aerobic activity, is one of the most important factors of fitness. The exact same exercise—for instance, going 3.5 miles per hour on a treadmill set at a 2 percent grade—might be moderate for a fit person but vigorous for someone who's been sedentary. So intensity is about how *you* feel when doing a particular exercise.

Although I give examples below of exercises that might place a "fairly fit" person into light, moderate, and vigorous intensity, that's just for example's sake—it may not apply to you. What determines your intensity is how hard your heart is beating and how hard you're breathing.

- *Light intensity.* Your heart rate is just a little higher than at rest, and you're breathing normally or just a little bit harder. For a fairly fit person, this would be walking from room to room, washing the dishes, supermarket shopping, or other chores that don't require much effort. It feels easy.
- *Moderate intensity.* Your heart rate is obviously higher, and you're breathing more quickly, but you're still able to carry on a conversation (although it's hard to sing). The workout is somewhat hard— it's physically challenging, but you're not pulling out all the stops. A brisk walk or mowing the lawn might be considered moderate for a fairly fit person.
- *Vigorous intensity.* Your heart is pumping hard, you're breathing quickly and deeply, and you are most likely sweating (perhaps profusely)—this is tiring! You can still speak, but not enough to carry on a real conversation. You can't say more than a few words without drawing a breath. You definitely can't sing. Running; a challenging game of tennis, basketball, or other sport; increasing the resistance on the elliptical or the speed/slope on the treadmill; a nonstop aerobic exercise class; or going uphill on a bike can usually push you into this zone.

If you haven't been doing even moderate-intensity activities, then ease into them. Even 10 minutes at a moderate intensity may be enough. When it gets easier, increase your minutes or the intensity. Gradually work up to vigorous intensity.

Strength Training

Free weights, machines, or exercise bands all do the same things: They make you stronger, tone and tighten your body, and help fight age-related declines in muscle. For examples of strength training moves, check out Bob Greene's *Total Body Makeover*. Another good resource: the Centers for Disease Control's site. They have videos showing you how to do the moves. And, there's even a strength training program (designed for older people, but the exercises are appropriate for all ages). I'll also post the links to the specific CDC web pages on ThePescetarianPlan.com.

Your guidelines:

- Do at least 6 exercises (total) for both upper and lower body, two to three times per week.
- Do 2 to 3 sets per exercise.
- Aim for 10 to 12 repetitions per set.

Flexibility Training (Stretching)

These exercises not only make it easier to reach up into a cabinet or touch your toes, they can also improve your posture, stability, and balance. Again, the CDC website and *Total Body Makeover* offer great examples.

- Do at least four types (stretching legs, back, arms) at least twice a week; you'll see the greatest gains if you do them daily.
- Hold your stretch for 10 to 30 seconds, until you feel slight discomfort. Older folks may see even more improvements in range of motion if stretches are held for 30 to 60 seconds.

SLEEP

While it may seem admirable to tough it out and operate on just five hours of sleep, you're better off proving your mettle in some other way. Otherwise, you may not feel so heroic when you've gained forty pounds and developed diabetes, heart disease, or any of the other conditions caused by chronic lack of sleep!

Experts say we need seven to nine hours of sleep, but 67 percent of Americans don't even log the seven-hour minimum on most nights, according to the most recent National Sleep Foundation survey. We all know the reasons: We are hooked on late-night TV, electronic toys, and smartphones; we try to finish up work and chores; or we stay out late having fun. Plus, there are medical reasons why we're not getting our forty winks: medications, menopause, insomnia, and aches and pains can keep us up. Stress, excessive caffeine, and a lack of exercise can also interfere with getting the requisite shuteye.

How bad for you is shortchanging sleep? Getting six hours or less has been linked to an increased risk of obesity, type 2 diabetes, heart disease, impaired cognitive function, slower reflexes, and premature death. Quite a sobering line-up!

If you're not getting the sleep you need, it's time to practice "good sleep hygiene," as they say in the biz. Some tips:

- Go to bed and wake up at the same time every day, including weekends.
- Set a relaxing bedtime routine (warm bath, low lights, listening to music, and so on).
- Turn off tech: The light from your computer, phone, TV, and e-reader can sabotage your sleep.
- Skip the pre-bed booze: While alcohol helps some people relax and fall asleep, your sleep quality throughout the night suffers. It actually prevents you from entering the deep, most restorative phases of sleep.
- Darken the room at night, but make sure that some light creeps in during the morning.
- Create a restful and restorative room: Keep it cool, dark, and quiet. It's not always possible to get all three, especially with small children. But do your best to create a peaceful environment that works for you. Consider investing in blackout shades, wearing an eye mask or ear plugs, or buying a white noise machine.
- Pick a comfortable, supportive mattress and use it for sleeping and intimacy only.
- Curb caffeine, which can pack a lasting punch; some people can feel its effects for up to twelve hours later.

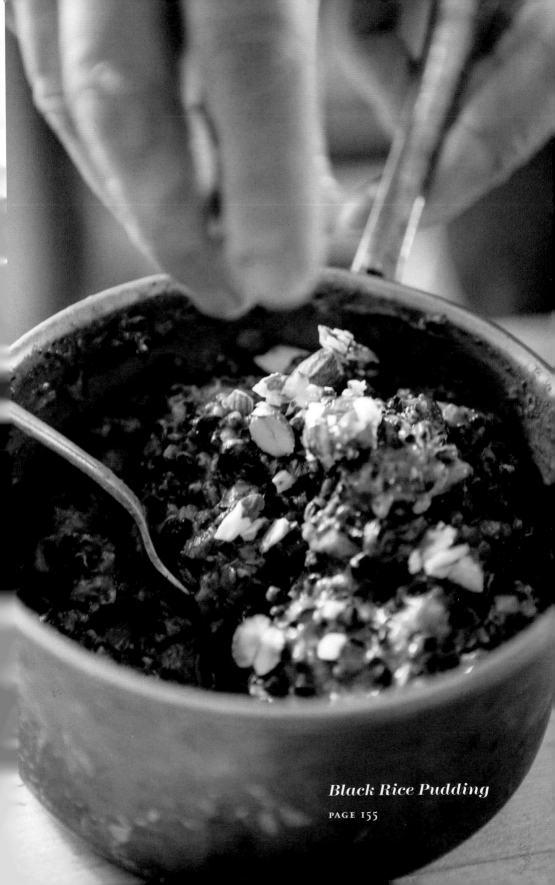

Black Rice Pudding

PAGE 155

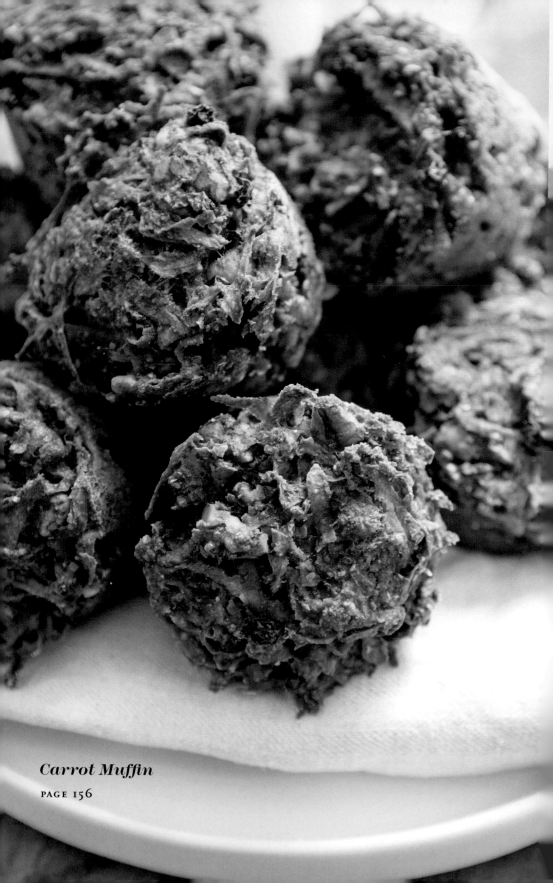

Carrot Muffin

PAGE 156

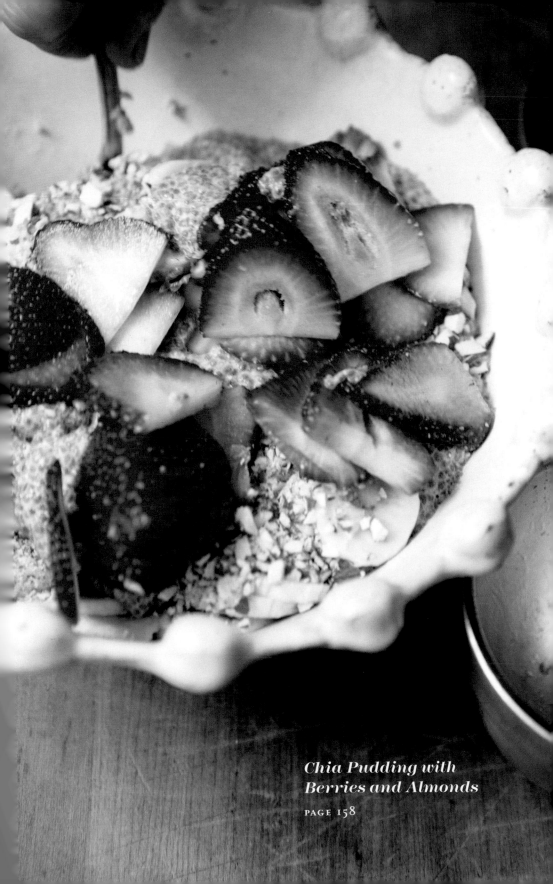

Chia Pudding with
Berries and Almonds

PAGE 158

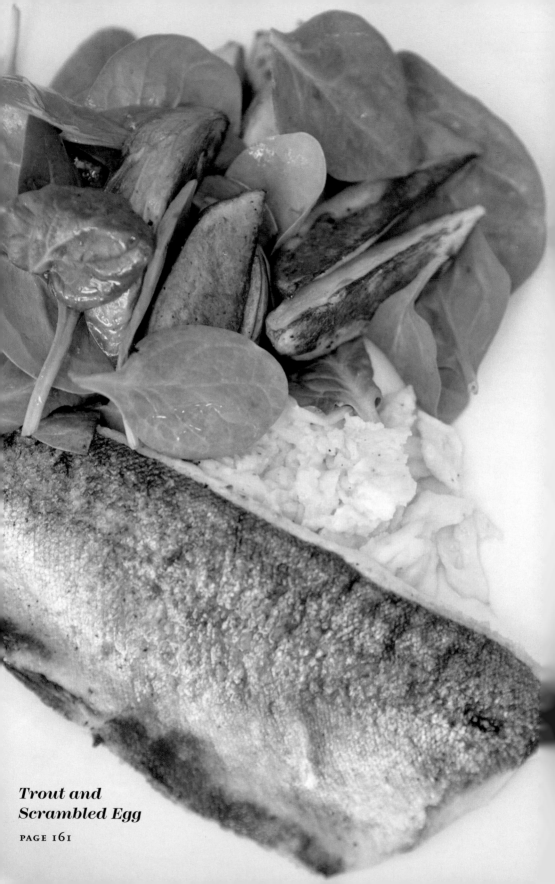

*Trout and
Scrambled Egg*

PAGE 161

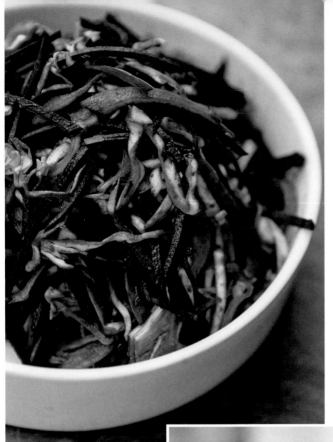

Beet Slaw

PAGE 165

*Brussels Sprouts
Marinated with
Sesame and
Rice Vinegar*

PAGE 169

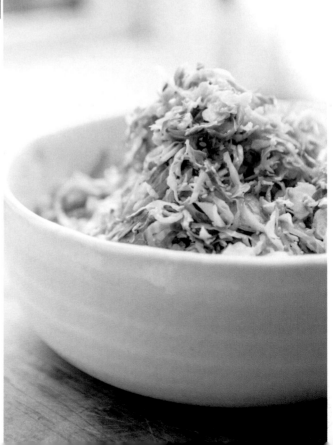

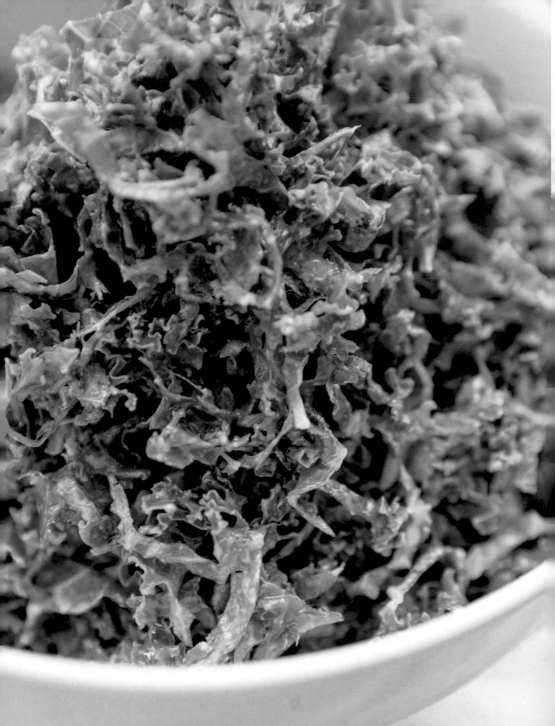

Kale Salad with
Sesame Dressing

PAGE 173

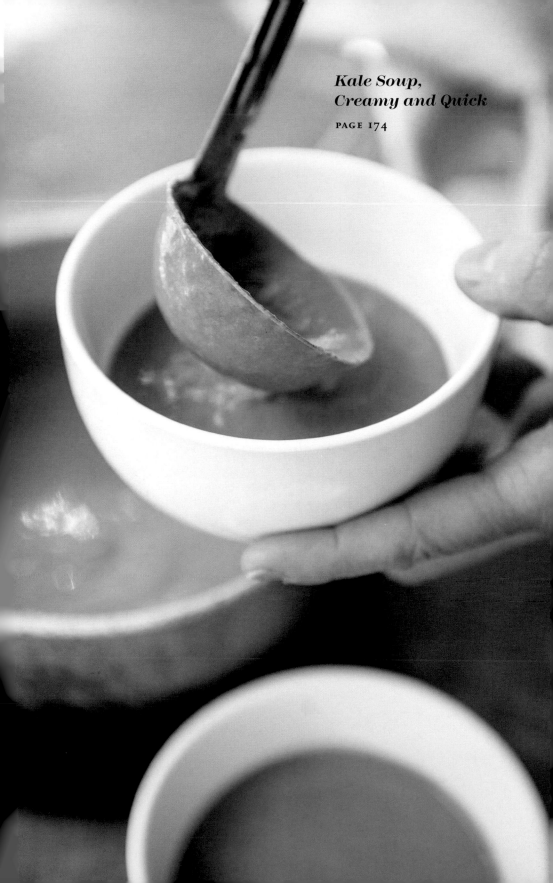

Kale Soup,
Creamy and Quick

PAGE 174

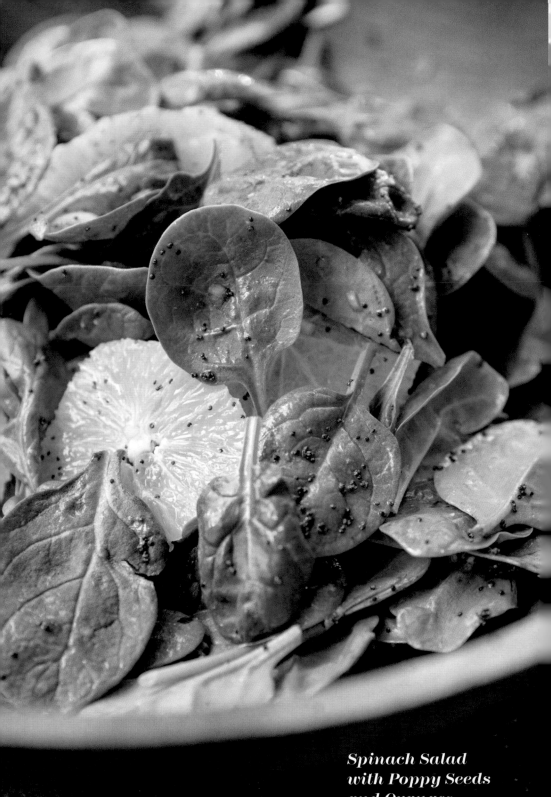

Spinach Salad
with Poppy Seeds
and Oranges

PAGE 179

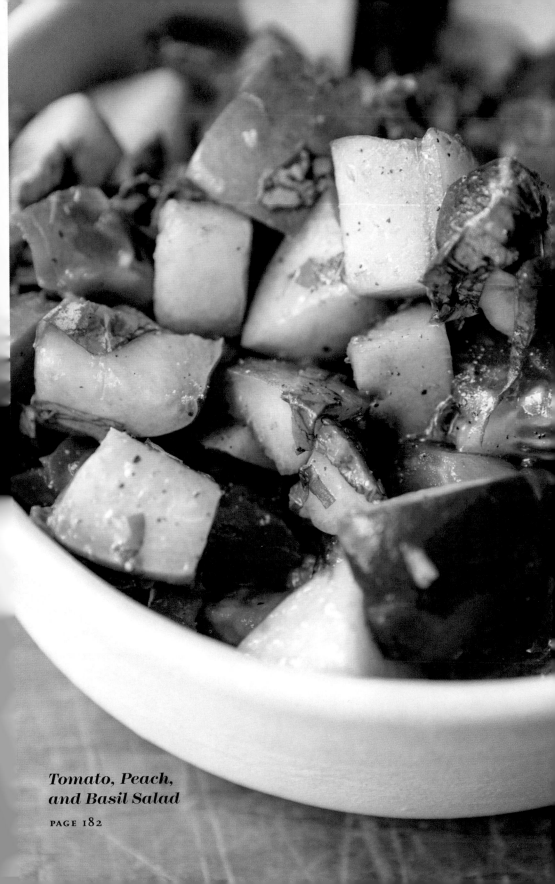

**Tomato, Peach,
and Basil Salad**

PAGE 182

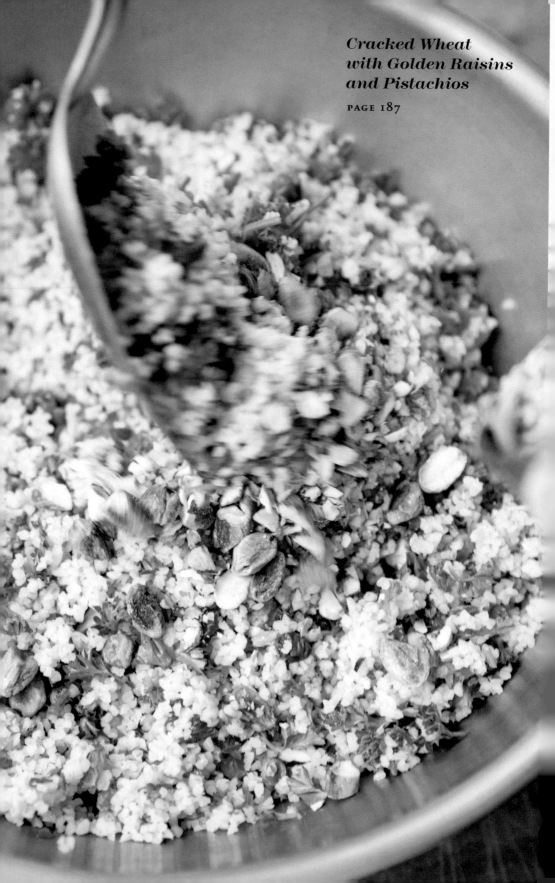

Cracked Wheat
with Golden Raisins
and Pistachios

PAGE 187

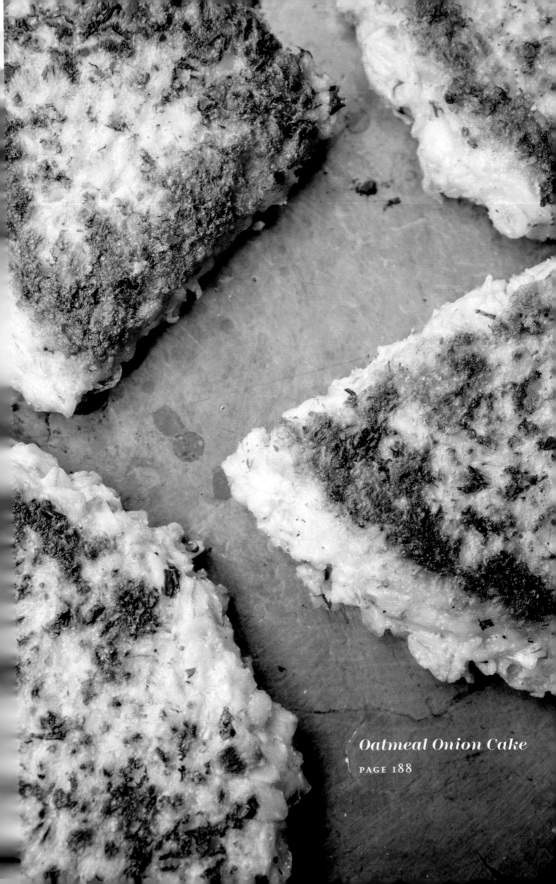

Oatmeal Onion Cake

PAGE 188

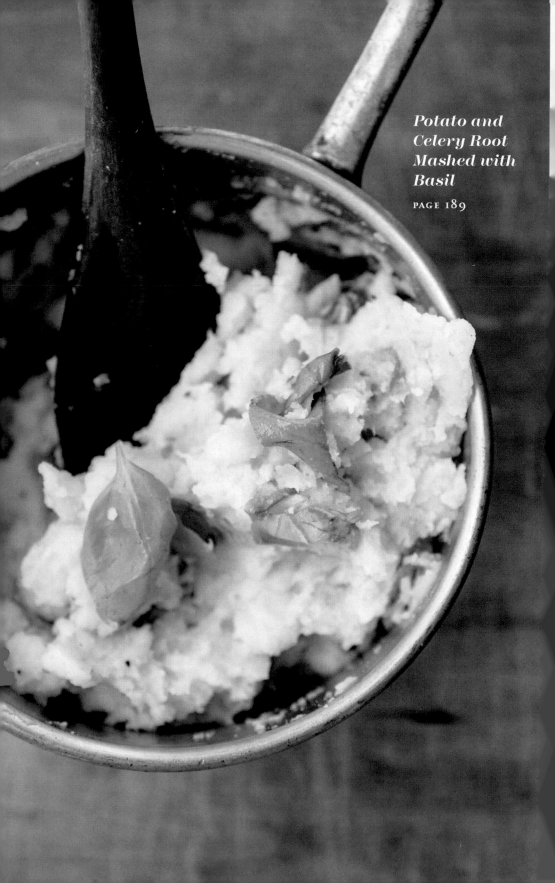

Potato and
Celery Root
Mashed with
Basil

PAGE 189

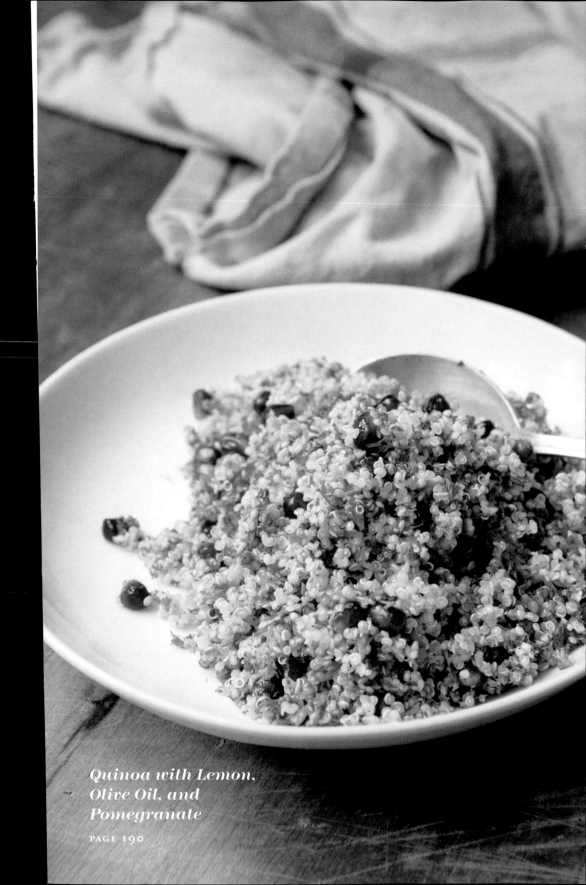

*Quinoa with Lemon,
Olive Oil, and
Pomegranate*
PAGE 190

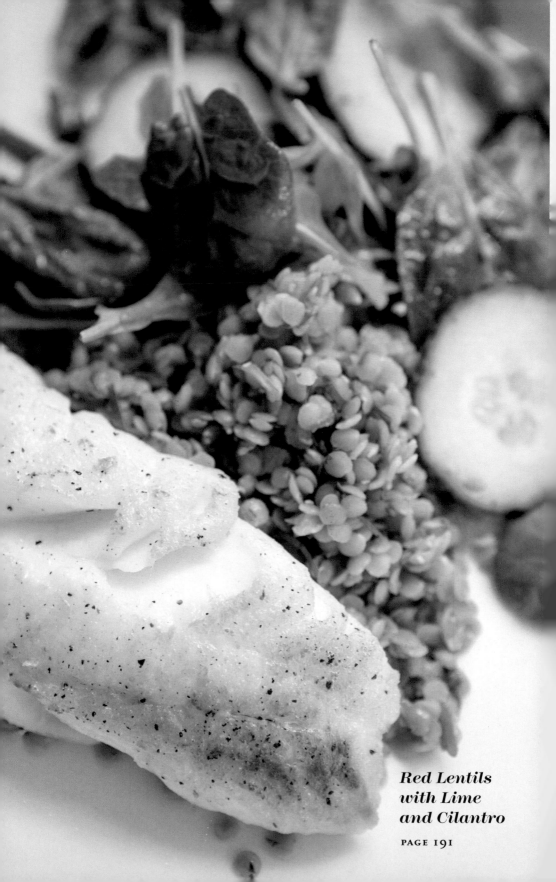

**Red Lentils
with Lime
and Cilantro**

PAGE 191

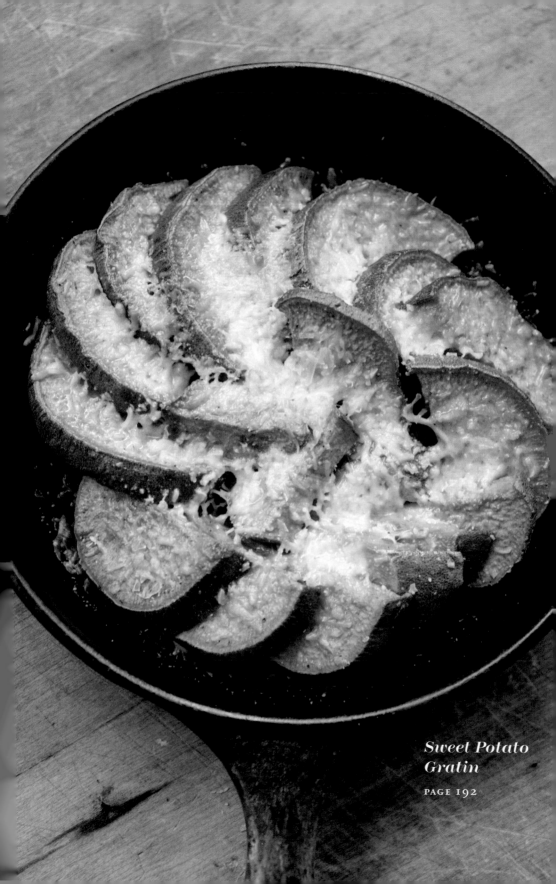

Sweet Potato
Gratin

PAGE 192

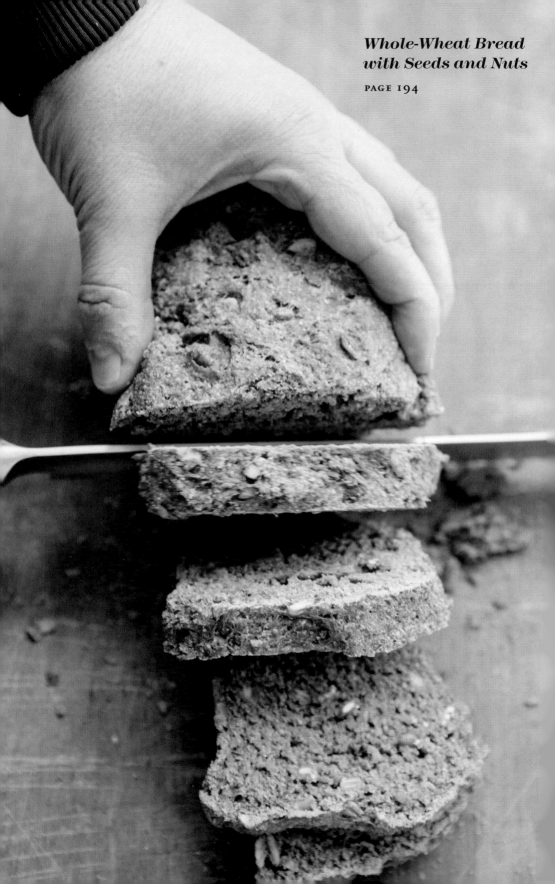

*Whole-Wheat Bread
with Seeds and Nuts*

PAGE 194

- Stop smoking. Nicotine is a stimulant, and smoking before bed can keep you up and make it hard to rouse in the morning.
- Exercise. Meeting the guidelines outlined in this chapter will make it easier to fall asleep and stay that way. The old thinking was that you should refrain from exercise at least three hours before bed, but recent research has shown that exercising before bed does *not* keep you up at night. The best practice is whatever works well for you.
- Have sex. Among its many benefits, sex can leave you feeling more relaxed and better able to fall asleep.

LOVE

If you've been working through the Seven Pescetarian Principles (chapter 5), you've become a *very* savvy eater. But even when you know just what you should (and shouldn't) be eating, you might still struggle with your weight. That's because the emotional and biological pull of food is so strong.

By *biological* I mean that your particular genetic makeup can make it harder to resist overeating; for instance, your levels of "appetite hormones" may make you feel hungrier and less full after a meal, particularly if you've recently lost weight. Or maybe you have a propensity for addiction, and food becomes your substance of choice. The types of food on the Pescetarian Plan, which are very filling for the calories and low in addictive elements like sugar and salt, can help circumvent your biology, as I explained in chapter 1. If you suspect you might be a food addict, take the addictive eating quiz on ThePescetarianPlan.com, which also includes advice on overcoming food addiction.

But a little different from true food addiction is emotional eating, although there is some overlap. It's not as much a biological drive as simply getting into the habit of using food to cope with stress, loneliness, depression, and even positive emotions such as excitement and joy. And boy, can that trip you up! If you're turning to food to cope in a big way, neither the Pescetarian Plan nor any other diet will work for you. Habitually reaching for the cookie and candy stash in your desk drawer when things get stressful at the office, stuffing your body with large portions at dinner to cheer yourself up, opening the fridge and chowing down when you're bored—all of this can be disastrous for your waistline and your health.

In research studies, people who successfully maintain their weight loss are *not* emotional eaters. Many were once but overcame the problem. You can, too. It would take another book to guide you through this issue, but fortunately, many good books on the topic are already out there. For instance, *The Life You Want: Get Motivated, Lose Weight, Be Happy*, which I cowrote with Bob Greene and Ann Kearney-Cooke, is an excellent guide. If you're a binge eater, an oldie but still top-of-the-line classic goodie is Christopher Fairburn's *Overcoming Binge Eating*. Judith Beck's *The Beck Diet Solution* also offers effective strategies to retrain your brain.

You might wonder why I'm calling this section "Love." Because finding the strength to overcome emotional eating involves love. For instance, if you're overwhelmed with demands from other people and food has become your sanctuary, you have to love and respect yourself enough to say no and reduce your stress. You have to love and respect yourself enough to stop calling yourself "fat" and "worthless" and treat yourself with compassion and sympathy and give yourself permission to carve out time to relax, to exercise, and to take care of yourself.

It's not just upping your self-worth; outside support can be tremendously helpful. Anything from hiring a babysitter or cleaning service to supportive friends and family all help reduce stress and make it easier to cope without abusing food.

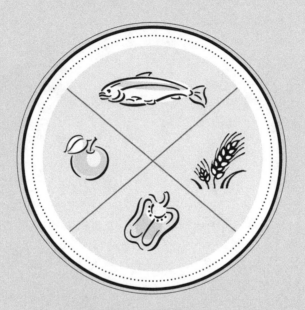

Pescetarian Cooking: Green, Clean, and Lean

Chapter 10

CATCHES TO REEL IN, CATCHES TO TOSS BACK

There may be a lot of fish in the sea, but if you're looking for the least polluted picks, you may not to be able to cast your net that wide. For instance, I haven't eaten swordfish in more than a decade, and there are a few other types of fish I've scratched off my list because they're likely to have high levels of mercury or other pollutants. Still, there are lots of "clean" choices in your local grocery store—and I'll help you find them.

When it comes to contaminants in wild fish, size matters. Small fish, like sardines and smelts, have very little mercury or other pollutants. But when big fish (a bluefin tuna can weigh up to one thousand pounds) gobble up large amounts of little fish, eventually the trace bits of mercury in these smaller fish start accumulating in their bodies. So the further up the food chain you go, the more contaminated the fish.

Your seafood-shopping bible is the "Catches to Reel In, Catches to Toss Back" chart in this chapter on page 121. The "Reel In!" section of that chart lists your seafood staples on *The Pescetarian Plan*. The chart is also posted on ThePescetarianPlan.com as well as an abbreviated version you can print out and take to supermarkets and restaurants. Or, you can always access it on your smartphone.

Here are general guidelines for choosing the purest seafood:

- Whenever possible, buy U.S., Canadian, or European seafood. Safety standards in these countries are generally tougher than in many others, so their seafood is generally cleaner. (Yes, "generally"— there are lots of exceptions.) At the seafood counter, ask about the country of origin—they should know. And better restaurants should be able to tell you as well.

    Because 91 percent of seafood eaten in the United States is imported, you may not always have domestic choices. Imports can be just as contaminant-free as the best U.S. fare, so if imported, follow guidelines on the "Catches to Reel In, Catches to Toss Back" chart (page 120).

- Choose small and medium-sized fish. Small (sardines, smelts) and medium (trout and flounder) generally have the lowest levels of mercury and other contaminants.

- Avoid large fish like shark, tilefish, swordfish, and bigeye tuna. They tend to have mercury levels over the safe limit established by the Food and Drug Administration and the Environmental Protection Agency.

- Eat shellfish, such as mussels, oysters, scallops, and shrimp, which tend to be very low in mercury and other chemicals. (Octopus and squid aren't technically shellfish, but they are cleaner, too.) Eat oysters from reputable markets or restaurants; they're more likely to come from clean waterways.

- As much as possible, choose wild salmon—fresh, frozen, or canned—over farm-raised. Depending on the farm, the fish could contain high levels of persistent organic pollutants (POPs), a class of chemicals described later in this chapter.

- Don't eat the greenish mushy stuff found inside crabs and lobster. It's an organ called the heptopancreas (also referred to as "crab butter," "mustard," or "tomalley"). POPs can concentrate in it.

- Before eating fish or shellfish caught in local lakes, bays, ponds, rivers, and other bodies of water, find out if they're safe. Start with the Environmental Protection Agency's (EPA) local fish advisory at fishadvisoryonline.epa.gov and click "Advisories Where You Live." Also, do an online search by typing in your county and state and "fish advisory." If in doubt, avoid it.

- Vary your seafood picks. Even if you stick to the "Reel In!" list of the cleanest seafood choices, it's smart to vary your choices just in case a particular fish at your local grocery is a little higher in contaminants than it should be. Plus, you get a wider variety of nutrients this way; for instance, you douse yourself with omega-3s when you have wild salmon, then get a day's worth of immune-boosting zinc from oysters.
- To buy the most eco-friendly seafood, choose from the "Most Environmentally Sustainable" column on the chart. Some seafood comes with a seal of approval from environmental groups—see page 139 in chapter 11 for more on that.

CONTAMINANTS IN SEAFOOD

The two main types of contaminants are mercury and persistent organic pollutants. Remember, I'll steer you to choices low in these contaminants. Here are the basics on this pair of pollutants.

MERCURY

If you've seen an old-fashioned thermometer or temperature gauge, you've seen mercury; it's the silver-colored liquid metal that rises with a fever or the summer heat.

Where it comes from: I was surprised to find out that about half of the mercury in water and land comes straight from nature. It's spewed out of volcanoes, comes off of disintegrating rocks, and is created after a forest fire. (Trees contain mercury; their roots take it up from the soil.)

The other half is man-made, and the levels are escalating. The culprits: car exhaust, other machines that burn gas, mining, and burning coal. Also, when batteries, fluorescent bulbs, or mercury-containing products are discarded, the contaminant seeps into the soil and water.

How it gets into seafood: Most of the mercury in the ocean starts out in one form (inorganic) but gets converted to a more toxic form (methylmercury) by bacteria living in the water. This, in turn, gets taken up by phytoplankton (single-celled algae), which are eaten by small sea creatures, which are consumed by fish, and so on. So it's methylmercury that winds up in seafood, getting more concentrated as you go up the food chain. The bigger the fish, the more mercury is concentrated in their bodies: A pound of swordfish contains about 77 times more mercury than a pound of sardines. Mercury tends to lodge in fish muscle, not fat.

Health effects: Unlike some metals, like iron or magnesium, your body has no use for mercury. It accumulates in tissues and hangs around for weeks or months before you excrete it. In excess, it can cause neurological damage, suppress immunity, and harm the heart. Fetuses, infants, and small children are much more susceptible to these ill effects than adults; overexposure can even dim intelligence.

Sounds dire, right? But here's the surprise twist: Studies consistently show that women who eat more fish—of any kind—have smarter babies. That's not thanks to mercury, of course; this just goes to show you how potent the brain-boosting powers of the omega-3s in fish are.

How to minimize exposure: Everyone, including pregnant and nursing women, should follow my three-times-a-week fatty fish recommendation. In fact, experts recommend that pregnant women get 200 mg of DHA—a type of fish oil—daily through fatty fish. Three weekly servings of just three ounces of fatty fish will cover this. Examples of fatty fish are on page 36.

That said, women who are pregnant, considering becoming pregnant, or lactating should stick to seafood in the "Reel In!" column—these are the low-mercury offerings. The same goes for small children. Everyone else can also have fish from the other sections of the chart, in the amounts recommended.

PERSISTENT ORGANIC POLLUTANTS

Where they come from: Unlike mercury, which comes from both nature and from factories, the class of chemicals called "persistent organic pollutants" (POP) is entirely our doing. Some POPs you may have heard of include dioxins, dioxin-like compounds, and polychlorinated biphenyls (PCBs). PCBs were once mixed into paints and sealants, added to cooling and insulating fluid for industrial transformers in electric plants, and used to create flame-retardant fabric. Production of PCBs was banned in the United States in 1977, and the European Union has heavily restricted its use since the mid-1980s. About a dozen other POPs have been either banned or production limited since then.

The good news is that levels of these contaminants in the environment are starting to fall. But all the existing POP-laden material is still being released into the ground and waterways—leaching out of hazardous waste sites, oozing out of areas where junk is dumped illegally, and leaking out of older electrical transformers. That means they're still polluting water and soil and accumulating in fish and animals and in our own bodies.

How they get into seafood: Wild fish get PCBs from eating smaller fish, in the same way mercury accumulates. It's all a matter of where they were fished from. Some bodies of water, like the Great Lakes, are notoriously polluted with POPs, whereas fish caught in the ocean, far from land, have much lower levels.

The chemicals are also in the fish oil given to farmed fish, like salmon and trout, which are "carnivorous" fish, meaning that they eat other fish. Unlike mercury, which infiltrates muscle, POPs accumulate in fat.

But POP levels in farm-raised salmon are declining, because the fish are now given vegetable oil sources of omega-3s and "finished off" with fish oils at the end of life. (Otherwise, salmon, trout, and other farmed fish wouldn't have enough omega-3s, cheating consumers out of this healthy fat.) This cuts POPs by up to 94 percent. But until large-scale studies come out showing that POP levels have dropped significantly, I've recommended in the chart on page 127 that you eat farmed salmon no more than six times per month. So far, studies indicate that farm-raised trout have lower POP levels than salmon (and are low in mercury), so this fish is on the "Reel In!" list.

Health effects: As with mercury, fetuses, infants, and children are most vulnerable to POPs' effects; they can cause low birth weight, developmental delays, hormonal imbalances, and other issues. Because some of these chemicals get into breast milk, nursing mothers need to limit their consumption of foods containing them. Some of these chemicals cause liver cancer in animals, and there's a high likelihood it can cause cancer in humans.

How to minimize exposure: Here's how to get enough fatty fish but keep POP levels low:

- Eat sardines, which are low in POPs (and mercury).
- Eat mostly wild-caught salmon (either fresh or canned).
- If you want to eat farm-raised salmon, have it no more than six times per month. (As I said, POP levels appear to be falling due to changes in the diet of farmed salmon, but until comprehensive studies emerge, it's best to be on the safe side.)

- Eat farm-raised trout, but don't make it your *only* fish. Their POP content really hasn't been studied much, so until comprehensive studies are published, play it safe and don't make trout your only fish staple.
- Avoid locally caught fish, especially trout, bluefish, and catfish, unless you've checked with authorities to confirm that they come from water that is not high in POPs. (See page 140 for how to find this information.)
- For extra precaution, remove skin from salmon and trout, as much of the POPs are in the skin. (I split the difference, eating the skin when it's crispy because I love it, and discarding it otherwise.)
- Along with fatty fish, have shellfish and "vegetarian" fish like tilapia and farm-raised catfish, which have virtually no PCBs because they're not consuming fish oil.

Catches to Reel In, Catches to Toss Back

Here's your guide to the types of seafood you can have often and those to limit or avoid.

Some notes on this chart:

- The chart is organized by *safety*: Seafood in the "Reel In!" column is the safest and purest, with little to no contaminants, such as mercury and PCBs. "Go Easy" items contain a little more mercury or other contaminants and so forth. The rest of the information (the three last columns) is about environmental sustainability. Most of the fish in the "Reel In!" column are being caught (or farmed) in ways that minimize their impacts on the environment. But once in a while, you'll find a fish like shad, which is perfectly safe but isn't sustainable.
- The cut-off points (Reel In!/Go Easy/Limit/Toss Back) are based on those of the Natural Resources Defense Council. This organization errs on the side of caution, basing their recommendations on mercury levels appropriate for pregnant women. So women who are not pregnant (or ever going to be) and adult men can probably get away with more servings from the last three groups. Unfortu-

nately, the research isn't clear on this yet, so we have to go with the information that's available so far.

- Sustainability information is adapted from Monterey Bay Aquarium Seafood Watch. For more detailed information on each type of fish, go to SeafoodWatch.org (you'll also find this link at ThePescetarian Plan.com). Blank spaces in the chart mean that the category does not apply to a particular species. For instance, Seafood Watch did not find a "Most Environmentally Sustainable" option for Alaskan pollock, but there is an "Acceptable Alternative."

- Species highlighted in gray are fatty fish rich in health-promoting omega-3s. Have any of these from the "Reel In!" column three times a week.

- Before going fishing or eating fish caught locally, check your local county or the EPA advisory (fishadvisoryonline.epa.gov and click "Advisories Where You Live") to ensure that they're safe to eat and not contaminated.

- You can find this same chart, as well as just the smaller "Reel In!" section on ThePescetarianPlan.com.

- For an explanation of "trawling," "longlining," "purse seining," and other fishing techniques, see page 135 in the following chapter.

Reel In!

These are the purest, cleanest choices and are your seafood staples on the Pescetarian Plan. For portion sizes, go to chapter 5. Remember to have three omega-3-rich seafood dishes weekly—*those choices are highlighted in gray.* The "Acceptable Alternative" column may have some environmental concerns but are a better option than those in the "Avoid" column.

Pescetarian Plan seafood staples	MOST ENVIRONMEN- TALLY SUSTAINABLE	ACCEPTABLE ALTERNATIVE	AVOID: **NOT** ENVIRON- MENTALLY SUSTAINABLE
ARCTIC CHAR	Farmed in the United States, Canada, Norway, Iceland	—	—

Pescetarian Plan seafood staples	MOST ENVIRONMENTALLY SUSTAINABLE	ACCEPTABLE ALTERNATIVE	AVOID: NOT ENVIRONMENTALLY SUSTAINABLE
CATFISH (U.S. farm-raised) (Avoid wild-caught, it may be high in contaminants.)	Farmed in the United States	—	—
CLAMS	Farmed worldwide	Wild surf clams from the Northeast and Mid-Atlantic	—
COD, ATLANTIC (also called scrod, white fish)	Hook-and-line caught from Iceland, Norway, Russia	Same regions, but caught by bottom longline, gillnet, trawl; Danish seine; or hook-and-line from Gulf of Maine in the United States	Trawl-caught from the United States or Canada
COD, PACIFIC (also called Alaska cod, gray cod, true cod)	Caught by bottom longline, jig, or trap from the United States	Trawl-caught from the United States	Imported wild-caught from the Pacific
Crab	Dungeness crab caught by trap from California, Oregon, Washington; Kona crab wild-caught from Australia; stone crab trap-caught from the U.S. Atlantic or Gulf of Mexico	Blue crab or king crab caught by trap from the United States; Kona crab wild-caught from Hawaii; Dungeness crab trap-caught from Alaska; Jonah crab trap-caught from the U.S. Atlantic; snow crab from Alaska or Canada	King crab from Russia
FLATFISH/FLOUNDER (includes dab, hirame, plaice, sole)	Wild-caught in the U.S. Pacific	—	Wild-caught in the U.S. Atlantic
HADDOCK (also called scrod)	Hook-and-line caught in the U.S. Atlantic	Trawl-caught in the U.S. Atlantic; wild-caught in the Icelandic Atlantic; Canadian haddock caught by bottom trawl	—

Pescetarian Plan seafood staples	MOST ENVIRONMEN- TALLY SUSTAINABLE	ACCEPTABLE ALTERNATIVE	AVOID: **NOT** ENVIRON- MENTALLY SUSTAINABLE
HERRING, ATLANTIC (also called sardine, slid, sperling, pilchard, brit)	—	Wild-caught in the U.S. Atlantic	—
HERRING, LAKE (also called northern cisco, tullibee)	—	Wild-caught in Lake Superior	—
MACKEREL, ATLANTIC (also called Boston mackerel, caballa, common mackerel, saba) NOTE: Not king mackerel, which is high in contaminants.	Wild-caught in Alaska	Wild-caught in the United States	
MACKEREL, PACIFIC	Insufficient sustainability information available on this fish		
MULLET, STRIPED (also called jumping mullet, jumping jack, Popeye mullet)	Wild-caught in the U.S. Atlantic or U.S. Gulf of Mexico	—	—
MUSSELS (blue, black, green)	Farmed worldwide	—	—
OYSTER	Farmed worldwide	Wild-caught in U.S. Gulf of Mexico and Canada	—
POLLOCK, ALASKA (also called imitation crab, surimi, kanikama)	—	Wild-caught in Alaska	—
POLLOCK, ATLANTIC (also called Boston bluefish, blue cod, blue snapper, coalfish, saithe)	Caught by gillnet or purse seine in Norway	Caught by Danish seine or trawl in Norway; caught by set gillnet in Iceland; caught in the United States or Canada	Caught by Danish seine or trawl in Norway

Pescetarian Plan seafood staples	MOST ENVIRONMENTALLY SUSTAINABLE	ACCEPTABLE ALTERNATIVE	AVOID: NOT ENVIRONMENTALLY SUSTAINABLE
SALMON, WILD-CAUGHT (canned, fresh, frozen)	Alaskan Chinook, coho, chum, keta, king, pink, red, silver, sockeye, and sake salmon caught by drift gillnet, purse seine, or troll	Coho salmon wild-caught in British Columbia; Chinook, coho, chum, keta, king, pink, red, silver, sockeye, or sake from California, Oregon, or Washington caught by drift gillnet, purse seine, or troll	—
SALMON ROE	Alaskan, caught by drift gillnet, purse seine, or troll	—	—
SARDINES, ATLANTIC	—	—	Wild-caught in the Mediterranean
SARDINES, PACIFIC	Wild-caught in the United States	—	—
SCALLOPS, BAY	Farmed worldwide	Diver-caught in the Mexican State of Baja California Sur in the Magdalena Bay	—
SCALLOPS, SEA	Diver-caught in Laguna Ojo de Liebre and Guerrero Negro in the Mexican state of Baja California Sur; dredge-caught in Alaska	Dredged from the U.S. or Canadian Atlantic; diver-caught in Sechura Bay, Peru	—
SHAD, AMERICAN	—	—	Wild-caught in the U.S. Atlantic

Pescetarian Plan seafood staples	MOST ENVIRONMENTALLY SUSTAINABLE	ACCEPTABLE ALTERNATIVE	AVOID: NOT ENVIRONMENTALLY SUSTAINABLE
SHRIMP/PRAWNS (Though technically different, markets and restaurants use the terms interchangeably.) NOTE: Because shrimp are high in cholesterol, limit to twice a week.	Freshwater prawns farmed in the United States; pink shrimp wild-caught in Oregon; shrimp farmed in recirculating systems or inland ponds in the United States; spot prawns wild-caught in the Canadian Pacific	Northern shrimp wild-caught in the U.S. and Canadian Atlantic; rock shrimp wild-caught in the United States; shrimp wild-caught in the U.S. Gulf of Mexico or south Atlantic; shrimp farmed in open-pen systems in the United States; shrimp farmed in fully recirculating systems in Thailand; spot prawn wild-caught in the U.S. Pacific	Imported shrimp (including from Mexico) farmed in open systems; imported wild-caught shrimp
SQUID (calamari) NOTE: Because squid is very high in cholesterol, limit to once a week.	Trawl-caught in the U.S. Atlantic	Wild-caught imported Argentine shortfin squid; wild-caught imported Japanese flying squid; wild-caught jumbo squid from the Gulf of California; Californian market squid caught by purse seine; shortfin squid trawl-caught from the U.S. Atlantic	—
TILAPIA	Farmed in the United States	Farmed in Brazil, Costa Rica, Ecuador, Honduras	Farmed in China, Taiwan
TROUT (lake) (also called char, laker, mackinaw, namaycush, salmon trout, togue)	—	Wild-caught from Lake Superior or Lake Huron	Wild-caught from Lake Michigan
TROUT, RAINBOW (also called golden trout, steelhead, steelhead trout)	Farm-raised in the United States		—

Pescetarian Plan seafood staples	MOST ENVIRONMENTALLY SUSTAINABLE	ACCEPTABLE ALTERNATIVE	AVOID: **NOT** ENVIRONMENTALLY SUSTAINABLE
WHITING (also called red, silver, ling, squirrel hake)	—	Wild-caught from the U.S. Atlantic	—
WHITE FISH, LAKE	Trap-netted in Lake Michigan; wild-caught in Lake Superior or Lake Huron	Wild-caught in Lake Erie; caught by set gillnet in Lake Michigan; round white fish wild-caught in Lake Huron or Lake Michigan	—

Go Easy

Eat no more than six ounces, no more than six times a month.

TYPE	MOST ENVIRONMENTALLY SUSTAINABLE	ACCEPTABLE ALTERNATIVE	AVOID: NOT ENVIRONMENTALLY SUSTAINABLE
BASS, BLACK (also called Atlantic sea bass, black perch, rock bass)	—	Wild-caught in the U.S. Mid-Atlantic	—
BASS, STRIPED (also called greenhead, rockfish, striper, Suzuki)	Hook-and-line caught in the U.S. Atlantic; farmed in the United States	Caught by gillnet or pound net in the U.S. Atlantic	—
HALIBUT	Wild-caught Pacific halibut (also called "Alaskan halibut") caught in the U.S. Pacific	California halibut caught by hook-and-line or bottom trawl; Greenland turbot (also called "Greenland halibut") wild-caught in the U.S. or Canadian Pacific	Atlantic halibut (also called "Hirame") wild-caught in the U.S. Atlantic; California halibut caught by set gillnet in the U.S. Pacific

TYPE	MOST ENVIRON-MENTALLY SUSTAINABLE	ACCEPTABLE ALTERNATIVE	AVOID: NOT ENVIRON-MENTALLY SUSTAINABLE
LOBSTER	California spiny lobster or red lobster wild-caught in California; Caribbean spiny lobster wild-caught in Florida; Spiny lobster wild-caught in Baja California or Mexico	American/Maine lobster trap-caught in the Northeast U.S. or Canada; Caribbean spiny lobster wild-caught in the Bahamas	Caribbean spiny lobster wild-caught in Brazil
MAHIMAHI (also called dorado, dolphinfish)	Troll or poll-and-line-caught in the U.S. Atlantic	Caught by longline in the United States; troll or pole-in-line caught in the U.S. Pacific, Hawaii; or imported	Imported longline caught
MONKFISH	—	—	Wild-caught in the U.S. Atlantic
ROCKFISH (also called rock cod, Pacific snapper, red snapper, Pacific Ocean perch)	—	Hook-and-line or jig caught in the Pacific	Trawl-caught in the Pacific
SABLEFISH (also called black cod, butterfish, gindara, sable)	Wild-caught in Alaska or the Canadian Pacific	Wild-caught in California, Oregon, Washington	—
SALMON, FARMED in the U.S. or South America*	Salmon farmed in tank (closed) systems in the United States	—	Salmon farmed in open-pens, worldwide
SNAPPER	—	Gray snapper wild-caught in Hawaii or elsewhere in the United States; pink, red, or ruby snapper hook-and-line caught in Hawaii; silk snapper wild-caught in the U.S. Gulf of Mexico, U.S. Atlantic, or U.S. Caribbean	Red snapper wild-caught in the U.S. Gulf of Mexico or wild-caught imported; vermillion snapper wild-caught in the United States
TUNA, canned, light: skipjack	Worldwide troll or pole-and-line	—	Worldwide caught by purse seine

* Although low in mercury, some studies show that farm-raised salmon have high levels of persistent organic pollutants (chemicals described on page 118). Those raised in the United States and South America tend to have lower levels, but even so, choose wild salmon as much as possible.

Limit

If you like the seafood on this list, limit to no more than 6 ounces three times per month.

TYPE	MOST ENVIRON-MENTALLY SUSTAINABLE	ACCEPTABLE ALTERNATIVE	AVOID: NOT ENVIRON-MENTALLY SUSTAINABLE
BLUEFISH	—	Wild-caught in the U.S. Atlantic	—
CHILEAN SEA BASS	—	—	Wild-caught in the Southern Ocean
GROUPER (also called mero, sea bass)	—	Black or red grouper wild-caught in the U.S. Gulf of Mexico; Hawaiian grouper hook-and-line caught in Hawaii	Wild-caught in the U.S. Atlantic; Gag, snowy, Warsaw, yellowedge grouper wild-caught in the U.S. Gulf of Mexico
SPANISH MACKEREL	Wild-caught in the U.S. Atlantic or U.S. Gulf of Mexico	—	—
TUNA, ALBACORE fresh, frozen, or canned (also called white)	Troll or pole-and-line caught in the U.S. or Canadian Pacific	Troll or poll-and-line caught elsewhere in the world; longline-caught in Hawaii	Longline-caught worldwide (except in Hawaii); wild-caught in the North Atlantic
YELLOWFIN TUNA, fresh, frozen, or canned (also called ahi, maguro, canned light)	Troll and poll-and-line caught in the U.S. Atlantic or Pacific	Longline-caught in the U.S. Atlantic or Hawaii; troll or pole-and-line caught worldwide except the U.S. Atlantic and Pacific	Wild-caught worldwide except troll or poll-and line; Longline-caught worldwide (except U.S. Atlantic and Pacific); worldwide purse seine caught

Toss Back

These species tend to be highest in mercury. In fact, the first four are so high that the Food and Drug Administration recommends that pregnant women, women of childbearing age, and small children avoid them entirely. Mercury levels in the remaining seafood on this list are sufficiently high that the Natural Resource Defense Council also recommends avoiding them. Until research clarifies the effects of these higher mercury levels on the rest of the population, it's probably wise for all of us to give them a pass.

> King mackerel
> Shark
> Swordfish
> Tilefish
> Marlin
> Orange roughy
> Bigeye tuna

IS RAW SEAFOOD SAFE TO EAT?

I love, love, love sushi, and if I were blissfully ignorant of the risks, I'd eat it all the time. But one of the curses of being a nutritionist is you learn just a little too much about food safety. As a result, I average just about one sushi meal per month, sticking to restaurants with really good reputations. Raw oysters are an even rarer (pardon the pun) occurrence for me.

Not that raw seafood is all that risky; you're more likely to get salmonella poisoning from chicken or vegetables, or *E. coli* poisoning from beef. And given all the sushi eaten in the United States, I haven't seen any reports that it's causing much food poisoning, so I'm cautiously concluding that it's usually safe. But because there is an element of risk, it's my duty to inform you about it.

THE ODDS ARE IN YOUR FAVOR

Odds are, you won't get seafood poisoning. You might be surprised to hear that you're more likely to get food poisoning from a vegetable than anything else. The Centers for Disease Control and Prevention (CDC) estimates that around nine million people get hit with food poisoning yearly; about half of these cases originate with a plant-based food. Vegetables are most often the culprit, followed by fruit and nuts. (The source is often the manure they're grown in, bacteria introduced during processing, or by people's hands during food preparation at a restaurant.)

The next most common sources: meat and poultry, which combined, cause 22 percent of cases. Dairy (usually unpasteurized milk) accounts for about 14 percent. Just 6 percent is due to any type of seafood (2.7 percent of cases are caused by fish, 3 percent by mollusks like clams, mussels, oysters, and scallops, and only 0.5 percent from crabs and lobsters).

Unfortunately, the CDC didn't parse out whether the seafood-related illnesses came from raw or cooked food. But raw seafood is riskier than cooked—in countries that eat more sushi, such as Japan and Australia, a higher percentage of foodborne illness comes from fish.

MINIMIZING RISKS

I hate to break it to you, fellow raw fish lovers, but the only way to truly kill off bacteria, viruses, and parasites (aka worms) is to cook them. (Cooking *won't* kill marine toxins, which are mainly an issue in tropical fish caught by sports fishermen or shellfish harvested from "red tide" areas or other areas where there has been serious algae bloom in the water.)

If you *are* going to eat it raw, the cardinal rule is refrigeration. If seafood is properly refrigerated every step of its journey from harvest to your home, then the odds are it'll be just fine. That's because a little bit of bacteria usually won't hurt you, but a lot will. Bacteria tend to multiply quickly at room temperature but very slowly in the cold.

That means you want seafood that has "followed the rules" by adhering to government and state regulations specifying how seafood is handled. For example, there are rules spelling out how quickly fish or shellfish must be refrigerated after harvesting and at what temperature. "Reputable markets and restaurants will buy seafood from reputable dealers that adhere to sanitation guidelines. So, the best way to reduce your risk of getting contaminated fish or shellfish is to buy from established supermarkets, fish markets, and restaurants," advises Doris T. Hicks, seafood technology specialist at Delaware Sea Grant in Lewes, Delaware. In other words, Safeway, Whole Foods, and the local seafood store are better bets than the guy selling his catches from the back of a truck!

A reputable sushi restaurant will go even further, freezing seafood that will be served raw at very low temperatures. This kills worms and other parasites. (That's why it's best to eat raw fish at a sushi restaurant—your home freezer might not get it cold enough.) As for ceviche—raw seafood marinated in lemon or lime juice—the juice acids aren't strong enough to kill parasites or bacteria. So you still need to start with fish that's been frozen at proper temperatures.

While fish tend to have garden-variety bacteria that usually aren't so harmful, oysters and clams can harbor a type of bacteria that occurs natu-rally in water and can be lethal in vulnerable people. It's called *Vibrio*. "Most people are *not* at risk for serious *Vibrio* infection," says Tori Stivers, seafood specialist at the University of Georgia Marine Extension Service and man-ager of the site SafeOyster.org. "If you're a basically healthy person to begin with, you may get mild gastroenteritis. However, the infection, particularly from one type, called *Vibrio vulnificus,* can be a lot more serious—even life-threatening—in people with weak immunity or with one or more high-risk conditions." (See "Raw Rules" below for a run-down of who's most vulner-able.)

Raw Rules

f you're going to eat raw oysters, clams, and other shellfish, or sushi, fish tartare, ceviche, and other raw seafood, here's how to minimize your risk:

- Buy oysters and clams from reputable, established markets, such as big chain supermarkets or well-established seafood markets instead of from your local fisherman. The former is most likely to buy from suppliers who followed proper handling procedures.
- Try post-harvest processed (also called "pasteurized" or "pressure-treated") oysters, which have either been subjected to freezing, heat, or high pressure, all of which drastically reduces levels of *Vibrio*. These oys-ters look and feel raw, but some raw oyster connoisseurs turn up their noses up at them. Ask for them at the seafood counter—if they're not in stock, you might be able to order them.
- Pass on locally caught oysters sold out of trucks and stands; they may not have been refrigerated properly.
- Eat freshly shucked shellfish; throw away any that have begun to open. (For more detailed tips on shellfish buying, see page 142.)
- Eat at sushi restaurants that are reputable (the same goes for restau-rants serving any type of raw fish). Responsible establishments will freeze seafood at the correct temperature and for the right amount of time to kill parasites.
- It's best not to make your own raw fish dishes at home; home freezers may not reach the low temperatures required to kill parasites.

Avoid raw seafood altogether if:

- You're pregnant. An infection could harm your fetus—it's not worth the risk. Pregnant women should also avoid smoked seafood (such as salmon, trout, and lox) found in the refrigerated section of supermarkets and delis. These items (as well as deli meats) can harbor *Listeria monocytogenes*, a bacterium that isn't inherent to fish but can latch on during processing or handling. Listeria can be very harmful—even lethal—to the fetus.

- Your immune system isn't up to par. This could be because you've had an organ transplant, have been diagnosed with kidney disease, HIV/AIDS, or cancer, or are in chemotherapy. The elderly, infants, and young children sometimes have reduced immunity. On the off chance that these groups of people do get an infection or parasite, it could be very hard for them to fight it off.

- You have liver disease (from hepatitis, cirrhosis, alcohol abuse, or cancer).

- You have diabetes.

- You have hemochromatosis (iron overload).

- You are traveling in a foreign country, especially a less developed one where seafood safety rules may be more lax.

Eat Seafood with Confidence

Learning about contaminants in food is scary stuff, but keep in mind that *every* food—beef, vegetables, chicken—has its contamination issues. When it comes to bacteria and other types of food poisoning, seafood is actually safer than most other foods. Seafood from the "Reel In!" list are very healthy choices, and you should enjoy them with confidence. Also keep in mind that on the Pescetarian Plan you're eating moderate—not excessive—amounts of seafood. Remember: Basically every study shows that fish eaters are healthier in virtually every way!

Chapter 11

ENVIRONMENTALLY FRIENDLY PESCETARIANISM

I*f you're like me, you want to feel good about what you* eat—and not only because you chose the healthiest options but the most earth-friendly ones, too. When I sit down to a seafood meal, I don't want anything on my conscience. So I do my best to choose fish and shellfish that are caught or farmed in environmentally sustainable ways. You'll find those catches in the "Catches to Reel In, Catches to Toss Back" chart in the previous chapter.

When you pick a sustainable piece of fish, you're doing the earth a much better turn than if you'd chosen beef, poultry, or most other land animals. But to "go fish" isn't necessarily to go green: Seafood has its own environmental issues, the main ones being overfishing and aquaculture pollution.

OVERFISHING

There *were* a lot of fish in the sea—but no longer. Wild fish are simply no match for modern fishing techniques. How can fish possibly reproduce quickly enough to replenish stocks scooped up by trawling, the practice of dragging nets that reach the size of football fields behind a boat? Trawling not only decimates target seafood populations, like pollock, flounder, and shrimp—it also presents challenges to populations of crabs, sharks, and other "bycatch," which get caught up in the nets and perish. Technologies like sonar (low-frequency sound waves), which track fish over vast expanses of ocean, pose another blow to fish populations because they uncover fish that would have remained hidden.

In fact, 85 percent of the world's fisheries (regions of the ocean, lakes, and other waterways where specific types of fish live) have been overfished, are on the verge of being overfished, or have collapsed, according to the ocean conservation organization Monterey Bay Aquarium. "Collapsed" means that a fishery has dropped to 10 percent of historically plentiful levels—a calamity from which fish populations may never recover.

A famous (or infamous) U.S. example is the collapsed. It cod population along the coast of New England. Cod fishing, which dates back four hundred years, is considered the first colonial industry. Up until about 1900, cod were caught by hook and line, a practice that doesn't make a real dent in their numbers. All of that changed with steam-powered trawlers (followed by even faster diesel engines), which not only destroyed the cod population but also severely damaged the haddock population. In 1930 alone, 70 to 90 million baby haddock were caught in cod trawler nets and were discarded or died at sea. By the 1970s, the cod population collapsed. It made a little comeback after fishing restrictions were set, and then collapsed again in the 1990s. Although sections of the New England coast are now off-limits to cod fishing, it's unclear whether these fish will ever repopulate.

So why is cod on my "Reel In!" list? (See page 121.) I recommend Pacific cod, whose population is "healthy and abundant," according to Monterey Bay Aquarium's Seafood Watch. This group also recommends Atlantic cod imported from Iceland and the Northeast Arctic (near Norway and Russia), where populations are well managed and levels are on the rise. The only U.S. Atlantic cod recommended—and not as a first choice—are those caught by hook and line in the Gulf of Maine. Because of better management practices, cod in this area are plentiful enough to allow fishing.

Fortunately, the tide may be turning on overfishing. "Countries like the U.S. are imposing and enforcing limits on the amount of fish that can be caught ['catch limits'] and there's increasing demand for seafood from better managed [read: more environmentally sustainable] fisheries. This means there's now economic incentive to produce sustainable seafood," notes Sheila Bowman, manager of culinary and strategic initiatives for the Monterey Bay Seafood Watch Program. And certifications like the Marine Stewardship Council, awarded to companies with sustainable fishing practices, while not perfect, have been helpful. According to a 2012 report by the United Nations Food and Agriculture Organization, 67 percent of U.S. fish stocks are being sustainably harvested, and just 17 percent are overexploited. The numbers look even better in New Zealand and Australia.

Some more good news: "Clams, mussels, and oysters are generally very sustainable—most are farmed and farmed responsibly," according to Bowman. In fact, because they filter water, they actually make water from their farms cleaner instead of contributing to waste pollution, as some fish farms do.

How We Reel Them In

If you've ever gone fishing the old-fashioned way—with just your rod and some bait—you know it can be slow going. You might be lucky to reel in three fish all day. If that's how seafood were caught, there wouldn't be an overfishing problem. But to meet a steadily increasing global demand for seafood, industrial fishing techniques harvest up to fifty tons or more!

Here are the main fishing practices—you'll see these terms mentioned on the "Catches to Reel In, Catches to Toss Back" chart on page 121.

Eco-friendly:

Poll fishing: A fishing poll line dangles bait or a lure in the water. There's no bycatch, accidental snaring of other fish, birds, turtles, and so on.

Trolling: This is similar to poll fishing, except the boat moves slowly while the bait or lure is in the water. The moving bait attracts fish like salmon and mahimahi. It's eco-friendly for the same reasons as poll fishing.

Harpooning: People still use this traditional fishing method, which requires brawn and skill to spear large fish like bluefin tuna and swordfish. There's no bycatch with this one either—it takes some doing just to catch one at a time!

Setting traps and pots: These cages, which sit on the ocean floor, are filled with bait that lure lobsters, crab, shrimp, and certain types of fish. They shut when the prey enter, holding them alive until fishermen come to claim the catch. There's little bycatch or disruption to the environment.

Harmful to ecosystems (but with some adjustments can be less so):

Longlining: These fishing lines can stretch fifty miles, containing hundreds or even thousands of baited hooks at regular intervals. They're either strung near the surface, to catch fish like tuna and swordfish, or on the sea floor, to attract cod and halibut. Unfortunately, they also wind up hooking sea turtles, sharks, and birds. Some scientists think that bycatch can be reduced if lines lie deeper in the water and use different types of hooks.

Purse seining: Fishermen drop large walls of netting that circle schools of sardines, tuna, and other fish, then pull the bottom of the net closed like a drawstring. Bycatch, such as dolphin, are a problem. This could be remedied if fishermen targeted a single species of fish that swims close together. This technique can range from responsible to environmentally destructive depending on which seafood is targeted.

Gillnetting: Picture a string of very large tennis nets close to the ocean floor, anchored down. When fish try to swim through them, they get trapped in the holes. These nets can also be suspended close to the ocean surface in order to catch top-dwelling fish. Like purse seines, these are a mixed bag environmentally. The best-case scenario: They catch the right fish, and the smaller fish pass through them unharmed. But use the wrong type of netting and there's a lot of bycatch.

Most destructive:

Trawling: Not to be confused with trolling (on page 135), this involves dragging nets that can be as big as football fields either along the ocean floor or somewhere between the bottom and the surface. It's used to catch pollock, cod, flounder, and shrimp but also traps bycatch, especially if dragged along the bottom. It's destructive to the ocean floor because the nets, heavy with fish, kill other fish, crabs, and other bottom-dwelling sea creatures. It pulls up coral, forests of sea plants, and in other ways destroys habitats.

Dredging: This is similar to trawling, except a heavy frame connects to a mesh bag that's dragged across the ocean floor instead of a more flexible net, so it's even more devastating as it crashes along the ocean floor.

HOW OUR WATERS BECOME POLLUTED

Most of us have fond memories of summer vacations at the beach. As much as we enjoy our oceans, lakes, gulfs, and seas, we also *need* them. They supply 50 percent of the oxygen we breathe—oxygen is constantly being released from the ocean into the atmosphere. (Microscopic organisms in water called phytoplankton—like trees and other "land plants"—absorb carbon dioxide and release oxygen.) Oceans also help regulate temperature. And, of course, they supply us with fish and shellfish, which are a major source of food for some populations.

But we haven't returned the favor. Instead we pollute our water, which harms and kills sea creatures. Oil spills can devastate marine life and birds, but the main source of pollution—80 percent of it—comes from the land. It's mostly runoff—rainwater carrying pollutants into sewers, creeks, and rivers, which eventually flow into the seas and ocean. This runoff contains pesticides, fertilizers, and animal waste from farms, ranches, and cars (that rainbow sheen you see in parking lot puddles is oil that has leaked from cars). Other pollutants take a more direct route—sewage treatment plants and factories spew waste and chemicals right into the water.

Fortunately, a number of nonprofit and nongovernmental organizations are working to save our waters and marine life. By supporting them, you can do your part to reverse the damage. To name a few: Defenders of Wildlife, Environmental Defense (formerly Environmental Defense Fund), Food and Water Watch, Greenpeace, the Monterey Bay Aquarium, the Ocean Conservancy, the Oceans Futures Society, Oceana, the Pew Institute for Ocean Science, the Sierra Club, the Wildlife Conservation Society, the Whale and Dolphin Conservation Society, and the World Wildlife Fund. The complete list with web links can be found on ThePescetarianPlan.com.

FISH FARMS—THE GOOD AND THE BAD

About half the seafood sold in the United States is farmed—not wild. You'd think fish farming (aquaculture) would be the ideal solution to overfishing. When it's done right, it can be. A well-managed fish farm leaves little environmental imprint and brings untainted fish to your plate.

But unfortunately, some fish farming practices actually *hurt* the environment. However, from my read on the state of the industry, farms are cleaning up and are becoming more eco-friendly. For instance, one issue is that wild forage fish, like sardines, could become depleted because they're harvested for fish food. Increased use of vegetarian feed sources, like soy protein and canola oil, are helping mitigate this problem.

Most fish farms are located in the ocean or other bodies of water. In the past, farmed fish were escaping into the wild, eating up the wild fish's food, and breeding with them, threatening biodiversity. But more secure fish pens have addressed the issue, at least in some countries. For instance, in the United States and Canada, annual escapes used to be in the 10,000 to 100,000 range. Since 2006, there have been no escapes in Washington, and almost none in Maine—these are the two biggest states for aquaculture. Fewer fish are escaping from farms in Norway, but I couldn't get reliable information on this issue in other regions.

Other environmental threats: waste and disease. Just as cattle and poultry produce waste, so do fish. This "fish poop" settles underneath the nets, along with uneaten fish feed. In excess, it can choke off seaweed, fish, and other marine life living in the mud. Meanwhile, farmed fish can spread disease to wild fish, such as sea lice, which causes them to get sick or die.

U.S. farms are now placed in areas where there's a quick current that doesn't allow as much debris to accumulate underneath. The Clean Water Act and other regulations have limited pollution from aquaculture in the United States. And less polluting forms of aquaculture, like closed containment farms, may eventually become more prevalent. As for what's going on internationally, the research is sparse, so I can't give you an up-to-date view.

One happy note: oyster, clam, and mussel farms actually clean up water. These "bi-valves" feed by filtering what's naturally in the water, so they don't require fish food.

Seafood Eco-Labels

I f you're shopping for fruit, vegetables, grains, beef, chicken, and other foods, the "USDA Organic" seal is a clear indication that the producers met certain environmental standards. There aren't yet organic standards for seafood, although they are in the pipeline. While we're waiting for the government to release them, a number of other organizations have filled the gap with their own labels.

Eco-labels for wild-caught fish take into account, among other things, the health of the fish stocks and how the seafood was caught. The two main labels come from the Marine Stewardship Council (MSC) and Friends of the Sea.

Aquaculture eco-seals reflect not only the environmental impact of the fish farm (such as pollution of the water and land) but the sustainability and safety of the fish feed. For instance, is the feed made from overfished sources? They may also look at the chemicals and antibiotics that were used. Friends of the Sea also has an aquaculture eco-label, and the other major seal is Best Aquaculture Practices.

You'll see these eco-seals on canned and frozen seafood, and grocery stores may display them right at the seafood counter. Some stores also have their own sustainability standards, hiring third-party inspectors to review fish farms or fishing outfits.

How useful are these seals? From my conversations with consumer and environmental groups, it's clear that most of these groups don't think the eco-seals or grocery store standards go far enough. Of all the seals, the Marine Stewardship Council seal seems to be the most well regarded.

One potentially bright spot is a certification used in Europe that's just starting to appear on farmed fish raised in the United States. Called the Aquaculture Stewardship Council, it's based on standards set by the respected environmental organization World Wildlife Fund. "Global demand for seafood is growing—in fact it's projected to double over the next forty years. Wild seafood is tapped out, so aquaculture is the only solution. We developed the most rigorous environmental standards to date," says Jose R. Villalon, vice president of Aquaculture for WWF-U.S. How it works: Independent certifiers award the ASC seal to farms that meet the standards.

HOW TO PICK A "GREEN" FISH

Ask before you buy. Quiz your waiter or the person behind the fish counter to find out whether the fish was farmed or wild-caught and where it came from. They might know how the fish was caught, but don't count on it. I've found that it's easier to get that info from a supermarket than a restaurant (either the waiters and chefs don't know, or they don't want to reveal). Also ask if the seafood carries an eco-label (see previous page for explanation of these terms).

Check the chart. Before purchasing, see where the seafood falls on the "Catches to Reel In, Catches to Toss Back" chart starting on page 121. And, no, you don't have to lug this book around with you to grocery stores and restaurants! You can print out a list, which is available at ThePescetarianPlan.com. Or, you can bring up the list on your smartphone.

Go Fish!

We're omnivores, meaning that our bodies were designed to eat both plants and animals. For all its issues, seafood is still the most environmentally smart source of animal protein—protein that not only helps you drop pounds and maintain a healthy weight, as I described in the first chapter, but also supplies you with the omega-3 fats that are so vital to your health.

With a little research—namely, referring to the "Catches to Reel In, Catches to Toss Back" chart in chapter 10—you can feel really good about your seafood choices. You're eating clean, nutritious, and environmentally sustainable sources of seafood. And when you turn the page, you'll see how to turn your catch into a delicious meal.

Chapter 12

SEAFOOD SHOPPING AND (FOOLPROOF) COOKING

Cooking a fish shouldn't be as difficult as hooking one! And yet, my dinner guests often ask me, "How do you get your fish to turn out so well?" Or they confess, "I don't do fish—it's too hard." My usual response: Start with good quality seafood, cook it gently, and be sure not to overcook it.

Believe it or not, seafood is actually a lot easier to cook than meat or poultry. I'm not sure where seafood got its hard-to-cook reputation. Think about how tricky it is to get chicken or beef (especially lean cuts) to turn out moist and tender. But follow the cooking instructions in this chapter, and even if you've never cooked seafood before (or have, but with poor results), your seafood will be cooked to perfection. Better yet, these skills are easy to attain.

SAVVY SEAFOOD SHOPPING

If you live on or near the ocean, it's easy to get good, fresh fish and other seafood. If you don't, fresh options may be more limited, but there's always the freezer case. No reason to turn your nose up at frozen—there are some high-quality offerings out there, in places that may surprise you, such as Costco.

Here's how to bring home the freshest catches:

1. ***At the fish counter, ask what's freshest.*** And don't take "Oh, they're all fresh" for an answer! Some are bound to have come in more recently than others. It's best to buy those, even if it means changing your dinner menu a little.

2. ***Observe the display.*** Seafood should either be refrigerated or sitting on a thick bed of fresh-looking ice that is not melting.

3. ***Look your fish in the eye.*** Obviously, this only applies to whole fish; the eyes should be clear and bulge out a little. Also check out the flesh, which should be firm and shiny with bright red gills and no milky slime.

4. ***Examine the fillets.*** Without the telltale head, you'll have to look for more subtle cues when buying fillets, such as lack of discoloration, darkening, and drying around the edges. Flesh should spring back when pressed. (Ask the fishmonger to do this, as you're probably not allowed to, for health reasons.)

5. ***Suss out the shrimp.*** If it's raw and still in the shell, it should be gray, not pinkish. If shelled (or partially shelled), look for gray flesh that is translucent and shiny.

6. ***Look for signs of life.*** Unlike fish, oysters, clams, mussels, crabs, and lobsters spoil rapidly after death, so they should be alive when you buy them.

   - If oysters, clams, and mussels are a little bit open, give them a tap. That should make them "clam up." If they don't close completely, they might be dead, so pass on these. If the store won't let you touch them, ask the person behind the counter to do it.
   - Touch the legs of crabs and lobsters; if you get movement, they're still alive. If not, they may not be, so don't buy them.
   - Don't buy any shellfish with cracked or broken shells.

7. ***Scan the tags and labels.*** Containers of live shellfish come with a tag stating the processor's certification number, indicating that they were harvested, transported, and processed according to national shellfish safety standards. Shucked shellfish should also have this information on the container's label.

8. *Use your nose.* While a salty, ocean breeze smell is fine, seafood should not smell fishy or give off a whiff of ammonia. That's a sign that it's past its prime. Some markets won't let you smell the fish, saying that it's against their health regulations. So if you get it home and it smells just a little fishy but otherwise looks good, it's probably fine. Cooking should get rid of the smell and kill off most everything that's not safe. (More on this in chapter 10.) However, if it really stinks, throw it away. (Keep your receipt to ask for a refund—and consider buying from a different location next time!)

9. *Buy it last, and keep it cold.* Seafood should be the last thing you put in your shopping cart, just before checking out. Keep it cold on its way back to your home, even if it means bringing ice packs to the store or asking for a bag of ice at the seafood counter.

At the freezer case:

1. *Skip the crystals.* Avoid frozen seafood with any coating of ice crystals on the bag or on the seafood itself. That's a sign that it's been defrosted and refrozen, which can mean a mushy texture or possibly bacterial contamination. It's easy enough to tell if it's in transparent packaging; with opaque packaging you can gently press the bag to feel for crystals and listen for their crunchy sound.

2. *Check for holes and tears.* This sounds obvious, but make sure the packaging isn't torn; even a little hole lets in bacteria.

3. *Buy it last, and keep it frozen* (see tip 9, above).

SAFE STORAGE AND PREP

Treat raw seafood just as you would raw poultry and meat (or how you *used* to treat them—you won't be buying these foods on the Pescetarian Plan!).

- Refrigerate or freeze it as soon as you arrive home.
- If you're not cooking fresh seafood within two days of purchasing it, then wrap it tightly in foil or plastic wrap and freeze it.

- Thaw frozen seafood overnight in the fridge—not out on the counter. If you forgot to take it out of the freezer, then seal it up tight and place it in cold water for a while. Or, just before cooking, zap it in the microwave on the "defrost" setting so it's still icy but pliable.
- When preparing raw seafood, make sure it doesn't contaminate the rest of your food. That means using a separate cutting board and knives for the raw seafood and the vegetables or other cooked foods.
- Wash your hands before and after handling raw seafood.
- Wash the cutting board and knives well with soap and hot water after using them.

COOKING SEAFOOD

If you're a novice at cooking seafood, there's really just one simple rule: *Don't overcook it.* Even experienced seafood cooks keep a close eye on their dish, especially in the last minutes of cooking. Depending on the variety and cut of your fish, your oven or stovetop, and your cookware, your seafood might take a little more or a little less time.

With that in mind, here are six basic techniques, information courtesy of our chef, Sidra Forman.

Pan-Roasting

Works best for: All fish, shrimp (shelled or unshelled), scallops, squid, and octopus. It's especially good with fish that have delicious skin when crisped, such as salmon, trout, and sardines.

HOW-TO:

1. Pat fish and shellfish dry with a paper towel and then, with fish that has skin, score the fish skin. Do this by making a row of X marks across the skin. This will ensure that the fish will not curl up and that the heat will distribute evenly throughout the fish in the pan. Using a sharp knife, take care to cut only the skin and leave the flesh of the fish intact. If the fillet does not have skin, there's no need to score it.

2. Next, coat the fish, shrimp, or other seafood in olive oil and season

with salt and pepper. The oil will help distribute the heat evenly and help prevent sticking to the pan.

3. Heat a heavy-bottomed skillet to high heat. Add a ¼ to ½ teaspoon of oil—that should be just enough to thinly cover the bottom of a 10- to 12-inch skillet. You can use canola oil spray—it's easy and withstands high temperatures. Let the oil get very hot—you can tell it's ready when you see the first sign of smoke.

4. Don't let it smoke for more than a moment—immediately add the seafood, gently shaking the pan as you do so.

For fish: Place fish skin side down. Once the skin is crispy and brown, about two to four minutes, use a flipping spatula (not made of rubber) to turn the fish over gently. Cook until the fish is just beginning to flake but the very center is still translucent, about two to four more minutes. Exact cooking times will depend on the thickness of your fish and the heat of your pan. If you like your fish more well-done, cook it a bit longer—but watch out! You run the risk of ending up with a dry fish.

For shrimp and scallops: Depending on their size, shrimp take one to two minutes on each side. They help you out by turning pink—that's the sign they're ready or very close to it. (You can remove one and cut it in half to see if it's cooked to your liking.) Sea scallops take about one minute on each side; bay scallops (which are smaller than sea scallops) take about 30 seconds on each side. They should be golden brown on both sides and have just turned opaque while still remaining moist. Use a pair of tongs to flip the shellfish—it's much easier than with a spatula.

For both fish and shellfish, you can check for doneness by slipping a very thin, small knife in the flesh and lifting gently. Remember that seafood continues to cook even after you remove it from the pan. The trick is to remove it moments *before* it is cooked to your liking. Let trial and error be your guide. The reward of perfectly crisped skin and flaky moist flesh is well worth the trouble.

Oven-Roasting

Works best with: Scallops, shrimp (shelled or unshelled), and all larger, meaty pieces of fish, such as catfish, salmon, and cod, both with and without skin.

Roast fish at either a high or low temperature; use high temperature for scallops and shrimp. No matter which temperature you choose, remember that the thicker and larger the cut is, the longer it'll take. That means a three-inch-thick piece of salmon will take more time to cook than a one-inch-thick cod fillet, even if they're both eight ounces.

One benefit of low-temperature roasting is that it's more forgiving when it comes to cooking time; an extra few minutes will not make a significant difference. You don't have that wiggle room at high temperatures; not only does the fish cook faster while in the oven, but because of the higher internal temperature it will also continue to cook longer once the fish is removed. Both methods can produce excellent results, so if you have the time, experiment with both. If not, stick to the high-temperature method, which will cut cooking times.

HOW-TO:

1. Preheat oven to 300°F for low-temperature roasting, 425°F for high-temperature roasting.
2. Coat the fish or shellfish in olive oil, salt, and pepper and top with fresh herbs, such as parsley, basil, or chives, if desired. If using a whole, gutted fish, oil the cavity as well and place the herbs (as well as a few thin slices of lemon, if you like) inside.
3. Place the seasoned seafood on a lightly oiled sheet pan. Even better, place it on oven (parchment) paper. At a low temperature, fish will take between 15 and 25 minutes, depending on the fish and your oven. Low temps aren't good for scallops and shrimp. At high temperature fish will usually take between 7 and 15 minutes, shellfish 3 to 6 minutes.
4. Remove fish from the oven when it is just beginning to flake but the very center is still translucent. You can slip a very thin, small knife into the fish and lift up gently to check. Shrimp is ready when it turns pink. Scallops are trickier—remove one from the oven, cut it in half, and check. The very center should be just barely translucent.

For fish with skin: A few minutes before it's done, set the broiler to high and place the fish, skin side up, two inches from heat source, to crisp the skin. This will take one to three minutes depending on your broiler.

Grilling

Works best with: All fish, although firm fish, such as wild salmon, are ideal. It's also a good way to cook shrimp (shelled or unshelled), squid (calamari), or octopus. Gas grills are easiest because you can regulate the temperature better. Both charcoal- and wood-burning grills take time and effort but offer amazing flavor. Much like pan-roasting, high heat is optimal to prevent sticking.

HOW-TO:

1. Scrape down the grilling surface to remove debris.
2. Heat the grill. You can tell that charcoal grills are ready when the briquettes are coated with white ash. A wood-burning grill is ready just after the high flames die down but the wood is still burning hot. For a gas grill, set to medium-high and let it get hot.
3. For fish with skin, such as trout or salmon, score the fillets by making the shallow X marks across the skin, as described under "Pan-Roasting" on page 144.
4. Coat the seafood in olive oil and season with salt and pepper.
5. If the fish has skin, place it skin side down directly on the surface of the grill. Once on the grill, let fish and other seafood cook for 2 minutes and then lift with a metal spatula, rotate 90 degrees, and gently set it down again, to create those professional-looking "X" grill marks!

   Flip again (very gently for fish!) with a spatula and repeat on the other side. Cook until the fish are just beginning to flake but the very center is still translucent, about 5 to 7 minutes total. After turning shrimp, it may only take another minute; for squid and octopus, another 2 to 3 minutes. Slip a thin small knife in the seafood and lift up gently to check your progress. Cooking time, as with any cooking method, depends on the type, shape, and size of the seafood as well as the heat of your grill.

Steaming

Works best with: All fish, especially thin delicate fish, such as flounder, mackerel, sole, and shellfish, including shrimp (shelled or unshelled), scallops, mussels, oysters, crabs, and clams. You can also steam whole fish or nearly any type of fillet.

HOW-TO:

1. Add water to the bottom of a steamer, place on the burner, and bring to a boil. If you think you're going to be doing this a lot, invest in a fish steamer, which is shaped to accommodate a long piece. Otherwise, just cut the fish to fit the steamer.

2. Season the seafood with salt, pepper, and herbs, if desired. You don't have to do this—the flavor can come from the herbs or the sauce you use after it's cooked.

3. Once the liquid is boiling, turn it down to a simmer, then add the seasoned seafood to the top of the steamer and cover.

   For fish: Cook until the fish is just beginning to flake but the very center is still translucent, about 3 to 7 minutes. Of course, the cooking time depends on type, size, and thickness of the fish.

   For scallops and shrimp: Shrimp are ready as soon as they turn pink. Sea scallops will cook in 2 to 3 minutes, and bay scallops will take only 1 to 2 minutes. Take care not to overcook!

   For crabs: Steam the crabs until the shell turns bright orange, about 20 to 25 minutes. For Maryland-style steamed crabs, coat with a light coating of Old Bay seasoning or your favorite dried spice mix just after you place the live crab in the steamer. (You can use the same spices for shrimp.)

   For clams, oysters, and mussels: Steam the cleaned shellfish until the shells open, about 5 to 7 minutes. If they were alive before cooking, they will all open; discard any that remain shut—these were probably dead when you bought them. Another easy method: Place them in an inch or two of boiling water or other cooking liquid, cover and cook until the shells open. Try enhancing the flavor of the liquid with a 50–50 mix of wine and water, with 1 tablespoon of finely chopped onions or shallots and 1 tablespoon of chopped herbs per cup of cooking liquid. Or try the Clams with Tomatoes and Garlic on Whole-Grain Pasta (page 217).

4. Serve sprinkled with herbs and lemon, or try the Salmon with Tahini and Toasted Nuts (page 230).

Steam, Bake, and Poach

While grilling, broiling, pan-searing, and barbecuing over hot coals are all quick and delicious ways to cook fish and shellfish, these shouldn't be your only cooking methods. That's because high-temperature cooking (including deep frying, which I never recommend) of protein-rich foods creates cancer-causing chemicals called heterocyclic amines (HCAs). Barbecuing over coals is the riskiest, because you're not only getting the HCAs but also other chemicals released into the cooking area when fat hits the coals. Those cancer-causing substances are called polycyclic aromatic hydrocarbons (PAHs). Interestingly, marinating the food before barbecuing and dousing it with marinade throughout can lower the amount of HCAs.

High-temp cooking can also create compounds called advanced glycation end-products. Aptly named "AGEs," these compounds, consumed in excess, can age you, causing sagging skin, cataracts, clogged arteries, and kidney and nervous system damage. People with diabetes who have out-of-control blood sugar produce these in high levels in their bodies. Whether you have diabetes or not, you can also accumulate too many AGEs through your diet. Protein-rich foods naturally contain AGEs, which rise dramatically when cooked at high temperatures.

So, while it's okay to cook at high temperatures, for longevity's sake, intersperse with steaming, poaching, and low-temperature roasting.

Poaching

Works best with: Meaty fish, such as cod and skinless salmon, as well as shrimp (shelled or unshelled) and scallops. Because the seafood is immersed in a liquid, it is a great method to infuse flavor with little to no oil. There are endless possibilities for flavorings, but lemon, wine, leeks, herbs, and garlic all work well. Also, see the recipes for Cod, Cauliflower, and Pea Curry (page 220) and Scallop Corn Chowder with Leeks (page 236).

HOW-TO:

1. Bring poaching liquid to a boil and then reduce heat to a simmer. Season seafood with salt and pepper and then add to liquid, making sure it's completely submerged. Keep at a simmer (if it boils, the seafood may get rubbery) until the fish is just beginning to flake but the very center is still translucent, about 3 to 7 minutes. Shrimp and scallops take about 2 to 3 minutes—shrimp is done when it turns pink and is opaque throughout. Scallops should be mostly opaque with a slightly translucent center.

Cast Iron Searing

Work best with: Scallops, salmon, or any other fish that tastes best rare in the center. This method involves high heat and short cooking times. The goal is a crispy, seared outside and a center that is rare or, if you don't like it rare, just barely done.

HOW-TO:

1. Make sure your cast iron skillet is clean, smooth, and in good condition. Bumps and pitting make for uneven cooking.
2. Put the pan on high heat and let it get very hot.
3. Ideally, your seafood is at room temperature before cooking. Rub with olive oil and season with salt and pepper.
4. Place the seafood in the pan and cook until very brown, about 30 seconds for scallops and 60 to 90 seconds for a fillet. Flip the seafood and brown the other side. If you like, slip a thin knife into the fish and lift up gently to see if the fish is flaking and scallops are mostly opaque but slightly translucent in the center.

Start Cooking!

We hope that you find these cooking methods straightforward and somewhat simple. I'll repeat the key rule again: Don't overcook! If you undercook, you can always cook it a little longer, but if you overcook, you're stuck!

With wonderful, fresh seafood, all you need to do is use any of these techniques, squirt a little lemon on the finished product, and maybe dust with fresh chopped herbs. If you are using frozen seafood, check out recipes like Cod Burger (page 218) and Salmon Seared with Fennel, Mushroom, and Sweet Red Pepper (page 228).

I predict that very soon, *your* dinner party guests will be asking, "How does your seafood turn out so perfectly?"

Chapter 13

PESCETARIAN RECIPES

In *developing recipes for this book, I challenged myself to* come up with foods that I hope will surprise and delight you—definitely not the same old same old, and definitely not "diet food."

And if you think you're too busy to cook, consider this: Most of these recipes take no more than 25 minutes to prepare, and many can be made in advance. There are both one-dish meals—like the Shrimp Taco Salad (page 240)—and others that only need to be paired with a simple salad, like the Scallop Corn Chowder with Leeks (page 236) or the Clams with Tomatoes and Garlic on Whole-Wheat Pasta (page 217). They've also been family-tested, so while all are interesting and flavorful, they are recipes that eaters of any age can enjoy. It's a collection of simple everyday recipes, most of which are quick enough for a weekday meal and delicious enough for entertaining.

When people hear "pescetarian," they often assume that it features a pretty limited menu of fish, fish, and more fish. But as you've learned throughout this book, plant-based foods are also a big part of the Pescetarian Plan.

So there are vegetarian main dishes as well as lots of recipes for side dishes based on vegetables, whole grains, and starchy vegetables as well as a number that include fruit. The idea is to pair these recipes with fish of all types. (Basic seafood cooking techniques are explained in chapter 12.) Have fun, mix and match, and come up with combinations of your own. Because each recipe comes with a "Pescetarian Portion" breakdown (for instance, 2 fruits, 2 fats), you can easily slip the recipes right into your diet. For ideas on how to fit these recipes into your Seven Pescetarian Principles, check out the guidelines in chapter 8. Also take a look at the meals in Appendix C; many are based on these recipes.

Keep in mind that your meals will only be as good as your ingredients. The way I shop to get the best ingredients for my money is to buy what's in season. For example, tomatoes and corn are most delicious—and afford-able—in the middle of summer, but not in winter. If a recipe calls for one vegetable but there's a similar ingredient that is either seasonal (or simply looks better once you get to the market), use it! Recipes should always be used as a starting point. Never buy a wilted bunch of spinach when there is a beautiful bunch of chard sitting next to it. The same goes for your fish selections: Find a good purveyor, and see what's freshest. Have no fear about substituting; just try to swap one fatty fish for another (such as salmon for arctic char) and the same for leaner fish (such as haddock for cod).

If you're a beginner cook, you'll gain confidence with every recipe you make. There's even a pantry section at the end of the recipe section to fill you in on how to make basic foods like salad dressing or from-scratch beans. You'll also become a pro at choosing ingredients; for instance, one encoun-ter with a too-hard or too-mushy avocado is about all it takes before you begin to figure out when they're just ripe! If you're already comfortable in the kitchen, I hope you will tweak these recipes to your liking. And I hope to surprise you with combinations and flavors you've never tried.

So dig in! You—and anyone else lucky enough to enjoy your cooking—should start seeing the rewards right away. A trimmer waistline, more en-ergy, and best of all, food you'll love.

—SIDRA FORMAN

BREAKFAST

~~~~

Black Rice Pudding

Black rice might not have made it to your grocery store yet, which is why brown rice is also an option in this recipe. But it is available online and worth the hunt. Delicious and a good source of anthocyanins—the same powerful antioxidants in blueberries—black rice nutritionally one-ups other types of rice.

SERVES: 4 • PREP TIME: 5 MINUTES • TOTAL TIME: 15 MINUTES (1 HOUR 15 MINUTES IF COOKING RICE FROM DRY)

3 cups cooked **black rice** (see p. 270 for cooking directions, or you can substitute **brown rice**)

4 cups **almond milk**

Dash of **salt**

2½ **bananas**, sliced

½ cup chopped **almonds**

1½ teaspoons **honey**

1. In a small saucepan, add rice, milk, salt, and banana, and bring to a boil. Stir and reduce heat to a simmer.

2. Cook for 10 minutes, stirring often.

3. While rice is cooking, combine almonds with the honey and set aside.

4. Top black rice with the almond mixture. Serve immediately or cover, refrigerate, and serve cold.

PER SERVING:		
Calories: 386	Total Sugar: 19 g	Cholesterol: 0 mg
Protein: 10 g	Total Fat: 13 g	Calcium: 501 mg
Carbohydrate: 63 g	Saturated Fat: 0.7 g	Sodium: 190 mg
Dietary Fiber: 8 g	Total Omega-3 Fat: 21 mg	

PESCETARIAN PORTIONS: 1 fruit serving; 1½ grain/starchy vegetable servings; 1 dairy serving; 2 fat servings (all as nuts/seeds)

Carrot Muffin

Satisfying and dense, these muffins are a good fuel to start the day. They're also so tasty that I find myself going back for half a muffin as a treat later in the day. You can make the batter, cover it, and refrigerate for a couple days before baking. Also, once baked, the muffins freeze well. Wrap them individually for a ready-to-go single breakfast serving; just add a glass of milk or soy milk.

SERVES: 12 • PREP TIME: 20 MINUTES • TOTAL TIME: 40 MINUTES

3/4 cup puréed **silken tofu** or 3 **large eggs**

3/4 cup **skim milk, almond milk**, or **soy milk**

3 tablespoons **honey**

1/4 cup **extra-virgin olive oil**

3 tablespoons **sugar**

1½ cup stone ground **whole-wheat flour**

1/3 cup **cracked wheat**, soaked in 1/3 cup boiling **water** for 5 minutes

3/4 cup **wheat bran**

1½ teaspoons **baking soda**

1½ teaspoons **baking powder**

1½ teaspoons **cinnamon**

4 cups shredded **carrot**

1½ cups chopped **walnuts**

3/4 cup **currants**

1. Preheat oven to 350°F.

2. In a large mixing bowl, combine the tofu or eggs, milk, honey, and olive oil.

3. Add the sugar, flour, cracked wheat, bran, baking soda, baking powder, and cinnamon. Mix until just combined.

4. Stir in the carrots, walnuts, and currants.

5. Place in 12 individual muffin tins and bake until a toothpick inserted in the center comes out clean, approximately 20 minutes.

PER SERVING:		
Calories: 299	Total Sugar: 17 g	Cholesterol: 47 mg
Protein: 8 g	Total Fat: 16 g	Calcium: 106 mg
Carbohydrate: 37 g	Saturated Fat: 2.0 g	Sodium: 270 mg
Dietary Fiber: 6 g	Total Omega-3 Fat: 1,400 mg	

PESCETARIAN PORTIONS: ½ fruit serving; 1 vegetable serving; 1 grain/ starchy vegetable serving; 3 fat servings (2 as nuts/seeds)

Chia Pudding with Berries and Almonds

Chia seeds are a staple on the Pescetarian Plan because they're so rich in omega-3 fats. In this recipe (which lasts in the refrigerator for a few days), chia takes center stage. You can also sprinkle the seeds on salads or over sliced fruit or add them to a smoothie. Grinding or soaking makes it easier for your body to wrangle those precious omega-3s from the seed.

SERVES: 4 • PREP TIME: 5 MINUTES • TOTAL TIME: 10 MINUTES

1	cup **chia seeds**
2 1/2	cups **almond milk**, **soy milk**, or **skim milk**
2	tablespoons chopped **almonds**
1	tablespoon **honey**
1/4	teaspoon **salt**
2	cups **berries**

Combine the chia, milk, almonds, honey, and salt in a bowl. Let sit for 5 minutes. Top with berries and serve immediately or cover and refrigerate until ready to serve. If you are letting the pudding sit or refrigerating it, you may need to add more milk to return it to a pudding consistency.

PER SERVING:		
Calories: 352	Total Sugar: 19 g	Cholesterol: 3 mg
Protein: 17 g	Total Fat: 18 g	Calcium: 572 mg
Carbohydrate: 44 g	Saturated Fat: 2.0 g	Sodium: 265 mg
Dietary Fiber: 20 g	Total Omega-3 Fat: 9,326 mg	

PESCETARIAN PORTIONS: 1 fruit serving; 1/2 dairy serving;
4 1/2 fat servings (all as nuts/seeds)

Granola

While I enjoy the crunchiness of this cereal as-is, Janis prefers it a little softened. She douses it with milk and lets it sit for 10 minutes before eating.

SERVES: 4 • PREP TIME: 15 MINUTES • TOTAL TIME: 45 MINUTES

2	cups cooked **quinoa**
½	cup **rolled oats**
1	tablespoon **honey**
2	tablespoons raw **pumpkin seeds**
2	tablespoons raw **sunflower seeds**
2	tablespoons chopped **walnuts**
2	tablespoons **unsweetened coconut flakes**
	Pinch of **salt**
2	tablespoons **golden raisins**

1. Preheat oven to 350°F.

2. On a sheet tray, combine thoroughly the quinoa, oats, honey, pumpkin seeds, sunflower seeds, walnuts, coconut flakes, and salt.

3. Bake, stirring often, until just golden brown and dry, 20 to 30 minutes. Remove from the oven and stir in the raisins.

4. This cereal keeps well for a couple of weeks in an airtight container.

PER SERVING:		
Calories: 282	Total Sugar: 8 g	Cholesterol: 0 mg
Protein: 10 g	Total Fat: 12 g	Calcium: 35 mg
Carbohydrate: 38 g	Saturated Fat: 2.3 g	Sodium: 49 mg
Dietary Fiber: 5 g	Total Omega-3 Fat: 400 mg	

PESCETARIAN PORTIONS: 2 grain/starchy vegetable servings;
2 fat servings (1½ as nuts/seeds)

Green Shake

I make a shake similar to this on most days, but it is never exactly the same. The specific ingredients depend on what I have on hand and what I am in the mood for. This recipe is a good template to help get the correct balance of fruit, vegetable, nuts, and milk for a nutritious start to your day.

SERVES: 1 • PREP TIME: 5 MINUTES • TOTAL TIME: 5 MINUTES

1	cup tightly packed **kale**
3	tablespoons chopped **cashews** or **almonds**
½	cup sliced **cucumber**
¼	cup diced **pineapple** or **strawberries**, fresh or frozen
1	pitted **date** or 1 tablespoon **honey**
½	medium **banana**
¾	cup **soy milk** or 1-percent **milk**
½	cup small **ice cubes**

1. Place kale, cashews, cucumber, pineapple, honey, banana, soy milk, and ice cubes in a high-speed blender.

2. Process until smooth, 1 minute, and serve immediately.

PER SERVING:		
Calories: 396	Total Sugar: 34 g	Cholesterol: 0 mg
Protein: 14 g	Total Fat: 15 g	Calcium: 356 mg
Carbohydrate: 59 g	Saturated Fat: 2.5 g	Sodium: 123 mg
Dietary Fiber: 7 g	Total Omega-3 Fat: 162 mg	

PESCETARIAN PORTIONS: 1½ fruit servings; 1 dairy serving; 1½ vegetable servings; 3 fat servings (all as nuts/seeds)

Trout and Scrambled Egg

It may seem odd, but for many people around the world, fish is a common breakfast food. You can substitute any of the fish recommended in *The Pescetarian Plan*—even canned sardines packed in water—if they are to your liking.

SERVES: 1 • PREP TIME: 10 MINUTES • TOTAL TIME: 25 MINUTES

> 1 small **potato**, cut into 8 wedges
> ½ teaspoon **extra-virgin olive oil**
> Freshly ground **black pepper** to taste
> 1 cup **spinach**
> 1 **egg**, scrambled
> 3 ounces **trout fillet**
> Dash of **salt**

1. Preheat oven to 375°F. Toss potatoes, ⅛ teaspoon of olive oil, and black pepper. Place on a sheet tray and bake until the potatoes are tender, approximately 10 minutes.

2. Remove from oven, toss in spinach, and set aside.

3. Heat 2 heavy-bottomed skillets over low heat. In a small bowl, combine the egg and black pepper. Put ⅛ teaspoon of olive oil in one pan, pour in the egg, and cook, stirring constantly until it reaches your desired doneness.

4. Place ⅛ teaspoon of olive oil in second pan and cook the fish until slightly browned, approximately 3 minutes. Flip and cook until the fish is just beginning to flake but the center is still translucent, 2 minutes.

5. Serve the spinach and potato mixture with the scrambled egg and fish. Just before eating, season the eggs and fish with a dash of salt.

PER SERVING:		
Calories: 304	Total Sugar: 2 g	Cholesterol: 257 mg
Protein: 24 g	Total Fat: 10 g	Calcium: 88 mg
Carbohydrate: 28 g	Saturated Fat: 3.0 g	Sodium: 326 mg
Dietary Fiber: 5 g	Total Omega-3 Fat: 500 mg	

PESCETARIAN PORTIONS: 1 vegetable serving; 1½ grain/starchy vegetable servings; ½ fat serving; 2½ protein servings

Whole-Grain Pancakes with Banana

Not just for breakfast! Because the pancakes themselves are not sweet, go ahead and serve them as a grain side paired with nearly any fish or vegetable.

SERVES: 4 • PREP TIME: 10 MINUTES • TOTAL TIME: 20 MINUTES

1	cup stone ground **whole-wheat flour**
2	tablespoons **rolled oats**
2	tablespoons **buckwheat flour**
1	cup **Greek nonfat yogurt**
3/4	cup **skim milk** or **soy milk**
1/8	teaspoon **baking soda**
1/4	teaspoon **baking powder**
1/8	teaspoon **salt**
	Canola oil cooking spray
2	medium **bananas**, sliced
1	tablespoon **maple syrup**
1/2	cup chopped **walnuts**

1. In a bowl, mix until just combined whole-wheat flour, oats, buckwheat flour, half a cup of yogurt, milk, baking soda, baking powder, and salt.

2. Heat a nonstick skillet over medium heat and spray with canola oil cooking spray. Make 8 pancakes, cook until browned, approximately 3 minutes, flip and cook until the other side is brown, 3 additional minutes.

3. Serve hot, topped with banana, maple syrup, walnuts, and the remaining half a cup of yogurt.

PER SERVING:		
Calories: 341	Total Sugar: 14 g	Cholesterol: 0 mg
Protein: 15 g	Total Fat: 12 g	Calcium: 182 mg
Carbohydrate: 49 g	Saturated Fat: 1.3 g	Sodium: 194 mg
Dietary Fiber: 7 g	Total Omega-3 Fat: 1,400 mg	

PESCETARIAN PORTIONS: 1 fruit serving; 2 grain/starchy vegetable servings; 1/2 dairy serving; 2 fat servings (all as nuts/seeds)

VEGETABLE SIDES

~~~~~

Arugula with Roasted Garlic Fig Dressing

Arugula is a staple in my refrigerator. I use it constantly in all sorts of salads, as a bed under a warm main dish, in smoothies, and in countless other ways. One of my all-time favorite combinations is arugula with fresh figs and roasted garlic. Because figs are in season only for a little while, I made this dressing with dry figs for all those months when fresh figs are not available.

SERVES: 4 • PREP TIME: 15 MINUTES • TOTAL TIME: 15 MINUTES

4 **dried figs**, stems removed and cut in half
4 roasted **garlic** cloves (see pantry)
2 tablespoons **red wine vinegar**
1 tablespoon **extra-virgin olive oil**
¼ teaspoon **salt**
Freshly ground **black pepper** to taste
8 cups **arugula**

1. In a small bowl, place the figs, cover with hot water, and let sit for 10 minutes. Drain the figs.

2. In a food processor or high-speed blender, combine the soaked figs, roasted garlic, vinegar, olive oil, salt, pepper, and ¼ cup of water. Process until smooth. Gently toss arugula with fig dressing and serve immediately.

3. You can make dressing in advance, cover, and refrigerate until ready to serve.

PER SERVING:		
Calories: 67	Total Sugar: 5 g	Cholesterol: 0 mg
Protein: 2 g	Total Fat: 4 g	Calcium: 84 mg
Carbohydrate: 8 g	Saturated Fat: 0.5 g	Sodium: 158 mg
Dietary Fiber: 2 g	Total Omega-3 Fat: 100 mg	

PESCETARIAN PORTIONS: ½ fruit serving;
2 vegetable servings; 1 fat serving

Beet Slaw

If you have not eaten or prepared a dish with raw beets before, no worries—they're as easy as carrots to peel and shred. This easy-to-love recipe is a perfect and quick complement to most of the fish dishes in this book—and to any piece of simply cooked fish. The slaw just gets better after it sits in the refrigerator for a couple days so I often make a double batch to last for a few meals.

SERVES: 4 • PREP TIME: 10 MINUTES • TOTAL TIME: 10 MINUTES

1	tablespoon **walnut oil** (can substitute **extra-virgin olive oil**)
2	tablespoons **sherry vinegar**
	Pinch of **sugar**
¼	teaspoon **salt**
	Freshly ground **black pepper** to taste
1	cup peeled and shredded **beets**
1	cup shredded **fennel**
1	cup shredded **cabbage**

1. In a small bowl, combine walnut oil, sherry vinegar, sugar, salt, and pepper.

2. In a large bowl, place beets, fennel, and cabbage. Toss thoroughly with vinegar mixture.

3. Serve immediately or cover and refrigerate until ready to serve.

PER SERVING:		
Calories: 58	Total Sugar: 3 g	Cholesterol: 0 mg
Protein: 1 g	Total Fat: 4 g	Calcium: 24 mg
Carbohydrate: 6 g	Saturated Fat: 0.3 g	Sodium: 187 mg
Dietary Fiber: 2 g	Total Omega-3 Fat: 400 mg	

PESCETARIAN PORTIONS: 1 vegetable serving; 1 fat serving

Beets with Onions, Balsamic Vinegar, and Rosemary

You can try this recipe with any root vegetable; you may have to reduce the cooking time by about 10 minutes for carrots and turnips and increase it by 5 to 10 minutes for rutabagas or parsnips. Just use a fork to test for doneness; once the vegetable is tender, add the balsamic and cook for an additional 5 minutes.

SERVES: 4 • PREP TIME: 10 MINUTES • TOTAL TIME: 40 MINUTES

2 medium **beets**, peeled and cut in quarter-inch cubes

1 **onion**, peeled and thinly sliced

2 tablespoons finely chopped **rosemary**

1 teaspoon **extra-virgin olive oil**

¼ teaspoon **salt**

Freshly ground **black pepper** to taste

1½ tablespoons **balsamic vinegar**

1. Preheat oven to 375°F.

2. Place beets, onions, rosemary, oil, salt, and pepper in a large bowl and mix thoroughly. Place on a sheet tray and cook for 15 minutes. Stir and cook until the beets are tender, approximately 10 more minutes. Add the balsamic vinegar and toss thoroughly.

3. Return to oven for an additional 5 minutes. Serve warm, at room temperature, or chilled.

PER SERVING:		
Calories: 49	Total Sugar: 5 g	Cholesterol: 0 mg
Protein: 1 g	Total Fat: 1 g	Calcium: 20 mg
Carbohydrate: 9 g	Saturated Fat: 0.2 g	Sodium: 181 mg
Dietary Fiber: 2 g	Total Omega-3 Fat: 0 mg	

PESCETARIAN PORTIONS: ½ vegetable serving

Broccoli, Quick Roasted with Cilantro, Ginger, and Garlic

It's the generous amount of fresh cilantro that really makes this dish. If you are a lover of cilantro, feel free to add even more! Or if you hate the herb (or don't have any around), you can substitute with parsley.

SERVES: 4 • PREP TIME: 10 MINUTES • TOTAL TIME: 20 MINUTES

4   cups **broccoli** florets
1   tablespoon finely chopped fresh **ginger**
1   tablespoon finely chopped **garlic**
1   tablespoon **sesame oil**
¼   teaspoon **salt**
    Freshly ground **black pepper** to taste
¼   cup roughly chopped **cilantro**

1. Preheat oven to 425°F.

2. In a large bowl, combine the broccoli, ginger, garlic, sesame oil, salt, and pepper. Mix thoroughly until broccoli is evenly coated with oil and seasonings.

3. Place the broccoli on a sheet pan and cook until edges are just browned, approximately 7 minutes. Serve hot, at room temperature, or chilled.

4. Just before serving, toss with the cilantro.

PER SERVING:		
Calories: 66	Total Sugar: 2 g	Cholesterol: 0 mg
Protein: 3 g	Total Fat: 4 g	Calcium: 48 mg
Carbohydrate: 7 g	Saturated Fat: 0.5 g	Sodium: 176 mg
Dietary Fiber: 3 g	Total Omega-3 Fat: 0 mg	

PESCETARIAN PORTIONS: 1 vegetable serving; 1 fat serving

Broccoli Salad

If you've never had a cashew-based sauce, you're in for a delightful surprise—it's wonderfully creamy. If your blender or food processor can't thoroughly purée the cashews, use store-bought cashew butter made from 100 percent cashews. A heaping ⅓ cup is the equivalent of ½ cup of chopped nuts. I toss this dressing with a variety of vegetables, including cauliflower, kale, and cabbage.

SERVES: 4 • PREP TIME: 5 MINUTES • TOTAL TIME: 5 MINUTES

½ cup chopped **cashews**

2 tablespoons **lemon juice**

2 teaspoons **extra-virgin olive oil**

¼ teaspoon **salt**

Red pepper flakes to taste

4 cups roughly chopped **broccoli** florets

1. In a blender or food processor, combine the cashews, 3 tablespoons of water, lemon juice, olive oil, salt, and red pepper flakes.

2. In a large bowl, combine the broccoli and the cashew mixture. Mix with your hands until the broccoli is thoroughly coated.

3. Serve immediately or cover, refrigerate, and serve chilled.

PER SERVING:		
Calories: 151	Total Sugar: 3 g	Cholesterol: 0 mg
Protein: 5 g	Total Fat: 11 g	Calcium: 51 mg
Carbohydrate: 12 g	Saturated Fat: 1.9 g	Sodium: 178 mg
Dietary Fiber: 3 g	Total Omega-3 Fat: 100 mg	

PESCETARIAN PORTIONS: 1 vegetable serving; 2½ fat servings
(2 as nuts/seeds)

Brussels Sprouts Marinated with Sesame and Rice Vinegar

If eating raw Brussels sprouts sounds odd to you, just think "baby cabbage." Also try this same recipe with other thinly sliced or shredded vegetables such as carrots, kale, cabbage, celery, cucumber, or turnips.

SERVES: 4 • PREP TIME: 5 MINUTES • TOTAL TIME: 20 MINUTES

- 4 cups **Brussels sprouts**, ends removed and thinly sliced
- 2 tablespoons **sesame seeds**
- 2 teaspoons **sesame oil**
- 1 tablespoon seasoned **rice vinegar**
- ⅛ teaspoon **salt**

1. Place the Brussels sprouts, sesame seeds, sesame oil, vinegar, and salt in a bowl and mix thoroughly.

2. Cover and let sit at room temperature for at least 15 minutes and up to 3 hours. Serve immediately or refrigerate and serve chilled.

PER SERVING:		
Calories: 88 Protein: 4 g Carbohydrate: 9 g Dietary Fiber: 4 g	Total Sugar: 2 g Total Fat: 5 g Saturated Fat: 0.7 g Total Omega-3 Fat: 100 mg	Cholesterol: 0 mg Calcium: 40 mg Sodium: 97 mg

PESCETARIAN PORTIONS: 1 vegetable serving;
1 fat serving (½ as nuts/seeds)

Brussels Sprouts, Pan Roasted

I should start keeping track of the number of people I've converted to Brussels sprouts with this simple dish! I think the reason for their change of heart (even happens to hardened Brussels sprout haters) is because this dish doesn't smell "sulfur-y," which can be an unpleasant side effect of cooking Brussels sprouts too long. So be very careful not to overcook!

SERVES: 4 • PREP TIME: 5 MINUTES • TOTAL TIME: 10 MINUTES

4 cups **Brussels sprouts**, halved
Canola oil cooking spray
¼ teaspoon **salt**
Freshly ground **black pepper** to taste

1. Heat a large heavy-bottomed skillet over medium-high heat.

2. Place the Brussels sprouts in a bowl, spray thoroughly with oil spray, and season with salt and pepper.

3. Spray the pan with oil and place the sprouts in the pan, cut side down; depending on the size of your pan, you may need to do this in a few batches. If the sprouts are small, cook until just browned, approximately 3 minutes, and remove from heat immediately. If the sprouts are large, flip to the other side for an additional 2 minutes. Take care not to overcook.

PER SERVING:		
Calories: 42	Total Sugar: 2 g	Cholesterol: 0 mg
Protein: 3 g	Total Fat: 1 g	Calcium: 37 mg
Carbohydrate: 8 g	Saturated Fat: 0.1 g	Sodium: 168 mg
Dietary Fiber: 3 g	Total Omega-3 Fat: 100 mg	

PESCETARIAN PORTIONS: 2 vegetable servings

Carrot and Cashew Soup

Traditional haute cuisine cream soups are just that: made from cream (and butter). Not here! Instead, healthy cashews are the key to the incredible texture and taste. Winter squash or pumpkin work well in lieu of carrots in this recipe. Just use already roasted squash or pumpkin, skip the first step, and start by blending vegetables with cashews and sage.

SERVES: 4 • PREP TIME: 10 MINUTES • TOTAL TIME: 20 MINUTES

3	cups peeled and roughly chopped **carrots**
¼	cup roughly chopped **cashews**
1	large leaf or 2 small **sage** leaves
¼	teaspoon **salt**
	Freshly ground **black pepper** to taste

1. In a large pot, place the carrots, cashews, and sage. Add 4 cups of water and bring to a boil. Reduce to a simmer and cook until the carrots are tender, approximately 7 minutes.

2. Place the carrot mixture in a high-speed blender and process until very smooth, 1 minute.

3. Before serving, reheat the soup and stir in salt and pepper. If the soup is too thick, add a few tablespoons of water.

PER SERVING:		
Calories: 87	Total Sugar: 5 g	Cholesterol: 0 mg
Protein: 2 g	Total Fat: 4 g	Calcium: 38 mg
Carbohydrate: 12 g	Saturated Fat: 0.7 g	Sodium: 213 mg
Dietary Fiber: 3 g	Total Omega-3 Fat: 0 mg	

PESCETARIAN PORTIONS: 1 vegetable serving; 1 fat serving (as nuts/seeds)

Cucumber with Fennel and Creamy Avocado Dressing

Cucumbers are a staple item in my fridge. I add them to salads, use them as a vehicle for spreads and dips, and have been known to bite into them whole as a snack between meals. The avocado dressing in this recipe turns an ordinary cucumber into something decadent-tasting, and it's great on nearly any raw vegetable or hardy green.

SERVES: 4 • PREP TIME: 10 MINUTES • TOTAL TIME: 10 MINUTES

2	cups sliced **cucumber** (taste the peel: if bitter, peel it; leave on if not)
1	large **fennel**, outer layer removed, quartered, cored, and thinly sliced against the grain
¼	teaspoon plus a dash **salt**
	Freshly ground **black pepper** to taste
½	medium **avocado**, peel and pit discarded
2	tablespoons fresh **lemon juice**
1	tablespoon finely chopped **chives**

1. In a large bowl, combine the cucumber and fennel, toss with ¼ teaspoon of salt and pepper, and set aside.

2. In a food processor, combine the avocado and lemon juice. Process until smooth, 20 seconds.

3. Add the avocado mixture to the cucumber mixture, combine thoroughly, add chives and a dash of salt, and serve immediately.

PER SERVING:		
Calories: 55	Total Sugar: 1 g	Cholesterol: 0 mg
Protein: 1 g	Total Fat: 3 g	Calcium: 40 mg
Carbohydrate: 8 g	Saturated Fat: 0.4 g	Sodium: 217 mg
Dietary Fiber: 3 g	Total Omega-3 Fat: 0 mg	

PESCETARIAN PORTIONS: 1 vegetable serving; ½ fat serving

Kale Salad with Sesame Dressing

This is probably the dish I make the most often. It works great as a side with pretty much anything. I use this same dressing on a variety of raw greens, such as collards and cabbage, but it is also great on cooked and chilled greens such as spinach and chard.

SERVES: 4 • PREP TIME: 10 MINUTES • TOTAL TIME: 10 MINUTES

2	tablespoons **tahini**
1	tablespoon **cider vinegar**
1	teaspoon **honey**
¼	teaspoon **salt**
	Freshly ground **black pepper** to taste
4	cups **kale**, very finely chopped and stem removed

1. In a large bowl, add the tahini, vinegar, honey, salt, pepper, and 1 tablespoon of water. Mix until smooth.

2. Add the kale, mix thoroughly with your hands, and serve immediately or cover and refrigerate until ready to serve.

PER SERVING:		
Calories: 84	Total Sugar: 1 g	Cholesterol: 0 mg
Protein: 4 g	Total Fat: 4 g	Calcium: 102 mg
Carbohydrate: 10 g	Saturated Fat: 0.6 g	Sodium: 177 mg
Dietary Fiber: 2 g	Total Omega-3 Fat: 151 mg	

PESCETARIAN PORTIONS: 1 vegetable serving; 1 fat serving (as nuts/seeds)

Kale Soup, Creamy and Quick

I like this easy-to-eat and easy-to-make soup as a start to a dinner, paired with a protein-rich salad for lunch or as a snack. Consider making a double batch and freezing individual portions. And look at the calcium—nearly twice as much as a cup of milk! (And Janis tells me that unlike spinach, the calcium in kale is very well absorbed.)

SERVES: 4 • PREP TIME: 10 MINUTES • TOTAL TIME: 15 MINUTES

4	cups **kale**, chopped and stem removed
1	cup thinly sliced **potato**
2	tablespoons chopped **onion**
4	cups **almond milk**
	Pinch of ground **nutmeg**
$\frac{1}{8}$	teaspoon **salt**
	Freshly ground **black pepper** to taste

1. In a medium pot, place the kale, potato, onion, milk, and nutmeg and bring to a boil, immediately reduce heat to a simmer, and cook for 10 minutes, stirring often.

2. Place the kale mixture in a high-speed blender. Process until very smooth, 1 minute.

3. Season with salt and pepper and serve hot.

PER SERVING:		
Calories: 109	Total Sugar: 7 g	Cholesterol: 0 mg
Protein: 7 g	Total Fat: 3 g	Calcium: 544 mg
Carbohydrate: 18 g	Saturated Fat: 0.1 g	Sodium: 255 mg
Dietary Fiber: 3 g	Total Omega-3 Fat: 100 mg	

PESCETARIAN PORTIONS: 1 vegetable serving; 1 dairy serving

Kale with Roasted Garlic

This simple oven-roasting method can be used with any green as well as most other vegetables. I wind up doing this practically every day, adjusting the cooking time according to the vegetable. I find that the best way to determine the cooking time is by tasting.

SERVES: 4 • PREP TIME: 5 MINUTES • TOTAL TIME: 15 MINUTES

8	cups **kale**, stems removed, leaves roughly chopped
4	roasted **garlic** cloves, chopped (see pantry)
2	teaspoons **extra-virgin olive oil**
	Red pepper flakes to taste
¼	teaspoon **salt**
	Freshly ground **black pepper** to taste

1. Preheat oven to 375°F.

2. Place the kale and roasted garlic on a sheet tray and toss thoroughly with oil. Season with red pepper flakes, salt, and pepper.

3. Cook until the edges are just starting to turn black, approximately 10 minutes. Let cool on pan; for crispy kale, serve as soon as possible.

PER SERVING:		
Calories: 91	Total Sugar: 0 g	Cholesterol: 0 mg
Protein: 5 g	Total Fat: 3 g	Calcium: 187 mg
Carbohydrate: 15 g	Saturated Fat: 0.4 g	Sodium: 204 mg
Dietary Fiber: 3 g	Total Omega-3 Fat: 300 mg	

PESCETARIAN PORTIONS: 2 vegetable servings; ½ fat serving

Mushrooms, Marinated

This is basically ceviche, lemony and refreshing. I like it on its own, but if the flavor is too intense for your taste, use it to top a piece of fish or tossed with salad greens, or reduce the lemon juice to 1 tablespoon.

SERVES: 4 • PREP TIME: 5 MINUTES • TOTAL TIME: 15 MINUTES

4 cups sliced **button mushrooms** (or other cultivated mushroom such as **cremini** or **portobello**)

2 tablespoons **lemon juice**

1 tablespoon finely chopped fresh **chives**

⅛ teaspoon **salt**

Freshly ground **black pepper** to taste

2 teaspoons **extra-virgin olive oil**

1. In a medium bowl, combine the mushrooms, lemon juice, chives, salt, and pepper.

2. Let sit at room temperature for 10 minutes. Drain out excess liquid, toss with olive oil, and serve immediately or cover, refrigerate, and serve chilled.

PER SERVING:		
Calories: 37	Total Sugar: 2 g	Cholesterol: 0 mg
Protein: 2 g	Total Fat: 2 g	Calcium: 6 mg
Carbohydrate: 3 g	Saturated Fat: 0.3 g	Sodium: 222 mg
Dietary Fiber: 1 g	Total Omega-3 Fat: 0 mg	

PESCETARIAN PORTIONS: 1 vegetable serving; ½ fat serving

Mushrooms, Oven Roasted with Green Onion and Thyme

Use this recipe with any mushroom variety. When I am lucky enough to get my hands on wild mushrooms, such as morels or chanterelles, this is my favorite way to prepare them. You can leave the mushrooms whole instead of slicing them, but the cooking time will increase.

SERVES: 4 • PREP TIME: 5 MINUTES • TOTAL TIME: 10 MINUTES

4	cups thinly sliced **mushrooms**, any variety
½	cup finely chopped **green onions**
1	tablespoon **thyme** leaves
¼	teaspoon **salt**
	Freshly ground **black pepper** to taste
	Canola oil cooking spray

1. Preheat oven to broil. Place the mushrooms, green onions, thyme, salt, and pepper on a sheet tray, spray with oil, and toss.

2. Place in the oven and cook until the edges are just starting to brown, approximately 5 minutes. Check the mushrooms often while cooking since the cooking time will vary depending on your oven. Serve hot or at room temperature.

PER SERVING:		
Calories: 24	Total Sugar: 2 g	Cholesterol: 0 mg
Protein: 2 g	Total Fat: 1 g	Calcium: 14 mg
Carbohydrate: 3 g	Saturated Fat: 0.1 g	Sodium: 151 mg
Dietary Fiber: 1 g	Total Omega-3 Fat: 0 mg	

PESCETARIAN PORTIONS: 1 vegetable serving

Seaweed Salad with Cucumber and Peanut Butter

Even if the idea of eating seaweed scares you, try this recipe! Its mild flavor will surprise you. And you're doing the oceans a favor—cultivating seaweed helps oxygenate and purify the water.

SERVES: 4 • PREP TIME: 10 MINUTES • TOTAL TIME: 10 MINUTES

1 cup **wakame** (about 1 ounce)

2 tablespoons **peanut butter**, no salt or sugar added

1 teaspoon **honey**

1 teaspoon **reduced-sodium soy sauce**

2 tablespoons **white vinegar**

2 cups sliced **cucumber**

1 cup grated **carrot**

½ **avocado**, diced, peel and pit discarded

1. Place the wakame in a bowl and cover with warm water, let soak for 5 minutes.

2. In a medium bowl, combine the peanut butter, honey, soy sauce, and vinegar.

3. Add the cucumber and carrot and toss with the peanut butter mixture.

4. Drain the wakame and add to the salad. Take care not to let the wakame sit too long or it will become mushy.

5. Mix thoroughly and top with the diced avocado.

PER SERVING:		
Calories: 109	Total Sugar: 4 g	Cholesterol: 0 mg
Protein: 3 g	Total Fat: 7 g	Calcium: 37 mg
Carbohydrate: 9 g	Saturated Fat: 1.0 g	Sodium: 163 mg
Dietary Fiber: 3 g	Total Omega-3 Fat: 100 mg	

PESCETARIAN PORTIONS: 1 vegetable serving; 1 fat serving (as nuts/seeds)

Spinach Salad with Poppy Seeds and Oranges

This classic combination of flavors goes perfectly with a simple piece of roasted fish and a whole-grain side. Citrus is at its best during colder months, so in the summer, substitute peaches or plums.

SERVES: 4 • PREP TIME: 15 MINUTES • TOTAL TIME: 15 MINUTES

4	oranges
2	tablespoons **poppy seeds**
1½	tablespoons **extra-virgin olive oil**
1	tablespoon freshly squeezed **orange juice**
1	tablespoon **sherry vinegar**
2	tablespoons very finely diced **red onion**
8	cups loosely packed **spinach**
¼	teaspoon **salt**
	Freshly ground **black pepper** to taste

1. With a sharp knife, peel the oranges, discarding all skin, including the white pith. Slice into thin wheels about ⅛-inch thick, set aside.

2. In a small bowl, combine the poppy seeds, olive oil, orange juice, and vinegar. Add onion and set aside.

3. Place the spinach and oranges in a large bowl. Dress with poppy seed mixture, season with salt and pepper, and serve immediately.

PER SERVING:		
Calories: 148	Total Sugar: 13 g	Cholesterol: 0 mg
Protein: 4 g	Total Fat: 7 g	Calcium: 177 mg
Carbohydrate: 20 g	Saturated Fat: 1.0 g	Sodium: 195 mg
Dietary Fiber: 5 g	Total Omega-3 Fat: 200 mg	

PESCETARIAN PORTIONS: 1 fruit serving; 2 vegetable servings;
1½ fat servings (½ as nuts/seeds)

Spinach with Olives and Preserved Lemons

This recipe uses two of the most important staples in my refrigerator: preserved lemons and roasted garlic. (Recipes for both are in the pantry section of this book, starting on page 267.) They're a great way to liven up fish or vegetable dishes, so use liberally!

SERVES: 4 • PREP TIME: 5 MINUTES (IF YOU HAVE LEMONS AND GARLIC PREPARED)
• TOTAL TIME: 5 MINUTES

  8 cups **spinach**

  1 tablespoon **extra-virgin olive oil**

1/2 cup **olives**, roughly chopped and pits removed

  3 tablespoons chopped **preserved lemons**
     (see pantry)

  2 finely chopped, **roasted garlic** cloves
     (see pantry)

1. Fill the bottom part of a steamer halfway with water and bring to a boil.

2. Place spinach in the top part of the steamer, cover and cook until just wilted, approximately 2 minutes. Take care not to overcook.

3. Place spinach in a large bowl, toss with olive oil, olives, lemons, and garlic. Serve immediately or cover, refrigerate, and serve chilled.

PER SERVING:		
Calories: 74	Total Sugar: 1 g	Cholesterol: 0 mg
Protein: 2 g	Total Fat: 5.711 g	Calcium: 83 mg
Carbohydrate: 6 g	Saturated Fat: 0.8 g	Sodium: 235 mg
Dietary Fiber: 2 g	Total Omega-3 Fat: 100 mg	

PESCETARIAN PORTIONS: 2 vegetable servings; 1½ fat servings

Summer Squash Salad with Lemon and Basil

With this side I suggest adding black pepper liberally. Pair the squash with a grilled whole fish, such as trout, or a steak-textured fish, such as mackerel or salmon.

SERVES: 4 • PREP TIME: 10 MINUTES • TOTAL TIME: 20 MINUTES

- 4 cups thinly sliced **summer squash (zucchini** or **yellow squash)**
- 2 tablespoons **lemon juice**
- 1 tablespoon **extra-virgin olive oil**
- ¼ cup roughly chopped fresh **basil**
- ⅛ teaspoon **salt**, plus a dash just before eating

  Freshly ground **black pepper** to taste

1. In a large bowl, combine squash, lemon juice, olive oil, basil, salt, and pepper.

2. Let sit at room temperature for 10 minutes and serve immediately or cover, refrigerate, and serve chilled.

3. Top with a dash of salt just before eating.

PER SERVING:		
Calories: 52	Total Sugar: 3 g	Cholesterol: 0 mg
Protein: 2 g	Total Fat: 4 g	Calcium: 28 mg
Carbohydrate: 4 g	Saturated Fat: 1.0 g	Sodium: 121 mg
Dietary Fiber: 1 g	Total Omega-3 Fat: 200 mg	

PESCETARIAN PORTIONS: 1 vegetable serving; 1 fat serving

Tomato, Peach, and Basil Salad

I've been making this salad for years and it's usually everyone's favorite dish of the meal no matter *what* I serve with it. Of course, starting with delicious, ripe, in-season tomatoes and peaches will always produce a better salad. If you can't snag the best produce, then let the salad marinate for at least 15 minutes at room temperature before serving.

SERVES: 4 • PREP TIME: 10 MINUTES • TOTAL TIME: 10 MINUTES

2	medium **tomatoes,** core removed and diced
2	medium **peaches,** pits removed and diced
¼	cup roughly chopped fresh **basil**
1	tablespoon **extra-virgin olive oil**
1	tablespoon **sherry vinegar**
¼	teaspoon **salt**
	Freshly ground **black pepper** to taste

1. In a large bowl combine tomatoes, peaches, basil, olive oil, vinegar, salt, and pepper.

2. Serve immediately.

PER SERVING:		
Calories: 72	Total Sugar: 8 g	Cholesterol: 0 mg
Protein: 1 g	Total Fat: 4 g	Calcium: 21 mg
Carbohydrate: 10 g	Saturated Fat: 0.5 g	Sodium: 149 mg
Dietary Fiber: 2 g	Total Omega-3 Fat: 0 mg	

PESCETARIAN PORTIONS: ½ fruit serving;
½ vegetable serving; 1 fat serving

Tomato Roasted with Garlic

I can't decide if I prefer this dish hot or cold—I really enjoy it either way. Decide for yourself by making a double batch, eating half hot out of the oven and refrigerate the remainder to enjoy cold the second day. Either way it will complement any simply prepared fish.

SERVES: 4 • PREP TIME: 10 MINUTES • TOTAL TIME: 25 MINUTES

4 medium **tomatoes,** cut in half, cored, and stemmed

2 teaspoons **extra-virgin olive oil**

1½ teaspoons finely chopped **sage**

1 tablespoon finely chopped fresh **garlic**

¼ teaspoon **salt**

Freshly ground **black pepper** to taste

1. Preheat oven to 425°F.

2. Place tomatoes on a sheet tray and rub with olive oil, sage, garlic, salt, and pepper.

3. Cook until skin blisters, approximately 15 minutes. Remove from the oven, let cool a little, then peel off the skin (it should come off easily).

4. Serve hot, cold, or at room temperature.

PER SERVING:		
Calories: 46	Total Sugar: 3 g	Cholesterol: 0 mg
Protein: 1 g	Total Fat: 3 g	Calcium: 21 mg
Carbohydrate: 6 g	Saturated Fat: 0.4 g	Sodium: 152 mg
Dietary Fiber: 2 g	Total Omega-3 Fat: 0 mg	

PESCETARIAN PORTIONS: 1 vegetable serving; ½ fat serving

GRAIN AND STARCHY
VEGETABLE SIDES

Black Rice with Sesame and Green Onions

I find that black rice is fun to serve to company because most people are unfamiliar with it. It's also called "forbidden rice" because in ancient China it was served only to the emperor and was considered off-limits to the general public. Pair this dish with a piece of roasted fish and a green vegetable for an easy everyday meal that's also elegant enough for entertaining.

SERVES: 2 • PREP TIME: 5 MINUTES • TOTAL TIME: 1 HOUR

1   cup **black rice**
2   tablespoons very finely chopped **green onion**
1   cup finely chopped **cilantro**
2   tablespoons **sesame seeds**
½   tablespoon **sesame oil**
½   tablespoon **rice vinegar** (sodium-free or "unseasoned")
⅛   teaspoon plus a dash of **salt**

1.   Place rice and 1¾ cups of water in a pot and bring to a boil, reduce heat to simmer, cover, and cook for 45 minutes. Turn off heat and let pot sit covered for an additional 10 minutes.

2.   Place rice in a bowl, fluff with a fork, add green onion, cilantro, sesame seeds, sesame oil, vinegar, and ⅛ teaspoon of salt. Mix thoroughly and serve immediately or cover, refrigerate, and serve chilled. Season with a dash of salt just before eating.

PER SERVING:		
Calories: 195	Total Sugar: 0 g	Cholesterol: 0 mg
Protein: 5 g	Total Fat: 6 g	Calcium: 7 mg
Carbohydrate: 34 g	Saturated Fat: 0.6 g	Sodium: 116 mg
Dietary Fiber: 4 g	Total Omega-3 Fat: 16 mg	

PESCETARIAN PORTIONS: 2 grain/starchy vegetable servings;
1 fat serving (½ as nuts/seeds)

Corn Salad

Make this only with tender fresh corn—preferably corn that's just been picked! That way you don't even have to cook it. That means you'll be serving this in the summer. (But surprisingly, while testing this recipe in the winter, I found decent fresh corn in a Washington, D.C., grocery store!) Feel free to toss this with arugula, cabbage, and additional fresh herbs such as chives, basil, or chervil.

SERVES: 4 • PREP TIME: 10 MINUTES • TOTAL TIME: 10 MINUTES

2 cups tender, sweet fresh **corn**, cut off the cob
1 cup finely chopped **parsley**
1 cup diced **cucumber**
1 tablespoon freshly squeezed **lime juice**
1 tablespoon **extra-virgin olive oil**
⅛ teaspoon **salt**
Freshly ground **black pepper** to taste

1. In a large bowl, thoroughly combine corn, parsley, cucumber, lime, olive oil, salt, and pepper.

2. Serve immediately or cover, refrigerate, and serve chilled.

PER SERVING:		
Calories: 106	Total Sugar: 3 g	Cholesterol: 0 mg
Protein: 3 g	Total Fat: 4 g	Calcium: 27 mg
Carbohydrate: 17 g	Saturated Fat: 0.6 g	Sodium: 93 mg
Dietary Fiber: 3 g	Total Omega-3 Fat: 0 mg	

PESCETARIAN PORTIONS: ½ grain/starchy vegetable serving;
½ vegetable serving; 1 fat serving

Cracked Wheat with Golden Raisins and Pistachios

This side is a natural at lunch or dinner, but it would also make a delicious breakfast with an egg or roasted fish fillet.

SERVES: 4 • PREP TIME: 10 MINUTES • TOTAL TIME: 20 MINUTES

1	cup **cracked wheat**
¼	cup **golden raisins**
½	cup chopped **pistachios**
1	tablespoon **extra-virgin olive oil**
1	cup chopped **parsley**
2	tablespoons freshly squeezed **lemon juice**
⅛	teaspoon **salt**
	Small pinch of **cayenne pepper**

1. In a large bowl, place cracked wheat and golden raisins, add 1 cup boiling water, cover with plastic wrap and let sit for 10 minutes.

2. Add pistachios, olive oil, parsley, lemon juice, salt, and cayenne. Serve immediately, chilled, or warm gently in the oven.

PER SERVING:		
Calories: 197	Total Sugar: 8 g	Cholesterol: 0 mg
Protein: 6 g	Total Fat: 11 g	Calcium: 49 mg
Carbohydrate: 23 g	Saturated Fat: 1.0 g	Sodium: 134 mg
Dietary Fiber: 5 g	Total Omega-3 Fat: 100 mg	

PESCETARIAN PORTIONS: ½ fruit serving; 1 grain/starchy vegetable serving; 3 fat servings (2 as nuts/seeds)

Oatmeal Onion Cake

The texture of oatmeal combined with the flavors of olive oil, oregano, and onion makes for a surprisingly rich-tasting side that pairs with any fish.

SERVES: 4 • PREP TIME: 10 MINUTES • TOTAL TIME: 25 MINUTES

1   cup **oatmeal**

2   tablespoons shredded **onions**

1   tablespoon chopped fresh **oregano**

1   teaspoon **extra-virgin olive oil**

¼   teaspoon **salt**

     Freshly ground **black pepper** to taste

     Canola oil cooking spray

1. Place 1¾ cups of water in a pot and bring to a boil. Add oatmeal, onions, and oregano, reduce to a simmer, and cook, stirring often, for 5 minutes. When the oats are finished cooking, stir in the olive oil and salt and pepper.

2. Coat a 9-inch pie plate with canola oil cooking spray. Pour the oats onto the plate and let sit until cool. Slice into 4 wedges.

3. Heat a heavy-bottomed skillet over medium heat. Coat the skillet with oil cooking spray, place oat cakes in skillet, and cook until they are browned on each side, approximately 3 minutes per side.

PER SERVING:		
Calories: 92	Total Sugar: 0 g	Cholesterol: 0 mg
Protein: 3 g	Total Fat: 3 g	Calcium: 24 mg
Carbohydrate: 15 g	Saturated Fat: 0.4 g	Sodium: 147 mg
Dietary Fiber: 2 g	Total Omega-3 Fat: 0 mg	

PESCETARIAN PORTIONS: 2 grain/starchy vegetable servings

Potato and Celery Root Mashed with Basil

The addition of celery root and basil results in a light but flavorful version of this traditional comfort food. You can turn it into a rich and creamy soup by adding water and puréeing in a high-speed blender.

SERVES: 4 • PREP TIME: 5 MINUTES • TOTAL TIME: 30 MINUTES

2	medium **potatoes**
2	cups peeled and cubed **celery root**
1	tablespoon **extra-virgin olive oil**
1/8	teaspoon plus a dash of **salt**
	Freshly ground **black pepper** to taste
1/2	cup roughly chopped **basil**

1. In a large pot, place potatoes and celery root and cover with water. Place on the stove over high heat and bring to a boil. Reduce heat to a rolling simmer and cook until potatoes and celery root are both tender, approximately 20 minutes.

2. Drain thoroughly and, using a wooden spoon, mash with the olive oil, salt, pepper, and basil. Serve hot and season with a dash of salt just before eating.

PER SERVING:		
Calories: 138	Total Sugar: 3 g	Cholesterol: 0 mg
Protein: 3 g	Total Fat: 4 g	Calcium: 50 mg
Carbohydrate: 24 g	Saturated Fat: 0.6 g	Sodium: 209 mg
Dietary Fiber: 3 g	Total Omega-3 Fat: 100 mg	

PESCETARIAN PORTIONS: 1 grain/starchy vegetable servings;
1/2 vegetable serving; 1 fat serving

Quinoa with Lemon, Olive Oil, and Pomegranate

Every year I come back to this dish when pomegranates are in season. The pairing of pomegranate and quinoa is one of my all-time favorite combinations.

SERVES: 4 • PREP TIME: 10 MINUTES • TOTAL TIME: 20 MINUTES

1	cup **quinoa**
½	cup chopped **mint**
1	cup chopped **parsley**
2	tablespoons fresh **lemon juice**
1	tablespoon **extra-virgin olive oil**
½	cup **pomegranate seeds** (use chopped **orange** sections if not available)
¼	teaspoon **salt**
	Freshly ground **black pepper** to taste

1. Rinse quinoa twice. Place quinoa in a pot and cover with water. Bring to a boil, reduce to a simmer, and cook for 5 minutes. Drain quinoa, rinse with cold water, and drain thoroughly.

2. Place quinoa in a large bowl and stir in the mint, parsley, lemon juice, olive oil, pomegranate, salt, and pepper. Serve immediately or cover with plastic wrap, refrigerate, and serve chilled.

PER SERVING:		
Calories: 207	Total Sugar: 2 g	Cholesterol: 0 mg
Protein: 7 g	Total Fat: 6 g	Calcium: 65 mg
Carbohydrate: 32 g	Saturated Fat: 0.8 g	Sodium: 160 mg
Dietary Fiber: 5 g	Total Omega-3 Fat: 200 mg	

PESCETARIAN PORTIONS: ¼ fruit serving; 1½ grain/starchy vegetable servings; 1 fat serving

Red Lentils with Lime and Cilantro

While red lentils and seared scallops are a classic combination, during recipe testing I subbed in roasted haddock and a green salad—delicious! I always have red lentils in my pantry and use them often—what other legume cooks from raw in less than 5 minutes?

SERVES: 4 · PREP TIME: 5 MINUTES · TOTAL TIME: 15 MINUTES

1	cup **red lentils**
2	tablespoons freshly squeezed **lime juice**
1	tablespoon **extra-virgin olive oil**
1/4	cup finely chopped **cilantro**
1/8	teaspoon plus dash of **salt**
	Freshly ground **black pepper** to taste

1. Place red lentils in a pot and cover with water. Bring to a boil and immediately reduce heat to a simmer. Stir the lentils to ensure that they cook evenly.

2. Cook lentils until just soft, approximately 3 minutes. Take care not to overcook because they will fall apart.

3. Drain lentils and rinse with cold water.

4. Place in a large bowl and gently toss with the lime juice, olive oil, cilantro, salt, and pepper.

5. Serve at room temperature or chilled. Season with a dash of salt just before eating.

PER SERVING:		
Calories: 202	Total Sugar: 1 g	Cholesterol: 0 mg
Protein: 13 g	Total Fat: 4 g	Calcium: 22 mg
Carbohydrate: 29 g	Saturated Fat: 0.5 g	Sodium: 117 mg
Dietary Fiber: 7 g	Total Omega-3 Fat: 0 mg	

PESCETARIAN PORTIONS: 2 grain/starchy vegetable servings; 1 fat serving

Sweet Potato Gratin

I'm always amazed at the depth of flavor in a well-roasted sweet potato. This dish works well with or without the cheese.

SERVES: 4 • PREP TIME: 5 MINUTES • TOTAL TIME: 25 MINUTES

    2   medium **sweet potatoes,** very thinly sliced
    2   teaspoons **extra-virgin olive oil**
  ¼   teaspoon **salt**
        Freshly ground **black pepper** to taste
    2   tablespoons grated **Parmesan cheese**

1.   Preheat oven to 375°F. Place sweet potatoes on a sheet tray and toss with olive oil, salt, and pepper.

2.   Roast until the potatoes are soft, 5 to 15 minutes depending on the thickness of the potatoes.

3.   Arrange sweet potatoes, slightly overlapping each other, in a 9-inch oven-proof skillet.

4.   Top with Parmesan cheese. Turn oven to broil and cook until deep golden brown. This will take 2 to 5 minutes depending on the strength of your broiler and the distance the food is from the flame.

PER SERVING:		
Calories: 86	Total Sugar: 3 g	Cholesterol: 2 mg
Protein: 2 g	Total Fat: 3 g	Calcium: 47 mg
Carbohydrate: 13 g	Saturated Fat: 0.8 g	Sodium: 219 mg
Dietary Fiber: 2 g	Total Omega-3 Fat: 0 mg	

PESCETARIAN PORTIONS: 1 grain/starchy vegetable serving; ½ fat serving

Whole-Grain Couscous with Rice Vinegar and Herbs

As with other couscous recipes in this book, you can use either the large pearl whole-grain couscous or the finer grain.

SERVES: 4 • PREP TIME: 5 MINUTES • TOTAL TIME: 15 MINUTES

1	cup **whole-grain couscous** (such as **whole-wheat** or **brown rice**)
2	tablespoons seasoned **rice vinegar**
2	tablespoons very finely chopped **chives**
¼	cup roughly chopped **basil**
1	tablespoon **extra-virgin olive oil**
	Freshly ground **black pepper** to taste

1. Prepare couscous according to package directions.

2. Place couscous in a large bowl and stir in vinegar, chives, basil, olive oil, and pepper. Serve immediately or cover, refrigerate, and serve chilled.

PER SERVING:		
Calories: 144	Total Sugar: 4 g	Cholesterol: 0 mg
Protein: 4 g	Total Fat: 4 g	Calcium: 15 mg
Carbohydrate: 24 g	Saturated Fat: 0.4 g	Sodium: 287 mg
Dietary Fiber: 3 g	Total Omega-3 Fat: 0 mg	

PESCETARIAN PORTIONS: 2 grain/starchy vegetable servings; 1 fat serving

Whole-Wheat Bread with Seeds and Nuts

Making bread takes time and patience, but it is well worth it! After much experimenting, I came up with this recipe that uses 100 percent whole-wheat flour.

SERVES: 8 • PREP TIME: 15 MINUTES • TOTAL TIME: 2 HOURS

3/4	cups warm **water**
1½	tablespoons fresh **compressed yeast** (can substitute 1 tablespoon **active dry yeast**)
2	tablespoons **extra-virgin olive oil**
2	tablespoons **molasses, maple syrup, honey,** or **sorghum syrup**
2	tablespoons **cracked wheat,** soaked for in 3 tablespoons boiling **water** for 10 minutes
2	tablespoons **sunflower seeds**
¼	cup cooked **wheat berries**
2	tablespoons chopped **walnuts**
2	cups plus stone-ground **whole-wheat flour**
½	teaspoon **salt**

1. In a large bowl combine water and yeast.

2. Add oil, molasses (or other sweetener), soaked cracked wheat, sunflower seeds, wheat berries, walnuts, 1 cup flour, and salt. Mix until thoroughly combined.

3. Add remaining flour and knead until smooth, add a little more flour if the dough is sticky.

4. Lightly coat a clean bowl with olive oil, place dough in bowl, and cover with a damp cloth.

5. Let dough sit in a warm spot until it doubles, approximately 40 minutes. Shape into a loaf and place in an oiled loaf pan.

6. Preheat oven to 375°F.

7. Put loaf in a warm place, cover with a towel, and let rise until it doubles, approximately 30 minutes.

8. Bake until top is browned and loaves sound hollow when tapped, approximately 30 minutes.

PER SERVING:		
Calories: 187	Total Sugar: 3 g	Cholesterol: 0 mg
Protein: 5 g	Total Fat: 7 g	Calcium: 26 mg
Carbohydrate: 29 g	Saturated Fat: 0.8 g	Sodium: 149 mg
Dietary Fiber: 4 g	Total Omega-3 Fat: 200 mg	

PESCETARIAN PORTIONS: 1½ grain/starchy vegetable servings;
1½ fat servings (½ as nuts/seeds)

VEGETABLE PROTEIN
MAIN DISHES

Black-Eyed Pea Stew

This soup is a favorite of mine—and not just because it's brimming with superfoods. It freezes beautifully, so you might consider making a double batch and storing a few portions for another day. Feel free to substitute mustard greens, chard, or another green for the kale or cracked wheat or a different whole grain for the barley.

SERVES: 4 • PREP TIME: 10 MINUTES • TOTAL TIME: 55 MINUTES (IF USING ALREADY COOKED BEANS)

	Canola oil cooking spray
1	medium **onion**, sliced
2	teaspoons **garlic**, minced
3/4	cup **barley**
1	cup finely chopped **sun-dried tomatoes** (not packed in oil)
1	tablespoon finely chopped fresh **oregano**
	Freshly ground **black pepper** to taste
	Red pepper flakes to taste
2	tablespoons **balsamic vinegar**
1	bunch **kale**, stems removed and roughly chopped
3	cups cooked **black-eyed peas**, dry (see pantry) or canned (preferably no salt added or low sodium), rinsed and drained
1/2	teaspoon **salt**

1. Heat a heavy-bottomed stock pot over medium heat. Spray with oil and add the onion and garlic. Cook until the onions are translucent, stirring often, 5 minutes.

2. Add 8 cups of water, barley, tomatoes, oregano, pepper, red pepper flakes, and balsamic vinegar. Bring to a boil. Reduce heat and simmer until barley is soft, approximately 30 minutes.

3. Add kale and peas and cook an additional 10 minutes. Serve immediately or cover, refrigerate, and reheat before serving.

PER SERVING:		
Calories: 365	Total Sugar: 12 g	Cholesterol: 0 mg
Protein: 19 g	Total Fat: 3 g	Calcium: 172 mg
Carbohydrate: 72 g	Saturated Fat: 0.5 g	Sodium: 366 mg
Dietary Fiber: 18 g	Total Omega-3 Fat: 300 mg	

PESCETARIAN PORTIONS: 3 grain/starchy vegetable servings;
1½ vegetable servings

Cabbage Stuffed with Tofu, Walnuts, Cracked Wheat, and Raisins in a Sweet and Sour Tomato Sauce

This dish is so hearty, satisfying, tasty—and family-friendly—that people will be surprised to find out it's vegan. This recipe is more involved and time-consuming than most in this book, but it's not difficult and is well worth it. You can prepare it up to two days in advance and then heat when ready to serve.

SERVES: 4 • PREP TIME: 15 MINUTES • TOTAL TIME: 50 MINUTES (IF USING ALREADY COOKED BEANS)

- 4 **tomatoes**, core removed and chopped
- 1 **onion**, finely chopped
- 1 tablespoon **cider vinegar**
- 1 tablespoon **honey**
- ⅛ teaspoon **cinnamon**
- ½ cup **cracked wheat**
- 1 14-ounce package firm **tofu**, thoroughly drained and crumbled
- ½ cup cooked **garbanzo beans**, dry (see pantry) or canned, no salt added, rinsed and drained
- ¼ cup **raisins**
- ¼ cup **pine nuts**
- ¼ teaspoon **salt**
  Freshly ground **black pepper** to taste
  Canola oil cooking spray
- 8 large **napa cabbage leaves**

1. Preheat oven to 375°F.

2. In a medium pot, combine the tomatoes, onion, vinegar, honey, and cinnamon. Bring to a simmer and let cook for 10 minutes.

3. While the tomatoes are cooking, place the cracked wheat in a large bowl and cover with ½ cup of boiling water. Cover with plastic wrap and let sit for at least 10 minutes.

4. Once the tomato mixture is cooked, place in a high-speed blender and process until smooth, 1 minute; set aside.

5. Once the cracked wheat has hydrated, add the tofu, garbanzo beans, raisins, pine nuts, salt, and pepper and mix thoroughly.

6. Place cabbage leaves on a sheet tray with 2 tablespoons of water. Place in oven until slightly softened, 3 minutes.

7. Lightly coat an oven-proof baking dish with canola oil cooking spray.

8. To stuff the leaves, place a leaf on a flat surface and place ⅛ of the cracked wheat mixture on the lower half of the leaf. Fold in the sides of the leaf and roll so that the filling is encased in the leaf.

9. Place the stuffed leaves in the baking dish, seam side down. Cover the leaves with the tomato sauce. Cook for 20 minutes and serve hot.

PER SERVING:		
Calories: 290	Total Sugar: 14 g	Cholesterol: 0 mg
Protein: 15 g	Total Fat: 11 g	Calcium: 281 mg
Carbohydrate: 38 g	Saturated Fat: 1.0 g	Sodium: 197 mg
Dietary Fiber: 7.14 g	Total Omega-3 Fat: 200 mg	

PESCETARIAN PORTIONS: 1 fruit serving; 1 grain/starchy vegetable serving; 2 vegetable servings; 1 fat serving (as nuts/seeds); 1 protein serving

Eggplant Stuffed with Lentils

This is such a great dish for entertaining, as you can make it in advance. If you are lucky enough to have any left over, I suggest eating it cold for lunch. It keeps for a few days tightly wrapped in the refrigerator.

SERVES: 4 • PREP TIME: 10 MINUTES • TOTAL TIME: 1 HOUR AND 5 MINUTES (IF USING ALREADY COOKED RICE)

1½	cups **green lentils**
2	medium **eggplants**
1	**onion**, sliced
2	teaspoons finely chopped **garlic**
1	tablespoon finely chopped **sage**
½	cup cooked **brown rice** (can substitute **cracked wheat**)
1	tablespoon **extra-virgin olive oil**
¾	teaspoon **salt**
	Freshly ground **black pepper** to taste
	Canola oil cooking spray
½	cup fresh **pomegranate seeds** (can substitute **currants**)
½	cup plain nonfat **Greek yogurt** or **vegan yogurt**

1. Place the lentils in a pot, cover with water, bring to a boil, reduce to a simmer, and cook until tender, 10 minutes. Drain the lentils and place in a food processor.

2. While the lentils are cooking, gut the eggplant by cutting them in half, scooping out the inside with a spoon, leaving the skin—with about a half inch of flesh—intact. Roughly chop the scooped-out flesh, and reserve.

3. Preheat oven to 375°F.

4. Add to the lentils in the food processor the onion, garlic, sage, the inside of the eggplant, rice, oil, salt, and pepper. Pulse on and off about 12 times until the lentil mixture is thoroughly combined, able to stick together but still has some texture.

5. Lightly spray an oven-proof baking dish with canola oil. Also spray the scooped-out eggplants with canola oil. Stuff the eggplant halves with the lentil mixture. Place stuffed side up in the baking dish and cook uncovered for 45 minutes.

6. Serve hot or chilled, topped with pomegranate seeds and yogurt.

PER SERVING:		
Calories: 410	Total Sugar: 12 g	Cholesterol: 0 mg
Protein: 25 g	Total Fat: 5 g	Calcium: 113 mg
Carbohydrate: 69 g	Saturated Fat: 0.7 g	Sodium: 460 mg
Dietary Fiber: 31 g	Total Omega-3 Fat: 100 mg	

PESCETARIAN PORTIONS: 3½ grain/starchy vegetable servings;
3 vegetable servings; 1 fat serving

Shiitake Quick Broth with Edamame and Brown Rice Noodles

This soup is fast, which makes it one of my go-to meals when I come in hungry from a long day. If you can find whole-grain Asian-style noodles, use them, but if not, any whole-grain noodle will do.

SERVES: 4 • PREP TIME: 10 MINUTES • TOTAL TIME: 35 MINUTES

- ½ pound **brown rice noodles**, Asian-style if available, cooked according to package directions
- 1 tablespoon **sesame oil**
- 8 medium **shiitake mushrooms**, stems removed and set aside, tops thinly sliced
- 1 tablespoon peeled and roughly chopped fresh **ginger**
- 2 peeled **garlic** cloves
- 1 medium **potato**, cut into about 8 pieces
- ½ teaspoon **salt**
- 3 tablespoons **wakame**
- 2⅔ cups frozen peeled **edamame**, cooked according to package directions
- 4 tablespoons **sesame seeds**, toasted
- ¼ cup thinly sliced **green onions**
- ¼ cup chopped **cilantro**

1. In a bowl, combine the noodles and sesame oil.

2. In a medium pot, place the shiitake stems, ginger, garlic, potato, and 5 cups of water. Bring to a boil, reduce to a simmer, and cook for 15 minutes.

3. Strain the broth and discard the vegetables.

4. Return the broth to the pot, add the salt and wakame, and heat thoroughly.

5. Add the shiitake slices and edamame, sesame, green onions, and cilantro. Serve immediately.

PER SERVING:		
Calories: 468	Total Sugar: 4 g	Cholesterol: 0 mg
Protein: 15 g	Total Fat: 14 g	Calcium: 106 mg
Carbohydrate: 74 g	Saturated Fat: 1.9 g	Sodium: 347 mg
Dietary Fiber: 8 g	Total Omega-3 Fat: 800 mg	

PESCETARIAN PORTIONS: 3 grain/starchy vegetable servings;
½ vegetable serving; 2 fat servings (1 as nuts/seeds); 2 protein servings

Tofu Sloppy Joe

This easy-to-love comfort food appeals to eaters of all ages.

**SERVES: 4 • PREP TIME: 10 MINUTES • TOTAL TIME: 20 MINUTES
(IF USING ALREADY COOKED BEANS)**

	Canola oil cooking spray
1	**onion**, finely chopped
1	large **sweet red pepper**, seeds removed and finely chopped
1	14-ounce container of firm **tofu**, thoroughly drained and crumbled
1½	cups chopped **tomato**
2	cups cooked **kidney beans** from dried (see pantry) or canned no salt, rinsed and drained
¼	cup **cider vinegar**
¼	teaspoon ground **cloves**
¼	teaspoon **cinnamon**
¼	teaspoon **mustard powder**
1½	teaspoons **brown sugar**
½	teaspoon **salt**
	Freshly ground **black pepper** to taste
	Cayenne pepper to taste
4	**whole-wheat hamburger buns**

1. Heat a large skillet over medium heat and coat with oil spray. Add the onion and sweet pepper. Cook for 3 minutes, stirring often.

2. Crumble in the tofu and cook, stirring often until browned, approximately 5 minutes.

3. Stir in the tomato, beans, vinegar, cloves, cinnamon, mustard powder, brown sugar, salt, pepper, and cayenne. Bring to a simmer and cook for 10 minutes.

4. Divide the mixture evenly across the 4 rolls and serve.

PER SERVING:		
Calories: 426	Total Sugar: 3 g	Cholesterol: 0 mg
Protein: 14 g	Total Fat: 14 g	Calcium: 99 mg
Carbohydrate: 64 g	Saturated Fat: 1.9 g	Sodium: 344 mg
Dietary Fiber: 8 g	Total Omega-3 Fat: 800 mg	

PESCETARIAN PORTIONS: 3 grain/starchy vegetable servings;
1 vegetable serving; 1 protein serving

Veggie Burger

I tried—and rejected—lots of recipes before hitting upon this favorite! It's especially delicious when cooked on an outdoor grill.

SERVES: 4 • PREP TIME: 10 MINUTES • TOTAL TIME: 25 MINUTES (IF USING ALREADY COOKED RICE AND BEANS)

2	cups cooked **black rice** (see pantry); can substitute **brown rice**
2½	cups cooked **white beans**, dry (see pantry) or canned, no salt added, rinsed and drained
¼	cup finely chopped **onion**
¾	cup **corn** kernels
½	cup shredded **carrot**
½	teaspoon **salt**
	Freshly ground **black pepper** to taste
	Canola oil cooking spray

1. Place about ¾ of the black rice, ¾ of the white beans, and ¾ of the onion in a food processor and process until smooth.

2. Place the mixture in a large bowl and mix in the remaining black rice, beans, and onion as well as the corn, carrot, salt, and pepper.

3. Form into four burgers.

4. Heat a heavy-bottomed skillet over medium heat, spray with oil, and cook the burgers, turning once until browned on both sides, approximately 7 minutes per side. Serve hot.

PER SERVING:		
Calories: 293	Total Sugar: 3 g	Cholesterol: 0 mg
Protein: 15 g	Total Fat: 1 g	Calcium: 110 mg
Carbohydrate: 58 g	Saturated Fat: 0.2 g	Sodium: 313 mg
Dietary Fiber: 10 g	Total Omega-3 Fat: 100 mg	

PESCETARIAN PORTIONS: 3 grain/starchy vegetable servings

Veggie Meatballs over Whole-Grain Spaghetti

If you have beautiful tomatoes available, you can save yourself some steps. Instead of making the sauce (steps 1 and 2), simply chop three tomatoes, toss with a teaspoon of olive oil, ⅛ teaspoon of salt, and freshly ground black pepper. Then pick the recipe back up at step 3.

SERVES: 4 • PREP TIME: 15 MINUTES • TOTAL TIME: 45 MINUTES

3	cups chopped **tomatoes,** fresh or canned
2	teaspoons **extra-virgin olive oil**
1	teaspoon **honey**
1	**onion,** finely chopped
2	teaspoons minced **garlic**
½	teaspoon **salt**
	Freshly ground **black pepper** to taste
1	**carrot,** peeled and grated
¼	teaspoon chopped fresh **oregano**
1	large **egg**
½	cup **whole-wheat bread crumbs**
⅓	cup **walnuts,** ground
¼	cup fresh **parsley,** chopped
1	tablespoon **Dijon mustard**
1	pound firm **tofu,** pressed (weighted with heavy pan to squeeze out water)
½	pound **whole-wheat spaghetti** (or other **whole-grain pasta**), cooked according to package directions
¼	cup grated **Parmesan cheese** (optional)

1. In a high-speed blender, combine the tomatoes, 1 teaspoon of olive oil, honey, half of the onion, 1 teaspoon garlic, ¼ teaspoon of salt, and black pepper. Blend until smooth, 30 seconds.

2. Place the tomato mixture in a pot, add ½ cup of water, and cook at a simmer for 25 minutes; set aside.

3. Heat a heavy-bottomed skillet over low heat and add ½ teaspoon of olive oil, the other half of the onion, the carrot, ¼ teaspoon of salt, pepper,

1 teaspoon of garlic, and oregano. Cook, stirring often until tender, 10 minutes.

4. In a large bowl, lightly beat the egg, then add bread crumbs, walnuts, parsley, and mustard.

5. Crumble the pressed tofu with your hands and add it to the bowl along with the sautéed vegetables. Mix well.

6. Preheat oven to 350°F. Form tofu mixture into 12 balls and place on an oiled baking sheet.

7. Bake until crisp and brown on the outside, approximately 30 minutes.

8. While meatballs are cooking, mix the pasta into the tomato sauce. To serve, divide the pasta into four portions, top each with hot meatballs and Parmesan cheese if desired.

PER SERVING:		
Calories: 476	Total Sugar: 12 g	Cholesterol: 51 mg
Protein: 25 g	Total Fat: 16 g	Calcium: 412 mg
Carbohydrate: 67 g	Saturated Fat: 3.2 g	Sodium: 508 mg
Dietary Fiber: 5 g	Total Omega-3 Fat: 900 mg	

PESCETARIAN PORTIONS: 3 grain/starchy vegetable servings;
½ vegetable serving; 2 fat servings (1½ as nuts/seeds); 2 protein servings

Whole-Wheat Couscous with Root Vegetables and Garbanzo Beans

This dish is all about the steamer. Feel free to substitute the best available produce. Just take care to adjust the cooking time—if necessary—because some vegetables cook more quickly than the root vegetables in this dish.

SERVES: 4 • PREP TIME: 10 MINUTES • TOTAL TIME: 25 MINUTES

¼	cup plus 1 tablespoon **tahini**
½	teaspoon minced **garlic**
2	tablespoons **lemon juice**
1	cup **whole-wheat couscous**
¼	cup toasted **pistachio nuts**
1	teaspoon **turmeric**
1	teaspoon **cumin**
	Cayenne pepper to taste
¾	teaspoon **cinnamon**
1	tablespoon plus 1 teaspoon **extra-virgin olive oil**
¼	teaspoon **salt**
	Freshly ground **black pepper** to taste
1	**onion**, peeled and cut into 8 wedges
1	medium **sweet potato**, cut in half the long way and each half cut into 4 long strips
2	medium **carrots**, peeled, cut in half the long way and each half cut into 2 long strips
1	medium **turnip**, peeled and cut into 8 wedges
4	cups **spinach**
1	cup cooked **garbanzo beans**, dry (see pantry) or canned, no salt added, rinsed and drained

1. Place the tahini, garlic, lemon juice, and ¼ cup plus 1 tablespoon of water in a food processor. Process until smooth and set aside.

2. Cook couscous according to package directions. Place couscous in a bowl and add the pistachios, turmeric, cumin, cayenne, cinnamon, 1 tablespoon of olive oil, an ⅛ teaspoon of salt, and black pepper. Combine thoroughly.

3. Fill the bottom part of a steamer halfway with water and bring to a simmer.

4. Place the onion, sweet potato, carrot, and turnip in a basket above the water, cover, and cook until tender, approximately 12 minutes. Add spinach and garbanzo beans and steam for an additional 2 minutes.

5. Remove vegetables from steamer, place in a large bowl, and season with 1 teaspoon of olive oil, ⅛ teaspoon of salt, and pepper.

6. To serve, divide the couscous onto 4 plates, top with vegetables and tahini sauce.

PER SERVING:		
Calories: 494	Total Sugar: 8 g	Cholesterol: 0 mg
Protein: 17 g	Total Fat: 19 g	Calcium: 158 mg
Carbohydrate: 70 g	Saturated Fat: 2.5 g	Sodium: 529 mg
Dietary Fiber: 11 g	Total Omega-3 Fat: 183 mg	

PESCETARIAN PORTIONS: 3 grain/starchy vegetable servings;
2 vegetable servings; 4½ fat servings (3½ as nuts/seeds)

Whole-Grain Pasta Baked with White Beans, Spinach, and Walnut Sauce

This a very rich and creamy pasta dish, thanks in large part to the walnuts. This one-dish meal definitely won't leave you feeling deprived!

SERVES: 4 • PREP TIME: 10 MINUTES • TOTAL TIME: 30 MINUTES

½	cup chopped **walnuts**
1	tablespoon finely chopped **onion**
1	tablespoon **extra-virgin olive oil**
1	teaspoon finely chopped **oregano**
¼	cup plus teaspoon **salt**
	Freshly ground **black pepper** to taste
½	pound dry **whole-grain penne** (or other shaped pasta)
2	cups cooked **white beans,** dry (see pantry) or canned, no salt added, rinsed and drained
8	cups **spinach**
	Canola oil cooking spray
½	cup tightly packed **whole-grain bread crumbs**

1. Preheat oven to 375°F.

2. Cook pasta according to package directions.

3. While pasta is cooking, place the walnuts, onion, 2 teaspoons of olive oil, oregano, salt, pepper, and ½ cup of water in a blender. Process until smooth, 1 minute.

4. In a large bowl, combine the walnut mixture, cooked pasta, white beans, and spinach.

5. Spray a large heavy-bottomed skillet with canola oil. Place the pasta mixture in the skillet. Place bread crumbs in a small bowl and toss with 1 teaspoon of olive oil.

6. Top pasta with bread crumbs and bake until top is browned, approximately 20 minutes.

PER SERVING:		
Calories: 508	Total Sugar: 2 g	Cholesterol: 0 mg
Protein: 23 g	Total Fat: 15 g	Calcium: 198 mg
Carbohydrate: 77 g	Saturated Fat: 1.8 g	Sodium: 341 mg
Dietary Fiber: 9 g	Total Omega-3 Fat: 1,500 mg	

PESCETARIAN PORTIONS: 3 grain/starchy vegetable servings;
2 vegetable servings; 3 fat servings (2 as nuts/seeds)

FISH/SEAFOOD
MAIN DISHES

~~~

Cornmeal Crusted Catfish with Cucumbers

Although catfish is the traditional choice in the South, haddock or flounder works just as well. For an ultra-comfort food meal, pair it with the Oatmeal Onion Cake (page 188) and lighten things up by serving it with an arugula salad.

SERVES: 4 • PREP TIME: 10 MINUTES • TOTAL TIME: 20 MINUTES

- 4 cups sliced **cucumbers**
- ¼ teaspoon **salt**, divided
  Freshly ground **black pepper** to taste
- 2 tablespoons finely diced **red onion**
- 1 tablespoon **red wine vinegar**
- 1 tablespoon **extra-virgin olive oil**
  Pinch of **cayenne pepper**
- 1 pound U.S. farm-raised **catfish**
- 1 tablespoon **grainy mustard**, store-bought or homemade (see pantry)
- ¼ cup **cornmeal**

1. Place the cucumbers in a large bowl and toss with ⅛ teaspoon of salt and pepper. Add the red onion, red wine vinegar, 2 teaspoons of olive oil, and cayenne, combine thoroughly, and set aside.

2. Season both sides of the fish with remaining ⅛ teaspoon of salt and black pepper. Paint 1 side of the fish with a thin layer of grainy mustard and then coat with cornmeal.

3. Heat a large heavy-bottomed skillet over medium heat. Coat with the remaining teaspoon of olive oil. Cook the fish until the crust is golden brown, approximately 2 minutes, flip fish, and cook until just flaky, 3 additional minutes.

4. Serve topped with the cucumber mixture.

PER SERVING:		
Calories: 191 Protein: 18 g Carbohydrate: 5 g Dietary Fiber: 1 g	Total Sugar: 2 g Total Fat: 10 g Saturated Fat: 2.0 g Total Omega-3 Fat: 300 mg	Cholesterol: 62 mg Calcium: 27 mg Sodium: 373 mg

PESCETARIAN PORTIONS: 1 vegetable serving; 1 fat serving; 2 protein servings

Clams with Tomatoes and Garlic on Whole-Grain Pasta

This simple version of a classic dish is quick and a real crowd-pleaser. It's just as delicious with mussels instead of clams.

SERVES: 4 • PREP TIME: 10 MINUTES • TOTAL TIME: 25 MINUTES

Canola oil cooking spray

1 **onion**, sliced

1 teaspoon minced **garlic**, or to taste

½ teaspoon **salt**

3 pounds of **clams**, in shell, thoroughly scrubbed

1 teaspoon **red pepper flakes**

1 cup **white wine**

½ pound **whole-grain linguine**, cooked according to package directions

½ cup chopped **flat-leaf parsley**

4 cups halved **cherry tomatoes**

1. Heat a large pot with lid over low heat.

2. Spray with vegetable oil cooking spray and add the onion, garlic, and salt. Cook for 3 minutes, stirring constantly.

3. Add the clams, red pepper flakes, and wine.

4. Cover and simmer until the clams open, approximately 7 minutes. Discard those clams that do not open.

5. Add the pasta, parsley, and tomatoes. Cover and let simmer for an additional 3 minutes. Stir and serve immediately.

PER SERVING:		
Calories: 325	Total Sugar: 6 g	Cholesterol: 17 mg
Protein: 17 g	Total Fat: 2 g	Calcium: 89 mg
Carbohydrate: 56 g	Saturated Fat: 0.3 g	Sodium: 341 mg
Dietary Fiber: 3 g	Total Omega-3 Fat: 100 mg	

PESCETARIAN PORTIONS: 2 grain/starchy vegetable servings;
1 vegetable serving; 1 protein serving

Cod Burger

Any meaty white fish such as haddock or tilapia will work in this burger, as well as canned salmon. If you can't get your hands on a good piece of fresh fish, frozen thawed fish is fine here. During recipe testing, we paired it with the Beet Slaw (page 166)—a combo I highly recommend!

SERVES: 4 · PREP TIME: 10 MINUTES · TOTAL TIME: 25 MINUTES

⅓	cup **cracked wheat**
1½	pounds **cod**
1	teaspoon **lemon juice**
	Canola oil cooking spray
1½	cups cooked **white beans**, dry or canned, no salt added, rinsed and drained
½	cup chopped **parsley**
½	teaspoon **salt**
	Freshly ground **black pepper** to taste
2	teaspoons **olive oil**

1.   Place the cracked wheat in a bowl, cover with ⅓ cup of boiling water. Let sit until water is absorbed, 10 minutes.

2.   Preheat oven to 375°F.

3.   Place the cod on a baking dish, coat with lemon juice and vegetable oil cooking spray. Cook until the fish is just beginning to flake but the center is still translucent, approximately 7 minutes.

4.   While the fish is cooking, purée the white beans in a blender or food processor.

5.   Remove the fish from oven, let cool, and flake into a large bowl.

6.   Add the beans, parsley, cracked wheat, salt, and pepper and mix with your hands.

7.   Form into 4 burgers. Heat a heavy-bottomed skillet over medium heat.

8.   Coat the bottom of the pan with olive oil. Cook the burgers until browned on each side, approximately 4 minutes per side.

9.   Serve hot.

PER SERVING:

Calories: 295	Total Sugar: 1 g	Cholesterol: 73 mg
Protein: 39 g	Total Fat: 4 g	Calcium: 102 mg
Carbohydrate: 26 g	Saturated Fat: 0.7 g	Sodium: 391 mg
Dietary Fiber: 6 g	Total Omega-3 Fat: 400 mg	

PESCETARIAN PORTIONS: 1½ grain/starchy vegetable servings;
½ fat serving; 3 protein servings

Cod, Cauliflower, and Pea Curry

This curry is just as delicious with scallops or shrimp instead of cod. I suggest pairing it with brown rice and the Red Lentil salad (page 191).

SERVES: 4 • PREP TIME: 15 MINUTES • TOTAL TIME: 40 MINUTES

1 tablespoon **extra-virgin olive oil**

1 **onion**, sliced

1 teaspoon **cumin**

1 teaspoon **mustard powder**

½ teaspoon **turmeric**

1 tablespoon minced fresh **ginger**

1 teaspoon minced **garlic**

½ teaspoon **salt**

Freshly ground **black pepper**

Pinch of **cayenne**, or to taste

2 cups chopped **tomatoes**

2 tablespoons finely chopped **cilantro**

1 medium head **cauliflower**, broken into small florets, approximately half-inch pieces

1 pound **cod**, cut into cubes, about half an inch each

2 cups fresh or frozen **peas**

4 cups **spinach**

1. Heat a large heavy-bottomed stock pot over low heat. Add the olive oil and onion and cook until translucent, stirring often, 5 minutes. Add the cumin, mustard powder, turmeric, ginger, garlic, salt, black pepper, and cayenne. Cook for 1 more minute, stirring constantly.

2. Add the tomatoes, cilantro, and 4½ cups of water. Bring to a boil, reduce to a simmer, and cook for 10 minutes.

3. Add the cauliflower; return to a simmer and cook for 2 minutes.

4. Add the cod, peas, and spinach; stir and cover. Simmer for 4 minutes and serve immediately.

PER SERVING:		
Calories: 261 Protein: 29 g Carbohydrate: 27 g Dietary Fiber: 10 g	Total Sugar: 11 g Total Fat: 5 g Saturated Fat: 0.8 g Total Omega-3 Fat: 400 mg	Cholesterol: 49 mg Calcium: 123 mg Sodium: 430 mg

PESCETARIAN PORTIONS: 1 grain/starchy vegetable serving;
3 vegetable servings; 1 fat serving; 2 protein servings

Flounder Baked with Grapes and Almonds

Quick, easy, and elegant, this pairs perfectly with a side of whole-wheat couscous (although any whole grain would be a good complement).

SERVES: 4 • PREP TIME: 10 MINUTES • TOTAL TIME: 20 MINUTES

1	pound **flounder fillet**
1	tablespoon **extra-virgin olive oil**
¼	teaspoon **salt**
	Freshly ground **black pepper** to taste
1	cup halved **red grapes**
1	cup chopped and toasted **almonds**
2	tablespoons finely chopped **parsley**
1	tablespoon **lemon juice**

1. Preheat oven to 375°F. Place fish on a sheet tray and season with 1½ teaspoons of olive oil, ⅛ teaspoon of salt, and freshly ground black pepper.

2. In a bowl, combine the grapes, almonds, parsley, lemon juice, 1½ teaspoons of olive oil, ⅛ teaspoon of salt, and black pepper.

3. Place the fish in the oven and bake for 3 minutes, flip the fish, return to the oven until the fish is just beginning to flake but the center is still translucent, approximately 3 minutes. Take care not to overcook.

4. Remove from oven and serve immediately, topped with grape mixture.

PER SERVING:		
Calories: 298	Total Sugar: 7 g	Cholesterol: 54 mg
Protein: 27 g	Total Fat: 17 g	Calcium: 90 mg
Carbohydrate: 13 g	Saturated Fat: 1.7 g	Sodium: 239 mg
Dietary Fiber: 3 g	Total Omega-3 Fat: 300 mg	

PESCETARIAN PORTIONS: ½ fruit serving; 1 grain/starchy vegetable serving; 5 fat servings (4 as nuts/seeds); 2 protein servings

Haddock Tacos

Fun to eat and fun to make, this recipe will work well with any white fish.

SERVES: 4 • PREP TIME: 20 MINUTES • TOTAL TIME: 30 MINUTES

¼	cup freshly squeezed **lime juice**
1	tablespoon **white vinegar**
4	dashes **salt**
1	fresh **jalapeño pepper**, chopped finely
2	tablespoons **extra-virgin olive oil**
1½	pounds **haddock** or other **white fish**
1	cup shredded **cabbage**
1	**avocado**, peel and pit discarded, cubed
½	cup chopped fresh **cilantro**
1	**tomato**, diced
	Canola oil cooking spray
8	6-inch **corn tortillas**

1. In a bowl, combine 2 tablespoons of lime juice, vinegar, 2 dashes of salt, jalapeño, and 1 tablespoon of olive oil.

2. Place the fish on a flat plate and pour the lime juice mixture over the fish and let sit for 20 minutes.

3. While the fish is marinating, in a medium bowl, combine the cabbage, avocado, cilantro, tomato, the remaining 2 tablespoons of lime juice, the remaining 2 dashes of salt, and 1 tablespoon of olive oil. Set aside.

4. Heat a heavy-bottomed skillet over medium heat, spray with canola oil, and place the haddock in the pan.

5. Cook for 3 minutes, flip and cook until the fish is just beginning to flake but the center is still translucent, approximately 3 minutes.

6. To assemble, fill each tortilla with fish and cabbage.

PER SERVING:		
Calories: 365	Total Sugar: 2 g	Cholesterol: 92 mg
Protein: 32 g	Total Fat: 14 g	Calcium: 76 mg
Carbohydrate: 28 g	Saturated Fat: 2.1 g	Sodium: 548 mg
Dietary Fiber: 6 g	Total Omega-3 Fat: 400 mg	

PESCETARIAN PORTIONS: 1½ grain/starchy vegetable servings;
½ vegetable serving; 3 fat servings; 3 protein servings

Mackerel with Sweet Potatoes, Collard Greens, and Okra

This recipe calls for a grill, but if you don't have one—no problem! Just cook the fish under the broiler. Preheat, place the fish in an oven-proof pan a few inches under the heat source and cook 3 to 5 minutes depending on your broiler and the thickness of the fish. The fish is done when it is just beginning to flake but the center is still translucent.

SERVES: 4 • PREP TIME: 10 MINUTES • TOTAL TIME: 30 MINUTES

- 2 cups diced **sweet potatoes**
- 2 cups sliced **okra**
- ½ cup diced **onion**
- 2 teaspoons **extra-virgin olive oil**
- ¼ teaspoon **salt**
  Freshly ground **black pepper** to taste
- 2 cups thinly sliced **collard greens**
- 1 tablespoon **cider vinegar**
- 1 pound **mackerel** (not king mackerel), skin removed, cut into 4 portions

1. Preheat oven to 375°F. Light a grill (gas, wood, or coal) and bring to a medium-high cooking temperature. If you do not have a grill, see broiling instructions above.

2. Place the sweet potatoes, okra, and onion on a sheet tray and toss with 1 teaspoon of olive oil. Season with ⅛ teaspoon of salt and black pepper. Place in the oven and cook for 10 minutes.

3. Add the collard greens to the sweet potato mixture and stir thoroughly. Cook for an additional 5 minutes. Remove from the oven, toss with cider vinegar, and cover to keep warm until ready to serve.

4. Season the mackerel with 1 teaspoon of olive oil, ⅛ teaspoon of salt, and black pepper. Place on the grill until you can see grill marks, approximately 3 minutes, flip and grill for another 3 minutes.

5. Serve the mackerel on the sweet potato mixture.

PER SERVING:		
Calories: 339	Total Sugar: 4 g	Cholesterol: 79 mg
Protein: 24 g	Total Fat: 18 g	Calcium: 105 mg
Carbohydrate: 20 g	Saturated Fat: 4.0 g	Sodium: 293 mg
Dietary Fiber: 5 g	Total Omega-3 Fat: 3,100 mg	

PESCETARIAN PORTIONS: 1 grain/starchy vegetable serving;
1 vegetable serving; ½ fat serving; 4 protein servings

Salmon Salad

Although I tested this with canned salmon, it would, of course, be terrific with leftover cooked salmon! Using canned with bones makes this salad high in calcium; don't worry, the bones are so soft you barely feel them.

SERVES: 1 • PREP TIME: 5 MINUTES • TOTAL TIME: 5 MINUTES

¼ **avocado**, peel and pit discarded

1 tablespoon **lemon juice**

2 teaspoons **extra-virgin olive oil**

1 teaspoon **Dijon mustard**

Dash of **salt**

Freshly ground **black pepper** to taste

4 ounces canned **wild salmon**, with bones, no salt added

2 tablespoons sliced **celery**

2 tablespoons finely chopped **parsley**

1. In a medium bowl, combine the avocado, lemon juice, olive oil, mustard, salt, and pepper. Mash the avocado with the back of a fork and combine thoroughly with the other ingredients.

2. Flake the salmon and add it to the avocado mixture. Add the celery and parsley and serve immediately.

PER SERVING:		
Calories: 312	Total Sugar: 1 g	Cholesterol: 62 mg
Protein: 24 g	Total Fat: 22 g	Calcium: 265 mg
Carbohydrate: 5 g	Saturated Fat: 3.7 g	Sodium: 364 mg
Dietary Fiber: 3 g	Total Omega-3 Fat: 2,100 mg	

PESCETARIAN PORTIONS: 2 fat servings; 4 protein servings

Salmon Seared with Fennel, Mushroom, and Sweet Red Pepper

This very versatile recipe works well with many types of fish, including arctic char, catfish, haddock, scallops, tilapia, and trout. If you have fresh basil available, add a generous amount before serving.

SERVES: 4 • PREP TIME: 5 MINUTES • TOTAL TIME: 30 MINUTES

2	bulbs **fennel**, sliced
1	**onion**, sliced
1	**sweet red pepper**, seeds removed and sliced
2	cups sliced **white mushrooms**
1	tablespoon **extra-virgin olive oil**
¼	teaspoon **salt**
	Freshly ground **black pepper** to taste
1	pound **wild salmon**, fresh or frozen

1. Place the fennel, onion, sweet pepper, and mushrooms in a pot and toss with 1½ teaspoons of olive oil, ⅛ teaspoon of salt, and black pepper. Turn heat on low and cook, stirring often until vegetables are soft, approximately 20 minutes.

2. When the vegetables are nearly done, heat a heavy-bottomed skillet over medium heat.

3. Season the fish with 1½ teaspoons of olive oil, ⅛ teaspoon of salt, and black pepper. Place the fish in the hot pan and cook until browned, approximately 3 minutes, turn fish, and continue cooking until the fish is a little pink in the middle, 2 to 3 additional minutes depending on the thickness of the fish.

4. Serve the salmon immediately with the fennel mixture.

PER SERVING:		
Calories: 275	Total Sugar: 6 g	Cholesterol: 51 mg
Protein: 28 g	Total Fat: 11 g	Calcium: 118 mg
Carbohydrate: 18 g	Saturated Fat: 1.9 g	Sodium: 268 mg
Dietary Fiber: 5 g	Total Omega-3 Fat: 1,700 mg	

PESCETARIAN PORTIONS:

1½ vegetable servings; 1 fat serving; 4 protein servings

Salmon with Tahini and Toasted Nuts

Janis told me about this Middle Eastern dish from her childhood, and she was very happy with my interpretation! Traditionally it's made with white fish—you can sub in haddock or flounder.

SERVES: 4 • PREP TIME: 10 MINUTES • TOTAL TIME: 15 MINUTES

- ¼ cup **tahini**
- 3 tablespoons fresh **lemon juice**
- 1 teaspoon mashed **garlic**
- ¼ teaspoon **salt**
- ½ cup finely chopped **cilantro**
- 2 tablespoons roughly chopped toasted **walnuts**
- 2 tablespoons roughly chopped toasted **almonds**
- 1 tablespoon finely chopped **onion**
- 1 teaspoon **extra-virgin olive oil**
- Pinch of **cayenne**, or to taste
- Freshly ground **black pepper** to taste
- 1 pound **wild salmon** skin removed, fresh or frozen

1. In a bowl, combine the tahini, 2 tablespoons of lemon juice, 3 tablespoons of water, mashed garlic, and ⅛ teaspoon of salt; set aside.

2. In a separate bowl, combine the cilantro, walnuts, almonds, onion, olive oil, cayenne, black pepper, and ⅛ teaspoon of salt.

3. Fill the bottom of a steamer with water and bring to a boil.

4. Season fish with 1 tablespoon of lemon juice, place on a plate, and put it in the top of the steamer. Cover and cook, taking care to remove while fish is still pink inside, 3 to 4 minutes.

5. Remove the fish from steamer, top with the tahini mixture and then with the cilantro mixture.

6. Serve warm or at room temperature.

PER SERVING:		
Calories: 311	Total Sugar: 1 g	Cholesterol: 51 mg
Protein: 29 g	Total Fat: 20 g	Calcium: 78 mg
Carbohydrate: 6 g	Saturated Fat: 3.0 g	Sodium: 204 mg
Dietary Fiber: 1 g	Total Omega-3 Fat: 2,100 mg	

PESCETARIAN PORTIONS: 3 fat servings (3 as nuts/seeds);
4 protein servings

Sardines, Broiled with Green Onion on Arugula

When I was testing this dish, the comment I got most often was, "I had no idea I liked sardines." This is a beautiful and quick dish; pair it with the quinoa salad (page 190) for a memorable meal.

SERVES: 4 • PREP TIME: 5 MINUTES • TOTAL TIME: 10 MINUTES

¼ cup pitted **black olives**

1 teaspoon **sherry vinegar**

1 tablespoon **extra-virgin olive oil**

Freshly ground **black pepper** to taste

1 pound fresh **sardines**, scaled and gutted

2 **green onions**, green ends trimmed and cut in half long ways

1 **lemon**, cut into thin round slices

1 teaspoon **minced garlic**

6 cups **arugula**

1. Set oven to broil.

2. Place the olives, vinegar, 1 teaspoon of olive oil, pepper, and 1 tablespoon of water in a food processor or blender and process until smooth, 30 seconds; set aside.

3. Fill the sardines with the green onions and lemon slices.

4. Rub the outside of the fish with the minced garlic and 2 teaspoons of olive oil.

5. Place the sardines on a sheet tray and place under the broiler until the skin is browned and crispy, 3 to 5 minutes depending on the strength of your broiler and how close the fish is to the flame.

6. While the fish is cooking, place the arugula in a large bowl and toss with the olive mixture. Transfer the arugula to a serving dish.

7. Remove the fish from the oven, place on the arugula, and serve immediately.

PER SERVING:		
Calories: 188	Total Sugar: 1 g	Cholesterol: 128 mg
Protein: 25 g	Total Fat: 15 g	Calcium: 160 mg
Carbohydrate: 4 g	Saturated Fat: 2.0 g	Sodium: 220 mg
Dietary Fiber: 1 g	Total Omega-3 Fat: 1,500 mg	

PESCETARIAN PORTIONS: 1½ vegetable servings;
1 fat serving; 3 protein servings

Sardine Niçoise

The sardines in this elegant salad can be substituted with any leftover cooked, chilled, and flaked fish. And if you can find haricot verts, the more delicate, tender form of green beans, give them a try.

SERVES: 4 • PREP TIME: 10 MINUTES • TOTAL TIME: 20 MINUTES

¼	cup **lemon juice**
2	teaspoons **Dijon mustard**
1	tablespoon **extra-virgin olive oil**
¼	cup finely chopped **red onion**
	Dash of **salt**
	Freshly ground **black pepper** to taste
4	small **eggs**
½	pound **red potatoes**, cut into quarter-inch rounds
1	pound **green beans**, ends trimmed
4	cups **baby arugula**, **spinach**, or **Bibb lettuce**
2	tablespoons chopped **flat-leaf parsley**
1	**tomato**, chopped
3	3.75-ounce cans **sardines**, packed in water, preferably no salt added, drained

1. In a small bowl, combine the lemon juice, mustard, olive oil, red onion, salt, and black pepper. Set the dressing aside.

2. Bring 2 medium pots of water to a boil. Add the eggs to one pot and cook at a gentle boil for 5 minutes. Cool with running cold water.

3. Add the potatoes to the second pot and cook until tender, approximately 5 minutes. Using a slotted spoon, remove and then drain, pat dry, and set aside.

4. Add the beans to the boiling potato water, cook for 30 seconds, drain, run under cold water, and set aside.

5. Peel the eggs, cut in half, and set aside.

6. Toss the greens and parsley and arrange on four individual plates. Arrange the potatoes, beans, tomato, and sardines on top of the greens. Use a

spoon to drizzle the dressing over the salad, taking care to coat each of the ingredients.

7. Serve immediately, garnished with the eggs. Just before eating, sprinkle with a dash of salt.

PER SERVING:		
Calories: 256	Total Sugar: 7 g	Cholesterol: 213 mg
Protein: 22 g	Total Fat: 10 g	Calcium: 298 mg
Carbohydrate: 22 g	Saturated Fat: 2.5 g	Sodium: 306 mg
Dietary Fiber: 5 g	Total Omega-3 Fat: 1,000 mg	

PESCETARIAN PORTIONS: ½ grain/starchy vegetable serving; 3 vegetable servings; 1 fat serving; 2½ protein servings

Scallop Corn Chowder with Leeks

This chowder is also delicious with shrimp in lieu of the scallops.

SERVES: 4 • PREP TIME: 5 MINUTES • TOTAL TIME: 20 MINUTES

	Canola oil cooking spray
1½	cups sliced **leeks**
4	cups **almond milk** or **skim milk**
1	teaspoon chopped fresh **thyme**
3	cups **corn**, cut off the cob or frozen
1½	pounds **bay scallops**
⅛	teaspoon **salt**
	Freshly ground **black pepper** to taste

1. Heat a heavy-bottomed stock pot over medium heat.

2. Coat the stock pot with cooking spray and add the leeks. Cook, stirring often until the leeks are soft, 5 minutes.

3. Add the milk and thyme. Heat until the soup is just beginning to simmer, 5 minutes, stirring frequently.

4. Add the corn, scallops, salt, and pepper. Return to a simmer, let cook for 2 additional minutes, and serve immediately.

PER SERVING:		
Calories: 330	Total Sugar: 17 g	Cholesterol: 46 mg
Protein: 33 g	Total Fat: 3 g	Calcium: 545 mg
Carbohydrate: 45 g	Saturated Fat: 0.8 g	Sodium: 892 mg
Dietary Fiber: 4 g	Total Omega-3 Fat: 300 mg	

PESCETARIAN PORTIONS: 1 grain/starchy vegetable serving; 1 dairy serving;
½ vegetable serving; 2 protein servings

Seafood Stew

My guests have been known to pick up the bowl and slurp down every last drop of this wonderfully flavorful stew. No need to limit yourself to the seafood on this ingredient list; you can substitute anything good and fresh. The Potato and Celery Root Mashed with Basil (page 189) makes a perfect pairing.

SERVES: 4 • PREP TIME: 10 MINUTES • TOTAL TIME: 25 MINUTES

2	teaspoons **extra-virgin olive oil**
1	cup finely chopped **shallots**
1	bulb **fennel**, sliced
2	stalks **celery**, chopped
2	cups **white wine**
1	tablespoon chopped fresh **thyme**
6	ounces **shrimp**, fresh or frozen, peeled and deveined
6	ounces **sea scallops**, each cut into two equal circles
6	ounces **arctic char**, cut into 1-inch pieces
¼	teaspoon **salt**
	Freshly ground **black pepper** to taste
1	cup chopped curly **parsley**

1. Heat a large heavy-bottomed skillet over low heat. Coat the hot pan with olive oil and add the shallots, fennel, and celery. Cook, stirring often until soft, 5 minutes.

2. Add the wine, 2 cups of water, and thyme.

3. Bring to a boil, reduce to a simmer, and cook for 10 minutes.

4. Add the shrimp, scallops, and arctic char. Return to a simmer and cook for 1 minute.

5. Stir in salt, pepper, and parsley and serve immediately.

PER SERVING:		
Calories: 310	Total Sugar: 4 g	Cholesterol: 77 mg
Protein: 21 g	Total Fat: 4 g	Calcium: 102 mg
Carbohydrate: 15 g	Saturated Fat: 0.9 g	Sodium: 540 mg
Dietary Fiber: 4 g	Total Omega-3 Fat: 381 mg	

PESCETARIAN PORTIONS: 1 vegetable serving; ½ fat serving;
3 protein servings

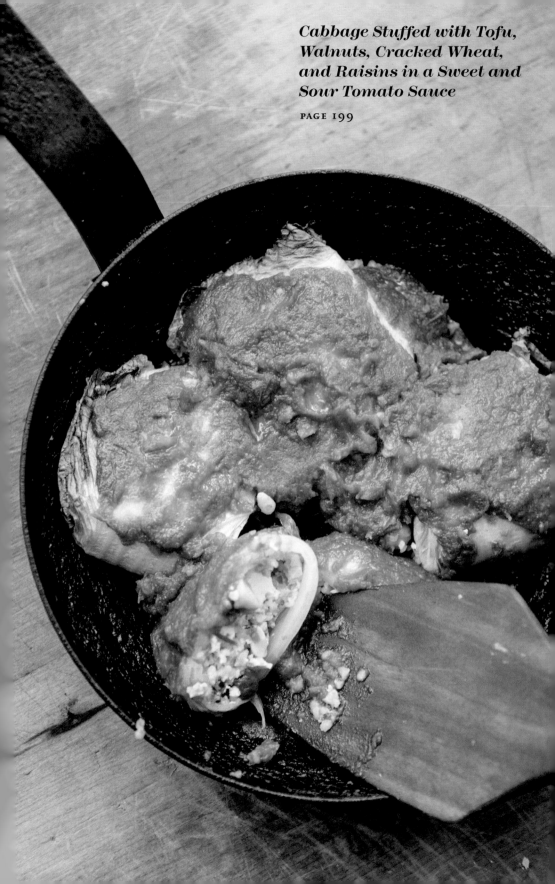

Cabbage Stuffed with Tofu,
Walnuts, Cracked Wheat,
and Raisins in a Sweet and
Sour Tomato Sauce

PAGE 199

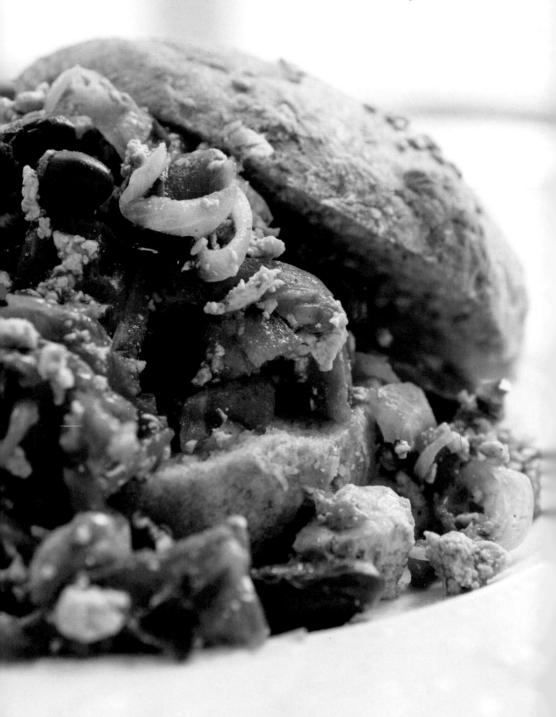

Tofu Sloppy Joe

PAGE 205

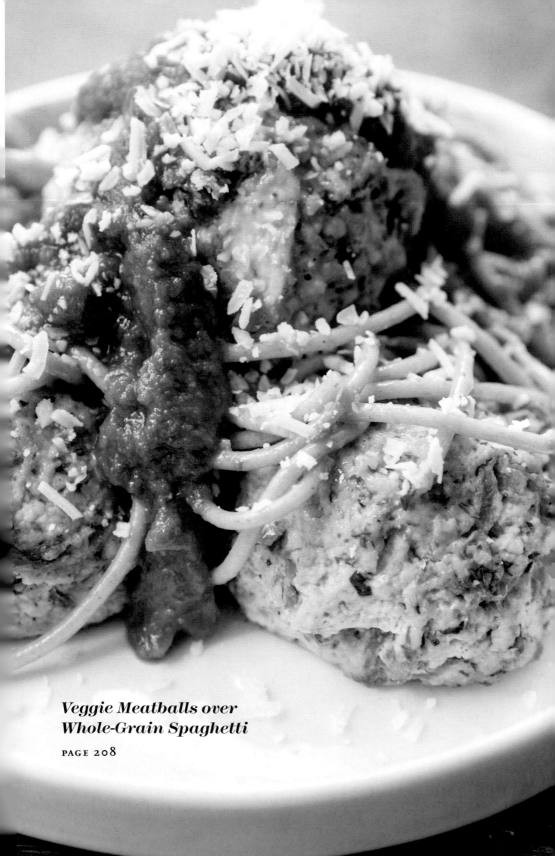

Veggie Meatballs over Whole-Grain Spaghetti

PAGE 208

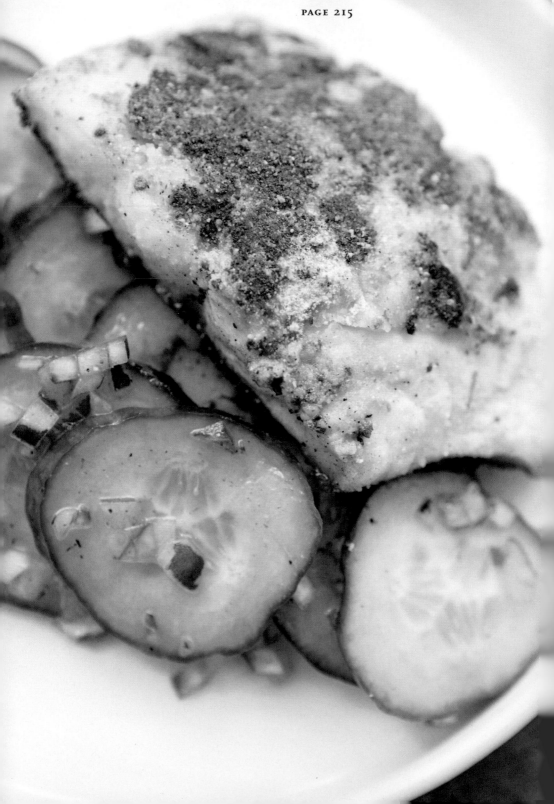

Cornmeal Crusted
Catfish with Cucumbers

PAGE 215

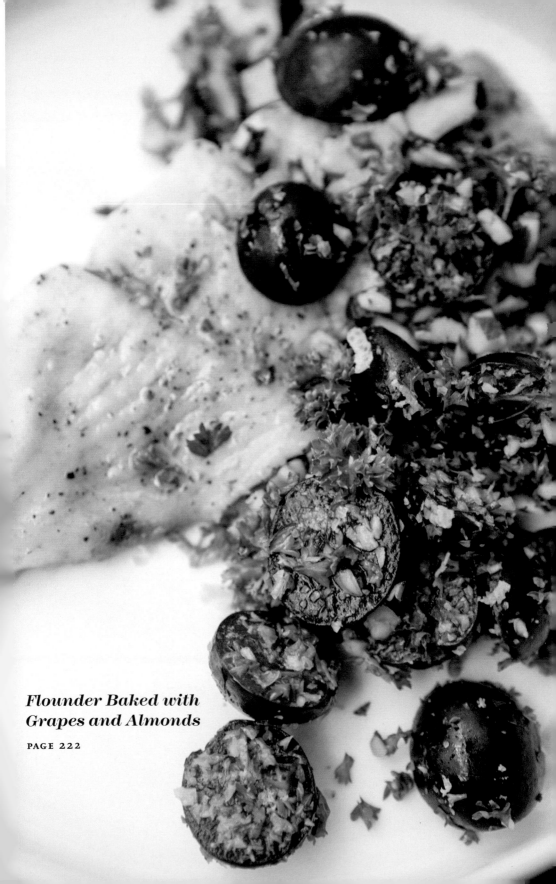

*Flounder Baked with
Grapes and Almonds*

PAGE 222

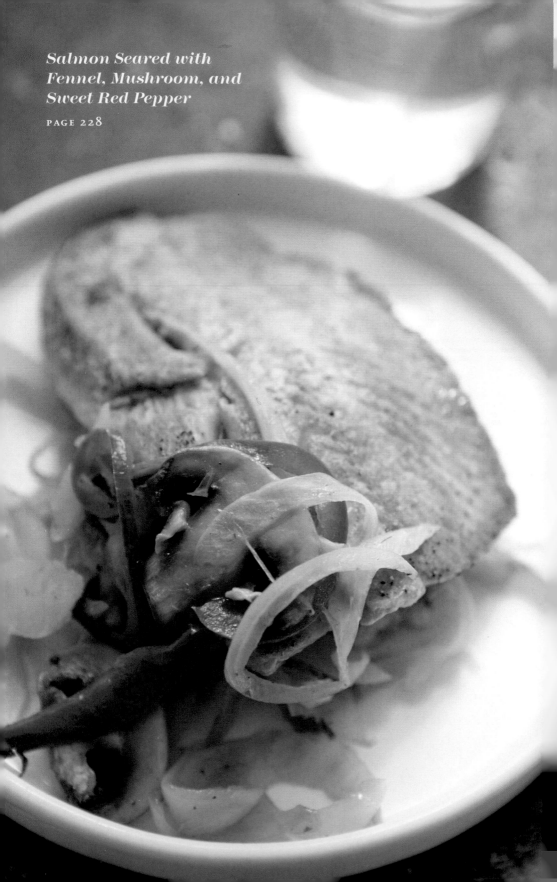

Salmon Seared with Fennel, Mushroom, and Sweet Red Pepper

PAGE 228

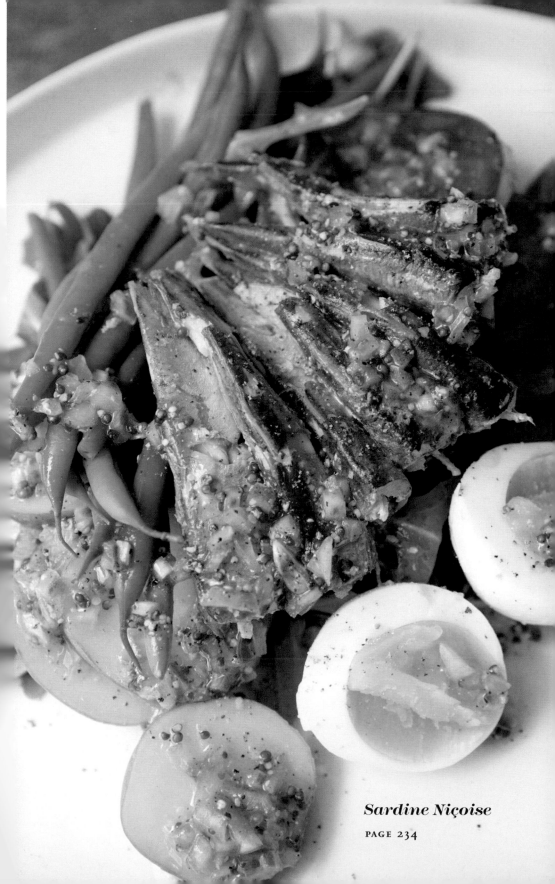

Sardine Niçoise

PAGE 234

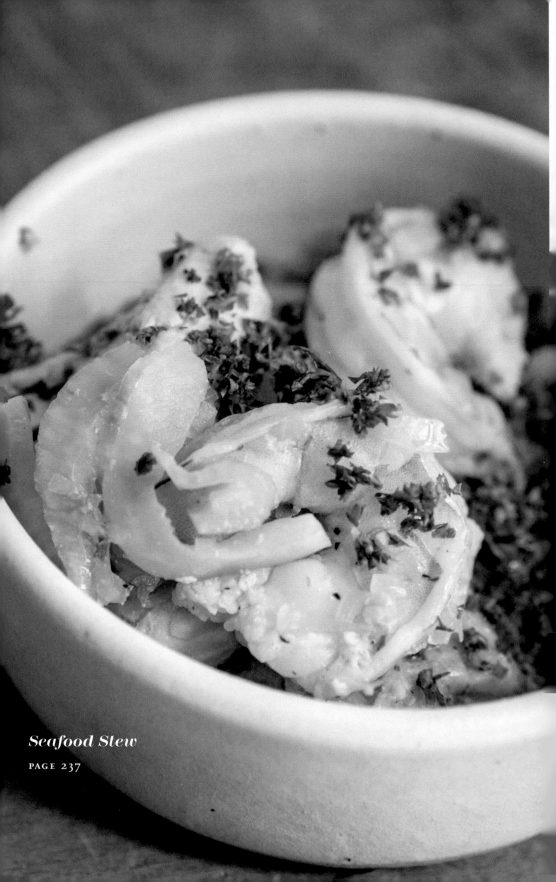

Seafood Stew

PAGE 237

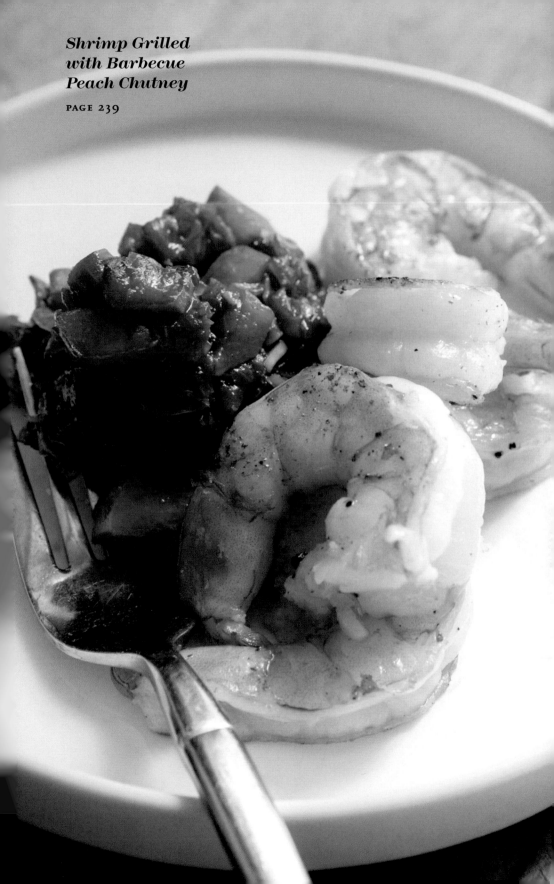

*Shrimp Grilled
with Barbecue
Peach Chutney*

PAGE 239

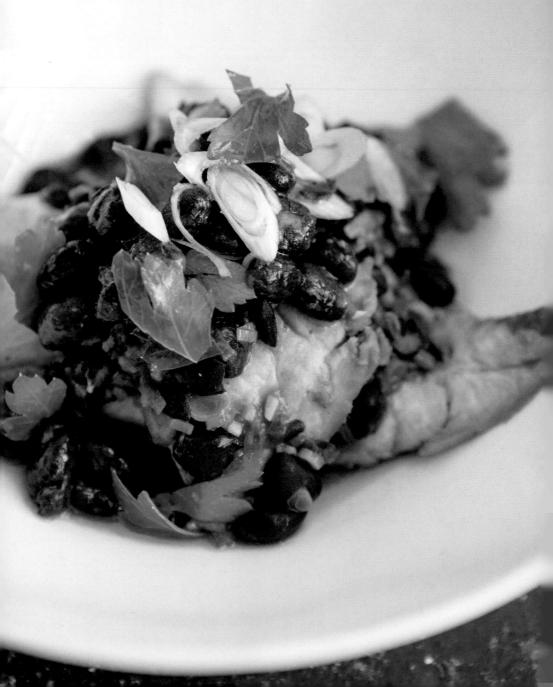

Tilapia with Black Beans, Green Onions, Garlic, and Ginger

PAGE 243

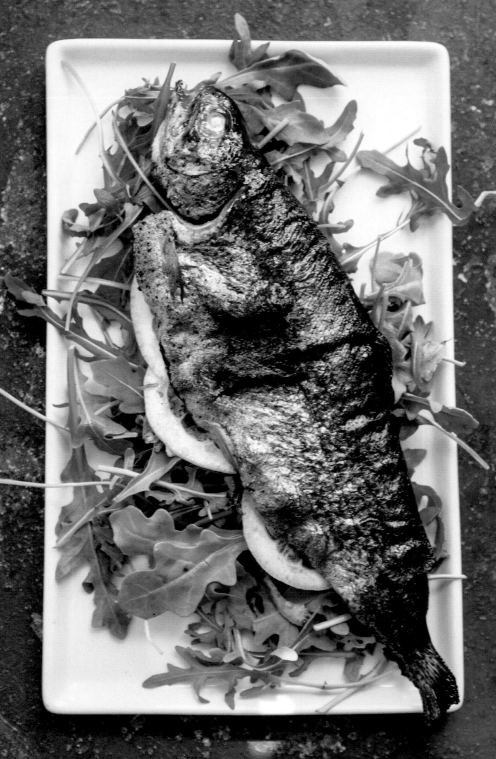

Trout, Whole with Thyme and Preserved Lemon

Trout, Whole with Thyme and Preserved Lemon

PAGE 247

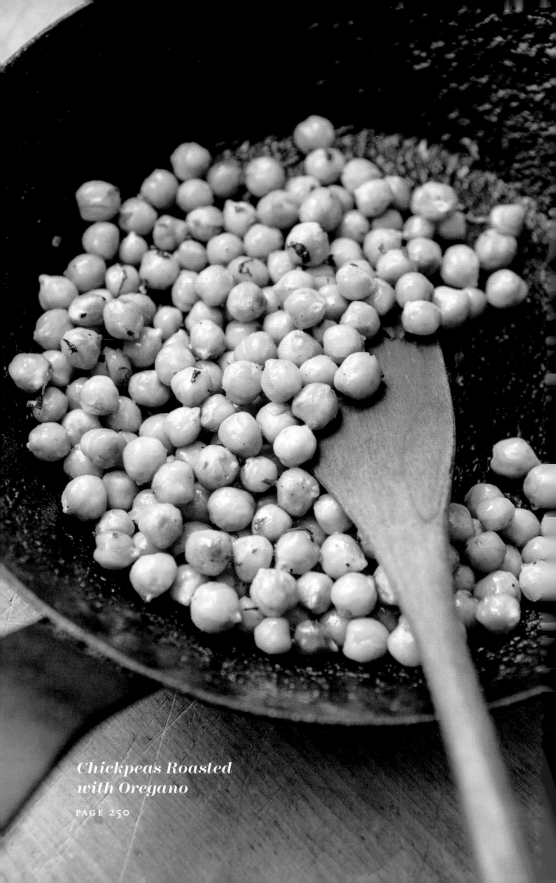

Chickpeas Roasted with Oregano

PAGE 250

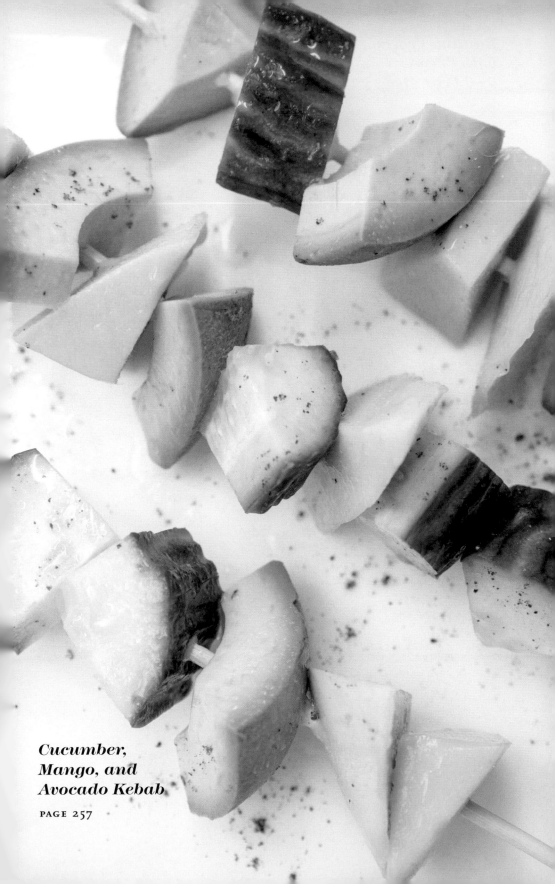

Cucumber,
Mango, and
Avocado Kebab

PAGE 257

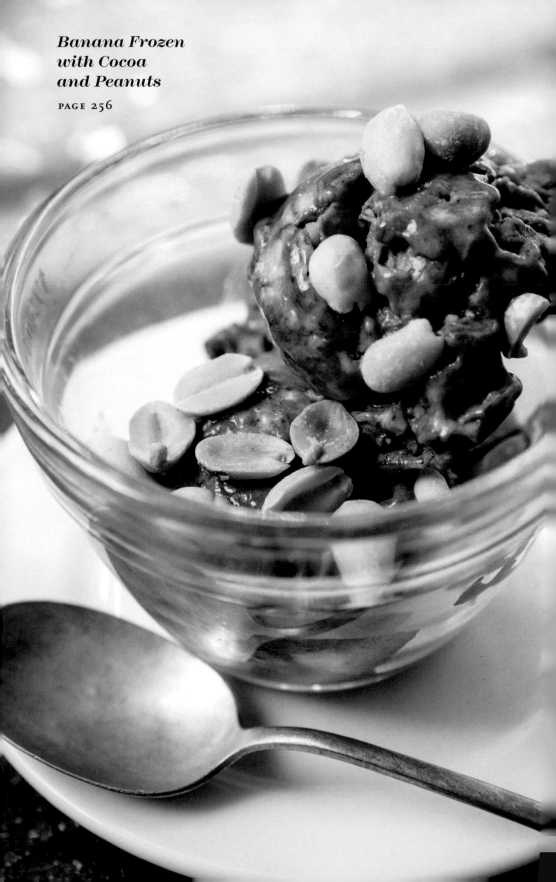

Banana Frozen
with Cocoa
and Peanuts

PAGE 256

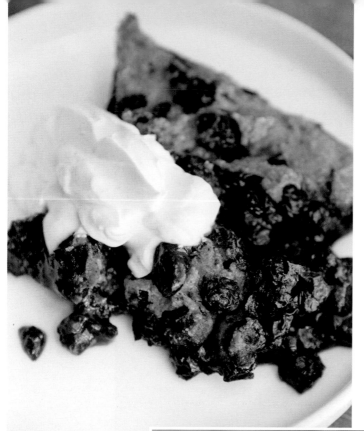

Blueberries Baked with Sweet Corn Cake

PAGE 259

Chocolate Cupcake with Mint Glaze

PAGE 260

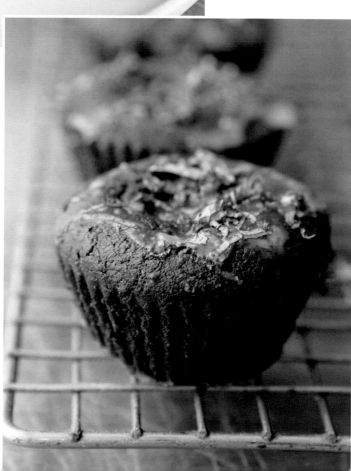

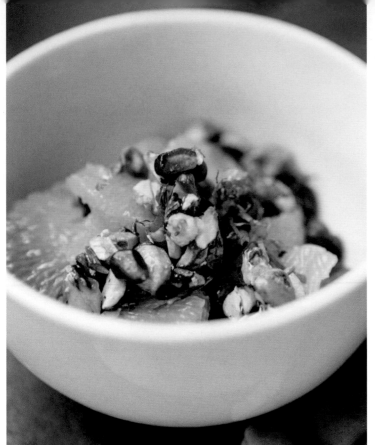

Oranges and Pomegranate with Candied Pistachio

PAGE 264

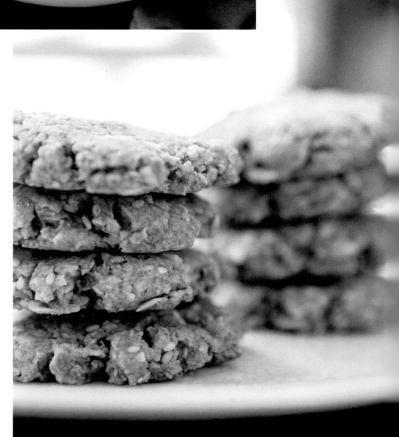

Sesame Coconut Cookies

PAGE 266

Shrimp Grilled with Barbecue Peach Chutney

The chunky chutney in this recipe would also taste great with catfish. If you have fresh parsley or cilantro, chop and add just before serving.

SERVES: 4 • PREP TIME: 10 MINUTES • TOTAL TIME: 30 MINUTES

3	**peaches**, chopped
1	**onion**, finely chopped
2	teaspoons mashed **garlic**
2	tablespoons **cider vinegar**
1	tablespoon **honey**
1	tablespoon **molasses**
	Large pinch of **cayenne pepper**
1½	pounds **shrimp**, shelled and deveined
2	teaspoons **extra-virgin olive oil**
⅛	teaspoon **salt**
	Freshly ground **black pepper** to taste

1. In a medium saucepan, place the peaches, onion, garlic, cider vinegar, honey, molasses, cayenne, and ¼ cup of water.

2. Bring to a boil, reduce heat to a simmer, and cook for 15 minutes, stirring often.

3. Place the shrimp in a bowl and toss with the olive oil, salt, and pepper.

4. Cook the shrimp until just pink, approximately 1 minute on each side on a grill or under the broiler.

5. Serve the shrimp with the peach sauce.

PER SERVING:		
Calories: 242	Total Sugar: 18 g	Cholesterol: 214 mg
Protein: 30 g	Total Fat: 4 g	Calcium: 126 mg
Carbohydrate: 23 g	Saturated Fat: 0.5 g	Sodium: 659 mg
Dietary Fiber: 2 g	Total Omega-3 Fat: 134 mg	

PESCETARIAN PORTIONS: 1 fruit serving; ½ fat serving; 4 protein servings

Shrimp Taco Salad

This dish is quick and easy, and it appeals to even the pickiest of eaters! You can also replace the shrimp with canned salmon or canned sardines. I suggest pairing it with a tomato salad or a fresh tomato salsa.

SERVES: 4 • PREP TIME: 5 MINUTES • TOTAL TIME: 5 MINUTES

2   **avocados,** skin and pits removed, flesh mashed with the back of a fork

3   tablespoons fresh **lime juice**

1/2 cup **reduced-fat sour cream** or **vegan sour cream**

Very finely chopped **fresh hot pepper** (such as jalapeño) to taste

Freshly ground **black pepper**

1   pound boiled **shrimp,** peeled and deveined

6   cups chopped **romaine lettuce**

1   cup sliced **cucumber**

11/2 cups baked **corn chips**

1   cup cooked **black beans,** dry or canned, low-sodium, rinsed and drained

1.   In a small bowl, combine the avocado, 2 tablespoons of lime juice, sour cream, and hot pepper.

2.   In a second small bowl, toss the shrimp with the remaining tablespoon of lime juice and freshly ground black pepper.

3.   In a large bowl, combine the romaine, cucumber, corn chips, and black beans. Dress with the avocado mixture, fold in the shrimp, and serve immediately.

PER SERVING:		
Calories: 429	Total Sugar: 2 g	Cholesterol: 205 mg
Protein: 38 g	Total Fat: 17 g	Calcium: 204 mg
Carbohydrate: 34 g	Saturated Fat: 4.4 g	Sodium: 496 mg
Dietary Fiber: 11 g	Total Omega-3 Fat: 785 mg	

PESCETARIAN PORTIONS: 1 grain/starchy vegetable serving;
2 vegetable servings; 2½ fat servings; 3 protein servings

Tilapia Fish Sticks

This crispy dish is mild and should appeal to eaters of all ages. You can also use the same method for cooking nearly any variety of fish.

SERVES 4 • PREP TIME: 10 MINUTES • TOTAL TIME: 25 MINUTES

	Canola oil cooking spray
2½	tablespoons **nonfat Greek yogurt**
1½	tablespoons **grainy mustard**, store bought or homemade (see pantry)
¼	teaspoon **salt**
1	tablespoon freshly squeezed **lemon juice**
2	cups finely ground **whole-wheat bread crumbs**
2	teaspoons finely chopped **parsley**
1¼	pounds **tilapia**
4	**lemon** wedges

1. Preheat oven to 450°F. Spray a baking sheet with canola oil and set aside.

2. In a medium bowl, combine the yogurt, mustard, salt, and lemon juice.

3. On a plate, combine the bread crumbs and parsley.

4. Coat the fish with the yogurt mixture and then gently roll the fish in the bread crumb mixture.

5. Place the coated fish on a baking tray and spray with vegetable oil cooking spray.

6. Bake until the fish is crispy on the outside and just beginning to flake, but the center is still translucent, 10 to 15 minutes.

7. Serve hot with a lemon wedge.

PER SERVING:		
Calories: 222	Total Sugar: 1.5 g	Cholesterol: 71 mg
Protein: 31 g	Total Fat: 4 g	Calcium: 36 mg
Carbohydrate: 13 g	Saturated Fat: 1.0 g	Sodium: 276 mg
Dietary Fiber: 2 g	Total Omega-3 Fat: 400 mg	

PESCETARIAN PORTIONS: 3 grain/starchy vegetable servings;
3 protein servings

Tilapia with Black Beans, Green Onions, Garlic, and Ginger

If you are in the mood for Asian flavors, this dish is for you! Catfish, haddock, arctic char, mackerel, or cod are also good choices. It's a natural with the Black Rice with Sesame and Green Onions (page 185).

SERVES: 4 • PREP TIME: 10 MINUTES • TOTAL TIME: 40 MINUTES

1 tablespoon **extra-virgin olive oil**

1 teaspoon finely chopped **garlic**

½ cup plus 1 tablespoon sliced **green onions**

½ teaspoon finely chopped fresh **ginger**

⅛ teaspoon **salt**

Freshly ground **black pepper** to taste

2 teaspoons reduced-sodium **soy sauce**

2 cups cooked **black beans**, dry or canned, no salt added

1 pound **tilapia**

2 tablespoons chopped **cilantro**

1. Heat a large heavy-bottomed skillet with a lid over low heat, add the olive oil, garlic, ½ cup of green onions, and ginger. Cook, stirring often until the green onions are soft, approximately 5 minutes.

2. Add the salt, pepper, soy sauce, black beans, and 1 cup of water. Cover and let simmer for 15 minutes.

3. Place the tilapia in a single layer on the black bean mixture and spoon some black beans over each piece of fish.

4. Cover and let cook until the tilapia is just beginning to flake but the center is still translucent, approximately 5 minutes. Take care not to overcook.

5. Serve topped with 1 tablespoon of green onions and the cilantro.

PER SERVING:

Calories: 262	Total Sugar: 0 g	Cholesterol: 57 mg
Protein: 31 g	Total Fat: 6 g	Calcium: 65 mg
Carbohydrate: 23 g	Saturated Fat: 1.2 g	Sodium: 223 mg
Dietary Fiber: 8 g	Total Omega-3 Fat: 300 mg	

PESCETARIAN PORTIONS: 1½ grain/starchy vegetable servings;
1 fat serving; 2 protein servings

Trout in Paper with Summer Squash, Green Onion, and Basil

This elegant dish also lends itself to scallops in lieu of the trout, or carrots in lieu of the squash.

SERVES: 4 • PREP TIME: 5 MINUTES • TOTAL TIME: 15 MINUTES

1½	cups thinly sliced **zucchini**
¾	cup thinly sliced **green onion**
1	tablespoon **extra-virgin olive oil**
¼	teaspoon **salt**
	Freshly ground **black pepper** to taste
1¼	pounds **trout** fillet cut into 4 equal pieces
4	pieces **parchment paper**, about 12 x 12 inches each
½	cup roughly chopped **basil**

1. Heat oven to 400°F.

2. In a bowl, combine the zucchini, green onion, 2 teaspoons of olive oil, ⅛ teaspoon of salt, and black pepper.

3. Season the fish on both sides with 1 teaspoon of olive oil, ⅛ teaspoon of salt, and black pepper.

4. Place ¼ of the zucchini mixture in the center of each of the pieces of parchment and then top each with 1 piece of fish. Fold the parchment paper over the fish to cover and tuck the ends under the fish to seal. Place packets on a sheet tray with sides.

5. Bake until the fish is just beginning to flake but the center is still translucent, 8 to 10 minutes. (Check one of the packets to ensure that you do not overcook.)

6. Top with basil and serve hot.

PER SERVING:		
Calories: 211	Total Sugar: 2 g	Cholesterol: 84 mg
Protein: 30 g	Total Fat: 9 g	Calcium: 119 mg
Carbohydrate: 2 g	Saturated Fat: 1.5 g	Sodium: 195 mg
Dietary Fiber: 1 g	Total Omega-3 Fat: 1,300 mg	

PESCETARIAN PORTIONS: ½ vegetable serving;
½ fat serving; 5 protein servings

Trout, Whole with Thyme and Preserved Lemon

This recipe is pretty foolproof if you do not overcook it. While I love it with preserved lemons, fresh lemon slices work just fine. For a quick meal, serve it over a bed of salad greens and a side of whole grains. Or, consider pairing it with the Tomato Roasted with Garlic (page 183), the Oatmeal Onion Cake (page 188), and a green salad.

SERVES: 4 · PREP TIME: 5 MINUTES · TOTAL TIME: 10 MINUTES

2	pounds whole **trout**, scaled, gutted, and cleaned (1 larger or 2 small fish)
¼	teaspoon **salt**
	Freshly ground **black pepper** to taste
3	tablespoons preserved **lemon** (see pantry), can also substitute fresh lemon slices
1	tablespoon fresh **thyme** leaves
¼	cup finely chopped **parsley**
2	teaspoons **extra-virgin olive oil**

1. Heat oven to 400°F. Season the trout inside with salt and pepper and fill with lemon, thyme, and parsley.

2. Close the fish and rub the outside with olive oil.

3. Place on a sheet tray and cook until the inside is flaky, approximately 10 minutes.

4. Turn oven to broil and cook until the skin browns, 2 to 5 additional minutes depending on the strength of your broiler and how close the fish is to the flame; serve immediately.

PER SERVING:		
Calories: 298	Total Sugar: 0 g	Cholesterol: 134 mg
Protein: 47 g	Total Fat: 10 g	Calcium: 163 mg
Carbohydrate: 1.5 g	Saturated Fat: 2.0 g	Sodium: 245 mg
Dietary Fiber: 1 g	Total Omega-3 Fat: 1,900 mg	

PESCETARIAN PORTIONS: ½ fat serving; 4 protein servings

SNACKS

~~~

150-CALORIE SNACKS

Black Bean Roll Up Wrapped in Romaine

Definitely not your run-of-the-mill snack! Feel free to use any type of bean you'd like.

SERVES: 1 • PREP TIME: 5 MINUTES • TOTAL TIME: 5 MINUTES

⅓ cup cooked **black beans**, dry (see pantry) or canned, no salt added

Dash of **salt**

1 tablespoon freshly squeezed **lemon juice**

2 tablespoons chopped **parsley**

1 tablespoon chopped **walnuts**

½ teaspoon **extra-virgin olive oil**

1 large **romaine leaf**

1. In a food processor or high-speed blender, combine the black beans, salt, lemon juice, parsley, walnuts, olive oil, and 1 teaspoon of water. Process until smooth, 30 seconds.

2. Spread bean dip on the romaine leaf and roll up lengthwise.

PER SERVING:		
Calories: 158	Total Sugar: 1 g	Cholesterol: 0 mg
Protein: 7 g	Total Fat: 7 g	Calcium: 62 mg
Carbohydrate: 18 g	Saturated Fat: 0.8 g	Sodium: 164 mg
Dietary Fiber: 6 g	Total Omega-3 Fat: 800 mg	

PESCETARIAN PORTIONS: 1 grain/starchy vegetable serving;

1½ fat servings (1 as nuts/seeds)

Chickpeas Roasted with Oregano

Enjoy! This is my new favorite snack.

SERVES: 1 • PREP TIME: 5 MINUTES • TOTAL TIME: 15 MINUTES

½ cup no-salt added canned **chickpeas**, drained, rinsed, and patted dry

½ teaspoon **extra-virgin olive oil**

1 teaspoon finely chopped **oregano**

Dash of **salt**

Freshly ground **black pepper** to taste

1. Heat oven to 425°F.

2. Place the chickpeas on a sheet tray and toss with the olive oil, oregano, salt, and pepper.

3. Cook until edges are brown, approximately 12 minutes.

4. Serve hot or at room temperature.

PER SERVING:		
Calories: 153	Total Sugar: 0 g	Cholesterol: 0 mg
Protein: 7 g	Total Fat: 2 g	Calcium: 77 mg
Carbohydrate: 22 g	Saturated Fat: 0.3 g	Sodium: 185 mg
Dietary Fiber: 5 g	Total Omega-3 Fat: 0 mg	

PESCETARIAN PORTIONS: 1½ grain/starchy vegetable servings;
½ fat serving

Peach Cinnamon Smoothie (A HIGH-CALCIUM SNACK)

Consider this recipe a starting point and substitute any in-season or frozen fruit.

SERVES: 1 • PREP TIME: 2 MINUTES • TOTAL TIME: 2 MINUTES

1 small **peach**

Pinch of **cinnamon**

⅔ cup **skim milk, almond milk**, or **soy milk**

2 teaspoons chopped raw **cashews**

¼ cup **ice** cubes

1. In a high-speed blender, combine the peach, cinnamon, milk, and cashews.

2. Process until smooth, 30 seconds. Add ice cubes and blend for an additional 15 seconds. Serve immediately.

PER SERVING:		
Calories: 141	Total Sugar: 19 g	Cholesterol: 3 mg
Protein: 8 g	Total Fat: 3 g	Calcium: 349 mg
Carbohydrate: 23 g	Saturated Fat: 0.7 g	Sodium: 86 mg
Dietary Fiber: 2 g	Total Omega-3 Fat: 0 mg	

PESCETARIAN PORTIONS: 1 fruit serving; ½ dairy serving;

1 fat serving (as nuts/seeds)

Strawberry Milk (A HIGH-CALCIUM SNACK)

This is an updated version of an old-time snack. It's even better with frozen strawberries because they make it thicker and icier.

SERVES: 1 • PREP TIME: 2 MINUTES • TOTAL TIME: 2 MINUTES

1	cup **milk** or **soy milk**
3/4	cup sliced **strawberries**, fresh or (even better) frozen
1/16	teaspoon **vanilla extract** or the inside of a quarter of a fresh **vanilla bean**
1/2	teaspoon **sugar**

1. In a high-speed blender, combine the milk, strawberries, vanilla, and sugar.

2. Blend until smooth, 30 seconds. Drink immediately.

PER SERVING:		
Calories: 148	Total Sugar: 14 g	Cholesterol: 0 mg
Protein: 8 g	Total Fat: 4 g	Calcium: 319 mg
Carbohydrate: 20 g	Saturated Fat: 0.5 g	Sodium: 120 mg
Dietary Fiber: 3 g	Total Omega-3 Fat: 100 mg	

PESCETARIAN PORTIONS: 1½ fruit servings; 1 dairy serving

Yogurt Avocado Dip (A HIGH-CALCIUM SNACK)

You can make this snack in no time, and it appeals to eaters of all ages. Mix it up by substituting sweet peppers, celery, or cucumber for the carrot.

SERVES: 1 • PREP TIME: 5 MINUTES • TOTAL TIME: 5 MINUTES

½	cup **plain nonfat Greek yogurt**
¼	ripe **avocado**, peel and pit discarded, flesh mashed with the back of a fork
2	teaspoons freshly squeezed **lime juice**
1	tablespoon finely chopped **cilantro**
	Dash of **salt**
	Freshly ground **black pepper** to taste
	Cayenne pepper, if desired
½	large **carrot**, cut on a slight angle into disks

1. In a food processor or high-speed blender, combine the yogurt, avocado, lime juice, cilantro, salt, pepper, and cayenne. Process until smooth, 30 seconds.

2. Use the avocado mixture as a dip with the carrot chips.

PER SERVING:		
Calories: 146 Protein: 13 g Carbohydrate: 13 g Dietary Fiber: 3 g	Total Sugar: 6 g Total Fat: 5 g Saturated Fat: 0.7 g Total Omega-3 Fat: 100 mg	Cholesterol: 2 mg Calcium: 219 mg Sodium: 92 mg

PESCETARIAN PORTIONS: ½ dairy serving; ½ vegetable serving;
1 fat serving

Yogurt, Banana, Peanut Butter Pop (A HIGH-CALCIUM SNACK)

I like to quadruple this recipe and make a bunch in advance. If well wrapped, these will last for months in your freezer.

SERVES: 1 • PREP TIME: 5 MINUTES • TOTAL TIME: 2 HOURS (INCLUDES FREEZING TIME)

- ½ cup **plain fat-free yogurt**
- ½ **banana**, sliced
- ½ teaspoon **honey**
- 1 teaspoon no-sugar-added **peanut butter**

1. In a blender, place the yogurt, banana, honey, and peanut butter. Process until smooth, 30 seconds.

2. Pour into a popsicle mold or a paper cup. Place a popsicle stick or a chopstick in the middle and freeze.

3. When ready to eat, remove from the popsicle mold or peel off the paper cup.

PER SERVING:		
Calories: 158	Total Sugar: 19 g	Cholesterol: 2 mg
Protein: 9 g	Total Fat: 3.3 g	Calcium: 250 mg
Carbohydrate: 25 g	Saturated Fat: 0.7 g	Sodium: 119 mg
Dietary Fiber: 2 g	Total Omega-3 Fat: 0 mg	

PESCETARIAN PORTIONS: 1 fruit serving; ¾ dairy serving;
1 fat serving (as nuts/seeds)

Apple with Spiced Sesame

If you're in a peanut butter rut, tahini is a nice change of pace. Sub in pears or oranges for the apple if you like.

SERVES: 1 • PREP TIME: 5 MINUTES • TOTAL TIME: 5 MINUTES

1	tablespoon **tahini**
1½	teaspoons **honey**
¼	teaspoon **cinnamon**
½	teaspoon **sesame seeds**
1	small **apple**, core removed and cut into 6 slices

1. In a small bowl, place the tahini, honey, cinnamon, sesame seeds, and 1 teaspoon of water. Stir until smooth.

2. Spread the tahini mixture on each of the apple slices.

PER SERVING:		
Calories: 209	Total Sugar: 24 g	Cholesterol: 0 mg
Protein: 3 g	Total Fat: 9 g	Calcium: 81 mg
Carbohydrate: 33 g	Saturated Fat: 1.3 g	Sodium: 20 mg
Dietary Fiber: 5 g	Total Omega-3 Fat: 100 mg	

PESCETARIAN PORTIONS: 1 fruit serving; 2 fat servings (all as nuts/seeds)

Banana Frozen with Cocoa and Peanuts

After tasting this recipe, Kate Headley, who photographed the recipes for this book, immediately went out and bought a food processor. Over the years, I have made different versions, but this cocoa powder and peanuts combo is my favorite. I always keep a bag of peeled bananas in my freezer for this recipe (and to toss into smoothies).

SERVES: 1 • PREP TIME: 5 MINUTES (IF BANANA IS FROZEN) • TOTAL TIME: 5 MINUTES

1 **banana**, cut into small pieces, placed in a plastic bag, and frozen

$1^1/_2$ teaspoons **cocoa powder**

14 dry-roasted salted **peanuts**

1. In a food processor, place the banana and cocoa powder.

2. Process on and off several times until creamy, stir in the peanuts, and serve immediately.

PER SERVING:		
Calories: 193	Total Sugar: 15 g	Cholesterol: 0 mg
Protein: 5 g	Total Fat: 8 g	Calcium: 17 mg
Carbohydrate: 32 g	Saturated Fat: 1.3 g	Sodium: 97 mg
Dietary Fiber: 5 g	Total Omega-3 Fat: 0 mg	

PESCETARIAN PORTIONS: 2 fruit servings; 2 fat servings (all as nuts/seeds)

Cucumber, Mango, and Avocado Kebab

So refreshing and flavorful, this has become one of my go-to snacks.

SERVES: 1 • PREP TIME: 5 MINUTES • TOTAL TIME: 5 MINUTES

⅓	**avocado**, peel and pit discarded, cubed
1	cup **mango**, cubed
1	cup **cucumber**, sliced
½	teaspoon freshly squeezed **lime juice**
	Small pinch of **cayenne pepper**, or to taste

1. Randomly place pieces of avocado, mango, and cucumber on a skewer.
2. Squeeze with lime and sprinkle with cayenne if desired.

PER SERVING:		
Calories: 196	Total Sugar: 27 g	Cholesterol: 0 mg
Protein: 2 g	Total Fat: 7 g	Calcium: 39 mg
Carbohydrate: 36 g	Saturated Fat: 1.1 g	Sodium: 9 mg
Dietary Fiber: 7 g	Total Omega-3 Fat: 100 mg	

PESCETARIAN PORTIONS: 2 fruit servings; 1 vegetable serving;
2 fat servings

DESSERT

~~~

Note: *Unlike the other recipes, the desserts don't have* Pescetarian portions attached. That's because on the Pescetarian Plan, you tally your daily treats by counting calories, not portions, as you do with grains, proteins, and the other food groups. (Details on page 75.)

Blueberries Baked with Sweet Corn Cake

You can substitute the blueberries with any other type of berry or with sliced pear or apple. Any version results in a homey, satisfying dessert. If you need a 100-calorie dessert, eat a half portion.

SERVES: 6 • PREP TIME: 10 MINUTES • TOTAL TIME: 30 MINUTES

- 4 cups **blueberries**
- 3 tablespoons **sugar**
- **Canola oil cooking spray**
- ½ cup **cornmeal**
- 1 teaspoon **baking powder**
- ¼ teaspoon **baking soda**
- ½ cup silken **tofu**, puréed
- ½ cup **soy milk**
- 1 tablespoon **extra-virgin olive oil**
- 4 tablespoons **low-fat sour cream** or **vegan sour cream**

1. Preheat oven to 350°F. In a medium bowl, toss the blueberries with 1 tablespoon of sugar.

2. Spray a small baking dish with canola oil cooking spray and fill with the blueberries.

3. In a medium bowl, combine 2 tablespoons of sugar, cornmeal, baking powder, baking soda, tofu, milk, and olive oil. Stir until thoroughly combined.

4. Top the blueberries with the cornmeal mixture and bake until golden brown, approximately 20 minutes.

5. Serve hot or at room temperature, topped with 1 tablespoon of sour cream per serving.

PER SERVING:		
Calories: 207	Total Sugar: 17 g	Cholesterol: 4 mg
Protein: 7 g	Total Fat: 7 g	Calcium: 215 mg
Carbohydrate: 32 g	Saturated Fat: 1.7 g	Sodium: 156 mg
Dietary Fiber: 4 g	Total Omega-3 Fat: 200 mg	

Chocolate Cupcake with Mint Glaze (Including a Gluten-Free Option)

It took a lot of tries to get this just right: rich, chocolatey, and amenable to either wheat- or gluten-free flour. I am a huge fan of chocolate and mint together, but these are still absolutely wonderful without the mint. You can substitute a sprinkle of cocoa powder or cinnamon instead.

SERVES: 12 • PREP TIME: 10 MINUTES • TOTAL TIME: 25 MINUTES

⅓	cup **extra-virgin olive oil**
⅛	teaspoon **vanilla extract** or inside of 1 **vanilla bean**
¾	teaspoon **cider vinegar**
¾	cup skim **milk, almond milk,** or **soy milk**
1	cup **all-purpose unbleached flour** (for gluten-free, substitute ½ cup gluten-free flour)
⅓	cup **almond meal**
⅓	cup **sugar**
⅓	cup **cocoa powder**
½	teaspoon **baking soda**
¾	teaspoon **baking powder**
	Dash of **salt**
1½	ounce **bittersweet chocolate**, chopped, or ¼ cup **bittersweet chocolate chips**
¼	cup **powdered sugar**
3	tablespoons finely chopped **fresh mint**

1. Preheat oven to 350°F.

2. In a medium bowl, combine the oil, vanilla extract, vinegar, and milk. Add flour, almond meal, sugar, cocoa powder, baking soda, baking powder, and salt. Stir until just smooth. Gently mix in the chocolate pieces or chips.

3. Coat a muffin tin or cupcake pan with vegetable oil cooking spray and divide batter evenly among 6 individual cups.

4. Bake until a toothpick inserted in the middle of the cake comes out clean, approximately 15 minutes.

5. While the cupcakes are cooking, combine the powdered sugar and 2 teaspoons of water in a small bowl, mix until smooth.

6. Once the cupcakes are finished baking, let cool slightly, remove from the pan, poke the tops a half-inch deep with a toothpick, and spoon the glaze over each cake. Finish the cupcakes by topping with the mint.

PER SERVING:		
Calories: 168	Total Sugar: 9 g	Cholesterol: 0 mg
Protein: 3 g	Total Fat: 9 g	Calcium: 52 mg
Carbohydrate: 21 g	Saturated Fat: 1.9 g	Sodium: 104 mg
Dietary Fiber: 2 g	Total Omega-3 Fat: 52 mg	

Grape Granita

This recipe seems like it couldn't work: Sorbet in seconds without an ice cream maker? But it does! It is a refreshing way to end any meal. Just make sure to plan in advance and have frozen grapes when you need them. I nearly always have a bag in my freezer ready to go.

SERVES: 4 • PREP TIME: 5 MINUTES (IF GRAPES ARE FROZEN IN ADVANCE) •
TOTAL TIME: 5 MINUTES

4 cups **grapes**

1. On a sheet tray, place grapes on a single layer and put in freezer. Leave until thoroughly frozen, at least 2 hours.

2. Place frozen grapes in a food processor and pulse on and off until the texture is sorbet-like, approximately 10 pulses.

3. Spoon into individual bowls and serve immediately.

PER SERVING:		
Calories: 104	Total Sugar: 23 g	Cholesterol: 0 mg
Protein: 1 g	Total Fat: 0 g	Calcium: 15 mg
Carbohydrate: 27 g	Saturated Fat: 0.1 g	Sodium: 3 mg
Dietary Fiber: 1 g	Total Omega-3 Fat: 0 mg	

Melon with Lemon Sauce

Hard to believe that this creamy, decadent lemon sauce is actually good for you! Honeydew is just a suggestion; use the best available fruit in season.

SERVES: 4 • PREP TIME: 5 MINUTES • TOTAL TIME: 5 MINUTES

1 cup thoroughly drained **silken** or **soft tofu**

1 tablespoon **lemon zest**

3 tablespoons fresh **lemon juice**

2 tablespoons **sugar**

2 cups cubed **honeydew** (can substitute other **melon**, **berries**, or **fruit**)

1. In a high-speed blender, combine the tofu, zest, lemon juice, and sugar. Process until completely smooth, 1 minute.

2. Pour the lemon mixture over the melon. Serve immediately or cover, refrigerate, and serve chilled.

PER SERVING:		
Calories: 108	Total Sugar: 17 g	Cholesterol: 0 mg
Protein: 5 g	Total Fat: 2 g	Calcium: 75 mg
Carbohydrate: 19 g	Saturated Fat: 0.4 g	Sodium: 21 mg
Dietary Fiber: 1 g	Total Omega-3 Fat: 200 mg	

Oranges and Pomegranate with Candied Pistachio

Don't be fooled by the simple ingredients; this is one exciting dessert! You can make it with any variety of orange or try it with grapefruit.

SERVES: 4 • PREP TIME: 10 MINUTES • TOTAL TIME: 10 MINUTES

2	**oranges**
½	cup fresh **pomegranate seeds** (can substitute **grapes** or **berries**)
1	tablespoon finely chopped **fresh mint**
3	tablespoons roughly chopped **pistachios**
1	teaspoon **honey**
	Pinch of **salt**

1. With a sharp knife, peel orange, discarding all skin, including the white pith. Slice into thin wheels, about ⅛-inch thick, and place in a medium bowl.

2. Add the pomegranate and mint.

3. In a small bowl, combine the pistachios, honey, and salt.

4. Place the orange mixture into 4 individual serving dishes. Top with the pistachio mixture and serve immediately.

PER SERVING:		
Calories: 108	Total Sugar: 5 g	Cholesterol: 0 mg
Protein: 3 g	Total Fat: 3 g	Calcium: 67 mg
Carbohydrate: 20 g	Saturated Fat: 0.4 g	Sodium: 60
Dietary Fiber: 5 g	Total Omega-3 Fat: 0 mg	

Pears Baked with Rosemary and Walnuts

If you've never had rosemary with fruit, I think you'll really enjoy this unexpected twist. No need to limit this recipe to pears—use apples, peaches, apricots, or whatever stone or core fruit is in season. If you're on the 1,500-calorie plan, a half portion of this dessert is the perfect 100-calorie treat.

SERVES: 4 • PREP TIME: 10 MINUTES • TOTAL TIME: 40 MINUTES

$\frac{1}{3}$ cup **walnuts**

$\frac{1}{3}$ cup **oatmeal**

1 tablespoon **honey**

$1\frac{1}{2}$ tablespoons **extra-virgin olive oil**

2 tablespoons **skim milk**

$\frac{1}{8}$ teaspoon **baking soda**

$\frac{1}{8}$ teaspoon **baking powder**

2 teaspoons chopped fresh **rosemary**

Dash of **salt**

Vegetable oil cooking spray

2 **pears**, cut in half, core removed

1. Preheat oven to 375°F.

2. In a food processor, combine the walnuts, oatmeal, honey, olive oil, milk, baking soda, baking powder, rosemary, and salt.

3. Spray a small oven-proof baking dish or skillet with vegetable oil cooking spray.

4. Place the pears cut-side up and fill them with the walnut filling.

5. Place in the oven and bake for 30 minutes. Serve hot or at room temperature.

PER SERVING:		
Calories: 205	Total Sugar: 14 g	Cholesterol: 0 mg
Protein: 3 g	Total Fat: 12 g	Calcium: 47 mg
Carbohydrate: 24 g	Saturated Fat: 1.4 g	Sodium: 99 mg
Dietary Fiber: 4 g	Total Omega-3 Fat: 900 mg	

Sesame Coconut Cookies

Here's a cookie you can feel really good about: It's whole-grain with very little sugar but still feels like a treat!

SERVES: 8 • PREP TIME: 5 MINUTES • TOTAL TIME: 20 MINUTES

½	cup	**whole-wheat flour**
3	tablespoons	**sugar**
¼	cup	**coconut flakes**
2	tablespoons	**sesame seeds**
⅛	teaspoon	**baking powder**
⅛	teaspoon	**baking soda**
2	tablespoons	**extra-virgin olive oil**
1	tablespoon	**tahini**
		Dash of **salt**

1. Combine the flour, sugar, coconut, sesame seeds, baking powder, and baking soda. Mix in the oil, tahini, salt, and 2½ tablespoons of water. Combine thoroughly using your fingers.

2. Preheat oven to 350°F.

3. Line a baking sheet with parchment paper. Divide the cookie batter into 8 parts. Wet your hands and roll each portion into a ball. Place cookies on the parchment paper and gently flatten with the palm of your hand.

4. Bake until cookies are just starting to turn golden brown, approximately 12 minutes.

5. Enjoy warm or at room temperature.

PER SERVING:		
Calories: 114	Total Sugar: 5 g	Cholesterol: 0 mg
Protein: 2 g	Total Fat: 7 g	Calcium: 17 mg
Carbohydrate: 11 g	Saturated Fat: 2.2 g	Sodium: 51 mg
Dietary Fiber: 2 g	Total Omega-3 Fat: 0 mg	

PANTRY

~~~~~

Beans

While there's nothing wrong with canned beans—especially the no-salt-added or low-sodium variety—they're never as tasty (or inexpensive) as when they're made from scratch. You'll notice the very wide range in cooking time; that's because there's such a great variety of beans that it's not possible to give exact instructions for each. But this is a good general guide for all varieties.

PREP TIME: 5 MINUTES • TOTAL TIME: 20 MINUTES TO 3 HOURS DEPENDING ON THE VARIETY AND FRESHNESS OF THE BEAN

DRIED BEANS

1. Rinse the beans (such as black, white, pinto, etc.) in a strainer and discard any discolored bean or material other than bean.

2. Place the beans in a large pot, cover with water—approximately 5 cups of water for every 1 cup of beans. Bring to a boil, reduce heat to low, and simmer. Make sure the beans stay covered with water during the cooking process. If necessary, add more water.

3. Test the beans often to see how quickly they are cooking. They should be tender but not mushy.

4. Use the beans immediately, refrigerate covered for 3 days, or freeze. If refrigerating or freezing, store the beans in their own liquid.

PREP TIME: 5 MINUTES • TOTAL TIME: 7 TO 20 MINUTES DEPENDING ON THE VARIETY OF BEAN

FRESH BEANS

1. Shell beans (such as lima, black-eyed pea, etc.), rinse in a strainer, and discard any discolored beans or any pieces of shell.

2. Place the beans in a large pot, cover with water—approximately 3 cups of water for every 1 cup of beans. Bring to a boil, reduce heat to low,

and simmer. Make sure the beans stay covered with water during the cooking process. If necessary, add more water.

3. Test the beans often to see how quickly they are cooking. They should be tender but not mushy.

4. Use the beans immediately, refrigerate covered for 3 days, or freeze. If refrigerating or freezing, store the beans in their own liquid.

Black Rice

Black rice is a staple in my kitchen. In addition to having a great taste and dramatic color, it's a whole grain and a true superfood, containing anthocyanins, which are powerful antioxidants.

YIELD: 3½ CUPS (8 SERVINGS) • PREP TIME: 2 MINUTES • TOTAL TIME: 1 HOUR

> 1   cup **black rice**

1. Place black rice and 1¾ cups of water in a covered pot.

2. Bring to a boil, stir, reduce heat to a simmer, cover, and cook for 45 minutes.

3. Turn off heat but leave the lid on the pot for an additional 10 minutes so that rice can finish cooking.

PER SERVING (⅓ CUP COOKED):		
Calories: 80	Total Sugar: 1 g	Cholesterol: 0 mg
Protein: 2 g	Total Fat: 1 g	Calcium: 7 mg
Carbohydrate: 17 g	Saturated Fat: 0.1 g	Sodium: 1 mg
Dietary Fiber: 1 g	Total Omega-3 Fat: N/A	

PESCETARIAN PORTIONS: 7 grain/starchy vegetable servings

Roasted Garlic

This is a core staple in my refrigerator because it's an easy way to give depth and flavor to so many different types of food. Use it smashed or whole. If you're a roasted garlic lover, you may want to double, triple, or quadruple the recipe. It keeps for at least 5 days if you store it covered in your refrigerator.

PREP TIME: 5 MINUTES • TOTAL TIME: 20 MINUTES

1	head **garlic**
¼	teaspoon **extra-virgin olive oil**

1. Preheat oven to 375°F. Separate the whole head of garlic into cloves, making sure that the papery skin remains on the individual cloves.

2. Lightly and evenly, coat the cloves with olive oil and place on a sheet tray.

3. Bake until the cloves are soft to the touch, approximately 15 minutes.

4. Remove from the oven and cool. Remove the papery skin from the garlic; it will peel off easily.

5. Look for a sprout running through the clove. Cut the clove in half lengthwise and remove the sprout with a small knife or your fingers. Occasionally, you will get a clove that does not have a sprout or is too small to remove.

Preserved Lemons

Use this on any type of fish and most vegetables to make an ordinary dish lively and interesting.

PREP TIME: 5 MINUTES • TOTAL TIME: 4 HOURS

4 **lemons**, very thinly sliced into rounds
¼ teaspoon **salt**
¼ teaspoon **sugar**
2 tablespoons **extra-virgin olive oil**

1. In a bowl, combine lemon, sugar, and salt. Toss and make sure ingredients are thoroughly combined. Let sit at room temperature for 4 to 8 hours.

2. Add olive oil and place in a container with a sealable top. Store in a refrigerator for up to 3 weeks.

Grainy Mustard

This mustard gets such rave reviews from guests, I should probably start selling it! I use it liberally with seafood, vegetables, salad dressings, sandwiches, and wraps.

YIELD: 1½ CUPS, SERVING SIZE: 1 TEASPOON • PREP TIME: 5 MINUTES •
TOTAL TIME: 1 WEEK

¼ cup **light mustard seeds**
¼ cup **dark mustard seeds**
3 tablespoons **mustard powder**
⅔ cup **water**
3 tablespoons **honey**
1 teaspoon **salt**

1. In a high-speed blender, blend the mustard seeds, mustard powder, water, honey, and salt until the ingredients are incorporated, 1 minute. Place in a glass jar, cover, and let sit in the refrigerator at least 1 week before serving.

PER SERVING:		
Calories: 8	Total Sugar: 1 g	Cholesterol: 0 mg
Protein: 0 g	Total Fat: 0 g	Calcium: 3 mg
Carbohydrate: 1 g	Saturated Fat: 0 g	Sodium: 37 mg
Dietary Fiber: 0 g	Total Omega-3 Fat: 0 mg	

┌─────────────────────┐
│ **SALAD DRESSINGS** │
└─────────────────────┘

Salad dressings aren't just for salads; toss with steamed greens and other vegetables or drizzle on cooked seafood for a light sauce.

Here are a few favorites.

Avocado Thick Dressing

SERVES: 4 • PREP TIME: 5 MINUTES • TOTAL TIME: 5 MINUTES

1	medium **avocado**, peel and pit discarded
¼	cup fresh **lemon juice**
⅛	teaspoon **salt**
	Freshly ground **black pepper** to taste
1	tablespoon finely chopped **chives**

In a food processor, combine the avocado, lemon juice, salt, and pepper. Stir in the chives.

PER SERVING:		
Calories: 60	Total Sugar: 1 g	Cholesterol: 0 mg
Protein: 1 g	Total Fat: 5 g	Calcium: 6 mg
Carbohydrate: 4 g	Saturated Fat: 0.7 g	Sodium: 76 mg
Dietary Fiber: 2 g	Total Omega-3 Fat: 100 mg	

PESCETARIAN PORTIONS: 1 fat serving

Mustard Vinaigrette

~~~~~~

SERVES 4 • PREP TIME: 5 MINUTES • TOTAL TIME: 5 MINUTES

 2 teaspoons **lemon juice**
 2 teaspoons **mustard**, store bought (no more than
    50 mg sodium per teaspoon) or homemade
    (see **Grainy Mustard**, page 273)
 2 teaspoons **balsamic vinegar**
 1 tablespoon plus 1 teaspoon **extra-virgin olive oil**

In a small bowl, combine the lemon juice, mustard, and balsamic vinegar.
Whisk in the olive oil.

PER SERVING:		
Calories: 49	Total Sugar: 1 g	Cholesterol: 0 mg
Protein: 0 g	Total Fat: 5 g	Calcium: 4 mg
Carbohydrate: 2 g	Saturated Fat: 0.6 g	Sodium: 30 mg
Dietary Fiber: 0 g	Total Omega-3 Fat: 0 mg	

PESCETARIAN PORTIONS: 1 fat serving

Nut Butter Dressing

SERVES: 4 · PREP TIME: 5 MINUTES · TOTAL TIME: 5 MINUTES

2   tablespoons **peanut butter** (or other **nut butter**), no salt or sugar added

1   teaspoon **honey**

1   teaspoon **reduced-sodium soy sauce**

2   tablespoons **white vinegar**

In a small bowl, combine the nut butter, honey, soy sauce, and vinegar. Mix until smooth. If the mixture is too thick, add water a half-teaspoon at a time until it reaches the desired thickness.

PER SERVING:		
Calories: 55	Total Sugar: 2 g	Cholesterol: 0 mg
Protein: 2 g	Total Fat: 4 g	Calcium: 4 mg
Carbohydrate: 3 g	Saturated Fat: 0.6 g	Sodium: 61 mg
Dietary Fiber: 1 g	Total Omega-3 Fat: 0 mg	

PESCETARIAN PORTIONS: 1 fat serving (1 as nuts/seeds)

Poppy Seed Dressing

SERVES: 4 • PREP TIME: 5 MINUTES • TOTAL TIME: 5 MINUTES

1½ tablespoons **extra-virgin olive oil**

1 tablespoon freshly squeezed **orange juice**

1 tablespoon **sherry vinegar**

⅛ teaspoon **salt**

Freshly ground **black pepper** to taste

2 tablespoons **poppy seeds**

In a small bowl, whisk together the olive oil, orange juice, vinegar, salt, pepper, and poppy seeds.

PER SERVING:		
Calories: 70	Total Sugar: 0 g	Cholesterol: 0 mg
Protein: 1 g	Total Fat: 7 g	Calcium: 64 mg
Carbohydrate: 2 g	Saturated Fat: 0.9 g	Sodium: 74 mg
Dietary Fiber: 1 g	Total Omega-3 Fat: 100 mg	

PESCETARIAN PORTIONS: 2 fat servings (1 as nuts/seeds)

APPENDIX A

~~~~~~~~~

Pescetarian Tracker

TIME OF DAY	SLEEP (NO. OF HOURS)	HUNGER SCALE * (BEFORE/ AFTER EATING)	FOOD AND DRINK (BE SPECIFIC AS IN "12 OUNCE SKIM LATTE WITH 1 TEASPOON SUGAR" OR "1 CUP BROWN RICE")	EXERCISE (TYPE, MINUTES OR NO. OF STEPS)	SITUATIONS/ EMOTIONS (IE. IN THE KITCHEN, STRESSED AT WORK, ETC.)

* Write down your hunger level before and after eating (i.e. 2/4). (1 = ravenous, 2= a little hungry 3= neither hungry nor full, 4 = a little full 5 = ugh! Too full).

GRAIN/STARCHY VEG _____   PROTEIN _____   WATER _____

FRUIT _____   FAT _____   TREATS (CALORIES) _____

VEGETABLES _____   DAIRY/SOY MILK _____   AEROBIC EXERCISE MINUTES _____

HOW TO USE YOUR PESCETARIAN TRACKER

Besides keeping you accountable (it's hard to "forget" that second giant chocolate chip cookie when it's staring at you in black and white in the "Food and Drink" column), this tracker serves another crucial function: identifying overeating triggers. It also shows you what you're doing *right*.

You'll notice that some days, things go well: You eat appropriate amounts of food—better yet, *healthy* foods—you work out, and you're full of energy. Other days may be just the opposite—you feel sluggish, you overeat (possibly binge), the food isn't very nutritious, and exercise never happens. And then there are the in-between days.

By filling out the "Time of Day," "Sleep," "Hunger," "Food and Drink," "Exercise," and "Situation/emotions" columns on your Pescetarian Tracker, you'll discover a *wealth* of information about what triggers those good, bad, or so-so days. Here are connections to look for:

Sleep. Both quality (disrupted vs. solid sleep) and quantity (number of hours) impact energy, appetite, and mood. Scan your Tracker for sleep connections. For instance, you might find that one night of skimping on Zs doesn't affect you much, but two nights in a row leave you lethargic, hungry, and sedentary.

Hunger. This one's usually obvious: Let yourself get too hungry and you overeat. The hunger scale, written at the bottom of your Tracker, goes like this:

1	=	Ravenous
2	=	A little hungry
3	=	Neither hungry nor full
4	=	A little full
5	=	Ugh! Too full.

Note your hunger level both *before* and *after* eating. So, you'd write in "1/5" if you went into a meal at "1" and got up from the meal a "5." Your goal: start eating at a "2" and leave the table at a "3" or "4."

Time of Day. How often do you eat? If you wait too long in between meals, you're going to see a lot of "1s" in your hunger scale column. If your meals are reasonably sized (something you're working toward in *The Pescetarian Plan*) hunger should kick in three to four hours after eating. When you're at a "2" have a meal or a snack. See Appendix C for snack suggestions.

Food and Drink. Use this information to:

1. Identify unhealthy foods. Eating too many sweets, fried foods, soda, and the like? Take note of them, and decide which ones you want to tackle first. Chapters 5 and 6 are your guides. If you're eating too many sweets and other treats, start limiting these foods (see page 61 for your daily treat calorie max). If your meals contain fried foods, meat, white bread, and the like, you might work on cleaning up one food group at a time. For instance, you could start with protein (page 55) and shift away from meat to fish.
2. Identify healthy foods. Eating fruits, vegetables, whole grains, fish, nuts, and other healthy foods? Give yourself a pat on the back, and vow to keep it up. Circle the meals and snacks you enjoyed, and make them again (and again).
3. Find out how your meals affect hunger, exercise, and even sleep. For instance, some meals are very satiating, meaning they keep you feeling full longer, for the calories. Others leave you hungry an hour later. Other meals sap energy—you might find they put the brakes on exercise even hours after eating them. Also, certain acidic or spicy foods or caffeinated beverages may make it harder to get to sleep, or may disrupt sleep.

Exercise. Tally up your weekly minutes of aerobic exercise. (Even if you fill out this log for just four days, record exercise minutes for seven days.) If it's not even close to the recommended 150 minutes (explained in chapter 9), don't be discouraged. We'll get you there! You can also track steps, using a pedometer. Ideally you'd hit 10,000 steps daily. Not there yet? Add 1,000 steps per day—hold that level for two weeks—then increase by another 1,000 steps per day for another two weeks, and so forth.

Also note any ripple effects of exercise—do you tend to eat more nutritiously after workout sessions? Sleep better?

Situations/emotions. Stress, loneliness, even exuberance can trigger overeating. Look for connections like heading to the vending machine after a tense encounter with your boss, or tearing into the bag of cookies at the end of a stressful day. Time of day can also be a trigger. For example, if you habitually have a coffee and doughnut at 10:30 A.M., that's just what you're going to crave at that hour. We all do a little emotional eating, but when it crosses the line, it'll be next to impossible to lose weight and keep it off. If you feel out of control around food, turn to chapter 9 for some useful tips.

Food Groups. The "Grain/Starchy Vegetables," "Fruit" and other foods groups at the bottom of the chart help you quickly assess how closely you're adhering to the Pescetarian Plan. As I explained in chapters 5 and 6, it takes a little studying up, but soon you'll know just what a portion of cereal, milk (or soy milk), fish, or other foods looks like. From your Food and Drink column, figure out how many portions of each food group you had. For instance, you had an egg? Write down "1" next to Protein. Later that day, you had a 4-ounce piece of salmon? Add "+4." If that's all the protein servings you had, then your total is "5." Do this for all the other food groups.

The exception is "Treats." Instead of food groups, you count up treat calories, which you can usually find on the back of the chocolate bar, box of cookies, or other packaged items. If there is no food label, use your best guess.

APPENDIX B

～～～

Weight and Inches Log

WEEK #	DATE	WEIGHT	WAIST (INCHES)	THIGHS (INCHES)	OTHER MEASUREMENT	OTHER MEASUREMENT

WEEK #	DATE	WEIGHT	WAIST (INCHES)	THIGHS (INCHES)	OTHER MEASUREMENT	OTHER MEASUREMENT

APPENDIX C

<hr style="width:15%">

Pescetarian Meals

This may be the most flexible plan you've ever tried. You choose the breakfast, lunch, dinner, snack, and treat—any combo will work. For a refresher on how the plan works, see chapter 8, starting on page 95.

BREAKFASTS

Breakfast stats: Breakfasts on the 1,500- and 1,800-calorie plans are approximately 390 calories; those on the 2,100 and 2,500 plan are approximately 440 calories. Breakfasts have at least 300 mg of calcium with no more than 425 mg of sodium. The ratio of omega-6 to omega-3 fats is, on average, 1 to 1.

A note on chia seeds and flaxseeds: Both are ultra-rich sources of ALA—the plant form of omega-3 described on pages 36 to 37. Sprinkling them on cereal or other foods is a great way to take in this healthy fat; they're both approximately 50 calories per tablespoon. You must grind flaxseeds to ensure that your body absorbs them, and preliminary research is showing the same may be true for chia (soaking or cooking in liquid may also help). Because both chia and flaxseeds tend to swell and even get a little slimy, I prefer adding the ground seeds to my spoon or fork just before taking a bite. They stay crunchy that way.

. . . .

Chia Pudding with Berries and Almonds with Sliced Banana

1,500- AND 1,800-CALORIE PLANS:

Chia Pudding with Berries and Almonds,
1 serving (page 158)

Top with ¼ of a sliced **banana**

2,100- and 2,500-calorie plans: Same as above, but top with an additional ¾ of a banana for a total of 1 sliced banana.

. . . .

Cereal, Fruit, and Milk

1,500- AND 1,800-CALORIE PLANS:

100% **whole-grain cereal** with no more than
5 g sugar/175 calories (such as 1 cup Kashi
7 Grain Flakes or a scant half cup of Ezekiel 4:9)

1   cup **nonfat milk** or **soy milk**
2   tablespoons **walnuts**
2/3   cup **blueberries** (or other **fruit**)

2,100- and 2,500-calorie plans: Same as above, but add a tablespoon of walnuts for a total of 3 tablespoons of walnuts.

. . . .

Black Beans, Salsa, and Eggs

1,500- AND 1,800-CALORIE PLANS:

Heat a 10-inch heavy-bottomed skillet; add:

2   teaspoons **olive oil**

Scramble one egg and one egg white in the olive oil.

When nearly set, move to one side of pan and in the empty space add:

½   cup **black beans**

Heat for 1 minute. Transfer eggs and beans to a serving plate. Top the beans with:

2   tablespoons fresh or jarred **salsa** (preferably no
    more than 100 mg sodium per 2-tablespoon
    serving)

1   tablespoon shredded **reduced fat cheddar** or
    other **cheese**

Serve with:

3/4   cup **nonfat milk** (plain or heated as part
      of a latte)

2,100- and 2,500-calorie plans: Same as above, but have an additional ¼ cup of black
beans for a total of ¾ cup of black beans and ¼ cup of nonfat milk for a total of 1 cup
of nonfat milk.

. . . .

Black Rice Pudding

1,500- AND 1,800-CALORIE PLANS:

Black Rice Pudding, 1 serving (page 155)

2,100- and 2,500-calorie plans: Stir in 1½ teaspoons of almond butter.

. . . .

Trout and Scrambled Egg with Almond Milk and Cantaloupe

1,500- AND 1,800-CALORIE PLANS:

Trout and Scrambled Egg, 1 serving (page 161): Serve with ¾ cup of
almond milk and ¾ cup of diced cantaloupe.

2,100- and 2,500-calorie plans: Same as above, but serve with an additional ¼ cup
of almond milk for a total of 1 cup of almond milk and an additional ½ cup of
diced cantaloupe for a total of 1¼ cups of diced cantaloupe.

. . . .

Yogurt, Fruit, and Chia

1,500- AND 1,800-CALORIE PLANS:

In a medium bowl, combine:

1   cup plain **nonfat Greek yogurt**

3   tablespoons **walnuts**

1 cup **strawberries**, halved (or other **fruit**)

2 tablespoons **granola** (from page 159 or store-bought)

1 teaspoon ground **chia seeds**

2,100- and 2,500-calorie plans: Same as above, but add another tablespoon of granola for a total of 3 tablespoons and another ½ teaspoon of chia seeds for a total of 1½ teaspoons of chia seeds.

· · · ·

Green Shake

1,500- AND 1,800-CALORIE PLANS:

Green Shake, 1 serving (page 160)

2,100- and 2,500-calorie plans: Add a tablespoon of nuts to the shake.

· · · ·

Crunchy Granola with Soy Milk

1,500- AND 1,800-CALORIE PLANS:

Crunchy Granola, 1 serving (page 159) with 1 cup **soy milk** or nonfat or 1% milk

2,100- and 2,500-calorie plans: Same as above, but add a tablespoon of nuts or seeds.

· · · ·

English Muffin, Almond Butter, and Pear

1,500- AND 1,800-CALORIE PLANS:

Spread half a toasted whole-grain English muffin (such as Ezekiel) with:

4 teaspoons **almond butter**

Top with:

slices from a small pear—have the rest of the pear with your breakfast

Serve with:

1   cup **nonfat milk** or **soy milk**, plain or as a latte

2,100- and 2,500-calorie plans: Same as above, but add half an English muffin for a total of 1 whole English muffin.

. . . .

Apple Oatmeal

1,500- AND 1,800-CALORIE PLANS:

Cook ¼ cup of steel-cut oats according to package directions using ½ nonfat milk (or soy milk) and ½ water (this will vary—you need more water for regular steel-cut oats and less for the quick-cooking type). In the last 5 minutes of cooking, add:

a small **apple**, chopped,

a dash of **nutmeg** and **cinnamon**

Top with:

1½   tablespoons **walnuts**

Serve with:

a total of 1 cup **nonfat milk** or **soy milk** in this breakfast (use some for the oatmeal).

2,100- and 2,500-calorie plans: Same as above, add another 1½ tablespoons of walnuts for a total of 3 tablespoons walnuts.

. . . .

Whole-Grain Pancake with Banana and Cafe au Lait

1,500- AND 1,800-CALORIE PLANS:

Whole-Grain Pancake with Banana, 1 serving (page 163) with ¾ cup coffee mixed with ¾ cup almond milk

---

2,100- and 2,500-calorie plans: Same as above, but top pancakes with a tablespoon of chopped walnuts.

. . . .

On the Run

¼ cup unsalted **almonds**

1 small **banana**

12 ounces **skim latte**

2,100- and 2,500-calorie plans: Same as above, but add another tablespoon of almonds for a total of ¼ cup of almonds plus 1 tablespoon.

. . . .

Carrot Muffin and Skim Milk

Carrot Muffin, 1 serving (page 156) with 1 cup skim milk

2,100- and 2,500-calorie plans: Same as above, but spread muffin with two teaspoons of peanut butter, no sugar added.

. . . .

French Toast with Berries

In a shallow, medium bowl, mix together:

3 tablespoons **egg whites**

3 tablespoons **soy milk** (regular or vanilla)

⅛ teaspoon **vanilla extract**

Dip 2 slices 100% whole-grain bread (80 calories per slice) into the egg mixture.

Spray a warm griddle with vegetable oil cooking spray.

Gently drop soaked bread onto griddle, cook 4 minutes on each side.

Top with:

2 teaspoons **maple syrup**

½   cup **blueberries** (or other **fruit**)

1   tablespoon **walnuts**

Serve with: ¾ cup nonfat milk or soy milk (plain or as a latte)

2,100- and 2,500-calorie plans: Same as above, but add another tablespoon of walnuts for a total of 2 tablespoons of walnuts.

HIGH-CALCIUM SNACKS

(For everyone at all daily calorie levels)

High-Calcium Snack stats: These snacks are approximately 150 calories and contain at least 200 mg calcium and no more than 175 mg sodium. The ratio of omega-6 to omega-3 fats is, on average, 1 to 1.

. . . .

Yogurt, Pistachios, and Pear

In a small bowl mix together:

1/2	cup **plain nonfat yogurt**
1/2	**pear**, chopped
10	**pistachio kernels**

. . . .

Peach Cinnamon Smoothie (page 251)

. . . .

Cucumber Yogurt

In a small bowl, combine:

3/4	cup **plain nonfat yogurt**
1	cup **cucumber**, chopped
1/2	teaspoon **grainy mustard**
1/2	teaspoon **olive oil**
1/2	teaspoon fresh **lemon juice**

. . . .

Strawberry Milk (page 252)

. . . .

Yogurt, Banana, Peanut Butter Pop (page 254)

. . . .

Latte and Almonds

Have a 12-ounce skim latte with 8 almonds.

. . . .

Greek Yogurt Dip

Dip:

$\frac{1}{2}$ cup **carrot sticks**

In:

$\frac{1}{2}$ cup **nonfat Greek yogurt**

Topped with:

1 teaspoon ground **chia seeds**
1 teaspoon **olive oil**
Dried **oregano** to taste

. . . .

Cheddar, Pear, and Walnuts

Have 1 ounce Cabot 75% cheddar with $\frac{1}{2}$ pear and 1 tablespoon walnuts (6 halves).

LUNCHES

Lunch stats: Lunch on the 1,500-calorie plan is 425 calories. On the 1,800- and 2,100-calorie plans it's 500 calories. On the 2,500-calorie plan, lunch is 600 calories. Lunches have no more than 575 mg sodium. The ratio of omega-6 to omega-3 fats is, on average, 1 to 1.

· · · ·

Sardines on Toast

1,500-CALORIE PLAN:

Mix together:

- 1 can (3.75 to 4.5) **sardines** packed in water, preferably low-sodium
- 2 tablespoons chopped **parsley**
- 1½ teaspoons **lemon juice**
- 1 tablespoon **olive oil**
- ⅙ teaspoon crushed **garlic** (or to taste)

Serve with:

- 1 slice **whole-wheat bread**

End meal with 1 kiwi (or other small fruit)

1,800- and 2,100-calorie plans: Same as above, but have another slice of bread for a total of 2 slices, and drizzle a teaspoon of olive oil on the toast.

2,500-calorie plan: To the 1,800 and 2,100 plan add 2 more kiwi for a total of 3 kiwi.

· · · ·

Kale Soup with Mozzarella, Tomato, and Avocado Sandwich

1,500-CALORIE PLAN:

Kale Soup, 1 serving (page 174)

Serve with sandwich:

2 slices **whole-wheat bread**

1 ounce **mozzarella cheese**

2 slices **tomato**

1/8 of an **avocado**

drizzle sandwich filler ingredients with
1½ teaspoons **olive oil** and top with
1 tablespoon chopped **basil**

1,800- and 2,100-calorie plans: End the meal with one medium apple.

2,500-calorie plan: End the meal with one large apple and one kiwi.

. . . .

Cod Burger with Walnut Salad

1,500-CALORIE PLAN:

Cod Burger, 1 serving (page 218)

Serve with walnut salad; toss together:

1½ cups **salad greens**

1½ tablespoons **walnuts**

1 teaspoon **olive oil**

Splash of **sherry vinegar**

1,800- and 2,100-calorie plans: Same as above, but make an open-faced cod burger on half of a whole-grain bun. Use 2 tablespoons walnuts on salad.

2,500-calorie plan: To the 1,800 and 2,100 plan, add the other half of the bun and add ½ teaspoon of olive oil for a total of 1½ teaspoons of olive oil on salad.

. . . .

Whole-Grain Couscous with Rice Vinegar with Greens and Sardines

1,500-CALORIE PLAN:

Whole-Grain Couscous with Rice Vinegar and Herbs, 1 serving (page 193)

Serve over a salad of greens and sardines; toss together:

1 3.75-ounce can of **sardines** packed in water, no salt added

2 cups **salad greens**

2 teaspoons **olive oil**

1/2 teaspoon **lemon juice**

Serve with:

1^{1}/2 cups **strawberry** halves

1,800- and 2,100-calorie plans: See above, but add 1½ tablespoons of walnuts to the couscous.

2,500-calorie plan: To the 1,800 and 2,100 plan, add ½ tablespoon of walnuts to the couscous for a total of 2 tablespoons, and add a teaspoon of olive oil to the salad for a total of 1 tablespoon.

. . . .

Red Lentils with Lime and Cilantro

1,500-CALORIE PLAN:

Red Lentils with Lime and Cilantro, 1 serving (page 191)

Serve in a warmed medium 6-inch corn tortilla stuffed with half an avocado and ½ cup of greens. End meal with one small apple for dessert.

1,800- and 2,100-calorie plans: Same as above, but stuff the lentil mixture into a warmed large 8-inch corn tortilla and top with 1½ tablespoons of reduced fat sour cream or vegan sour cream.

2,500-calorie plan: To the 1,800 and 2,100 plan, add another ½ tablespoon of reduced fat sour cream or vegan sour cream for a total of 2 tablespoons. Instead of one small apple, end the meal with 1¼ cups of grapes.

. . . .

Shiitake Quick Broth with Edamame and Brown Rice Noodles

1,500-CALORIE PLAN:

Shiitake Quick Broth with Edamame and Brown Rice Noodles, 1 serving (page 203)

1,800- and 2,100-calorie plans: Same as above, but add ⅓ cup of diced tofu to the soup.

2,500-calorie plan: To the 1,500 plan, add ½ cup diced tofu. End the meal with one large orange.

. . . .

Sardine Niçoise with Whole-Wheat Toast

1,500-CALORIE PLAN:

**Sardine Niçoise, 1 serving (page 234) with two slices of toasted
100% whole-grain bread. End the meal with 1 small piece fruit.**

1,800- and 2,100-calorie plans: Same as above, but instead of a small piece of fruit,
have a large piece of fruit.

2,500-calorie plan: In addition to the 1,800 and 2,100 plan, drizzle 2½ teaspoons of
olive oil on the toast.

. . . .

Black Rice with Arugula Shrimp Salad

1,500-CALORIE PLAN:

Black Rice with Sesame and Green Onions, 1 serving (page 185)

Serve with arugula shrimp salad; toss together:

4	ounces precooked **shrimp** (or steam them yourself, see chapter 12 for cooking how-to)
2	cups **arugula**
2	teaspoons **olive oil**
½	teaspoon **lemon juice**
	Dash of **salt**

1,800- and 2,100-calorie plans: Same as above, but have an additional ½ serving of
black rice salad for a total of 1½ servings of black rice salad.

2,500-calorie plan: To the 1,800 and 2,100 plan, add one ounce of shrimp for a total of
5 ounces of shrimp, and add one teaspoon of olive oil for a total of 1 tablespoon of
olive oil and adjust lemon juice in dressing to taste.

. . . .

On-the-run

1,500-CALORIE PLAN:

1	large **banana**
1	cup plain **nonfat Greek yogurt**

2 tablespoons **almonds**

1 cup baby **carrots**

Slice banana into yogurt and stir in almonds. Serve carrots on the side.

1,800- and 2,100-calorie plan: Same as above, but have an additional 1 ½ tablespoons of almonds for a total of 3½ tablespoons of almonds.

2,500-calorie plan: To the 1,800- and 2,100 plan, add an additional half a cup of Greek yogurt for a total of 1½ cups of plain nonfat Greek yogurt.

· · · ·

Tuna Salad Sandwich

1,500-CALORIE PLAN:

Mix together:

1 5-ounce can of **light (skipjack) tuna**, preferably no-salt-added

1 tablespoon + 1 teaspoon **mayonnaise**

2 tablespoons each: chopped **celery** and **carrot**

1½ to 2 teaspoons **mustard** (to taste), preferably no more than 50 mg sodium/teaspoon, such as Gulden's

1 teaspoon each: **olive oil** and **lemon juice**

Serve on two slices of whole-grain bread (about 70 calories each)

With: 2 stalks celery

1,800- and 2,100-calorie plan: Same as above, but end the meal with a medium orange.

2,500-calorie plan: Same as the 1,800 and 2,100 plan, but have 1½ tablespoons of nuts with the orange.

· · · ·

Garbanzo Bean, Red Pepper, Pumpkin Seed, and Olive Salad

1,500-CALORIE PLAN:

Mix together:

1   cup canned, rinsed, and drained **garbanzo beans** (**chickpeas**), preferably no salt added, such as Eden Foods brand

1   cup chopped **red pepper** (or **other vegetable** of your choice)

⅓   cup chopped **cilantro**

3   **olives**, roughly chopped

1   tablespoon chopped **green onion**

1   tablespoon **pumpkin seeds** (or other **seeds** or **nuts**)

In a small bowl, combine, then add to bean mixture:

1½   teaspoons **olive oil**

1   teaspoon **lemon juice**

Sprinkle with a dash of salt.

1,800- and 2,100-calorie plans: Same as above, but add two tablespoons of garbanzo beans and a teaspoon of olive oil for a total of 2½ teaspoons of olive oil.

2,500-calorie plan: Same as the 1,800 and 2,100 plan, but end the meal with one large piece of fruit.

. . . .

Salmon Salad

1,500-CALORIE PLAN:

Top one slice (70–80 calories) 100% whole-grain bread with:

1   serving **Salmon Salad** (page 227)

Serve with:

at least 1 cup of **celery** stalks and baby **carrots**

1,800- and 2,100-calorie plans: Same as above, but end the meal with a piece of fruit.

2,500-calorie plan: Same as the 1,800- and 2,100 plan, but use an additional half an avocado (sliced) in the salmon salad.

. . . .

Open-Faced Peanut Butter and Apple

1,500-CALORIE PLAN:

Spread 1 slice 100% whole-grain bread with:

2   tablespoons **peanut butter**

slices from a small **apple**

Serve with:

The rest of the **apple**

1   cup **nonfat milk** or **soy milk** (preferably calcium-enriched)

- -

1,800- and 2,100-calorie plans: Same as above, but add one slice of 100% whole-grain bread for a total of 2 slices of bread.

- -

2,500-calorie plan: To the 1,800 and 2,100 plan, add a tablespoon of peanut butter for a total of 3 tablespoons of peanut butter.

- -

. . . .

Cannellini Bean Spread on Toast

1,500-CALORIE PLAN:

Mash together:

½   cup plus 1 tablespoon canned **cannellini beans**, no salt added or low sodium, drained

1½   teaspoons **lemon juice**

½   teaspoon **olive oil**

1   tablespoon chopped **basil** (or other **herb**)

2   **olives**, chopped

Dash of **salt**

Spread mixture on:

2   slices (70–80 calories each) 100% **whole-grain bread**

Top with:

1 tablespoon crumbled **feta cheese**

½ **avocado**, sliced

1,800- and 2,100-calorie plans: Same as above, but drizzle 2½ teaspoons of olive oil on the bread.

2,500-calorie plan: Same as the 1,800 and 2,100 plan, but have 1¼ cups of berries or chopped fruit.

FRUIT OR VEGETABLE SNACKS

(for those following the 2,100-calorie and the

2,500-calorie plans only)

Fruit/Vegetable Snack stats: 200 calories, no more than 100 mg sodium. The ratio of omega-6 to omega-3 fats is, on average, 1 to 1.

. . . .

Apple with Spiced Sesame (page 255)

. . . .

Two bananas

. . . .

Mango and pistachios

Have a heaping cup of mango slices sprinkled with 22 pistachios

. . . .

Banana Frozen with Cocoa and Peanuts (page 256)

. . . .

Cucumber, Mango, and Avocado Kebab (page 257)

. . . .

Grapes and Almonds

Have one cup of grapes with two tablespoons of almonds

DINNERS

Dinner stats: The 1,500-calorie plan dinner is 500 calories; it's 600 calories on the 1,800- and 2,100-calorie plans, and 700 calories on the 2,500-calorie plan. Dinners contain no more than 750 mg sodium. The ratio of omega-6 to omega-3 fats is, on average, 1 to 1.

. . . .

Shrimp Taco Salad with Fresh Salsa

1,500-CALORIE PLAN:

Shrimp Taco Salad, 1 serving (page 240), plus 2 tablespoons black beans

Top with fresh salsa, mix together:

½ cup chopped **tomato**

½ teaspoon chopped **onion**

¼ teaspoon chopped **jalapeño** (or to taste)

1 teaspoon **lime juice**

1,800- and 2,100-calorie plans: Same as above, but add an extra ½ cup of black beans to the salad for a total of ½ cup plus two tablespoons.

2,500-calorie plan: Same as the 1,800 and 2,100 plan, but end the meal with a medium piece of fruit.

. . . .

Salmon with Tahini and Toasted Nuts with Quinoa with Lemon, Olive Oil, and Pomegranate and a Salad

1,500-CALORIE PLAN:

Salmon with Tahini and Toasted Nuts, 1 serving (page 230) with Quinoa with Lemon, Olive Oil, and Pomegranate, 1 serving (page 190)

Serve with a salad, mix together:

2 cups **mixed greens**

2 teaspoons **olive oil**

1 teaspoon **balsamic vinegar**

⅛ **avocado**, chopped

1,800- and 2,100-calorie plans: Same as above, but end the meal with a cup of strawberries with a tablespoon of chopped pecans.

2,500-calorie plan: Same as the 1,800 and 2,100 plan, but chop ⅓ of an avocado in the salad, and end the meal with an additional cup of strawberries for a total of 2 cups of strawberries.

. . . .

Tofu Sloppy Joe with Side Salad and Berries

1,500-CALORIE PLAN:

Tofu Sloppy Joe, 1 serving (page 206)

Serve with a side salad, toss together:

2	cups **greens**
½	cup **cucumber**
2	teaspoons **olive oil**
1	teaspoon **vinegar**
	Dash of **salt**

End the meal with:

½	cup **berries**

1,800- and 2,100-calorie plans: Same as above, but top the salad with two tablespoons of chopped pecans. End the meal with an additional ½ cup berries for a total of 1 cup of berries.

2,500-calorie plan: Same as the 1,800 and 2,100 plan, but add a tablespoon of chopped pecans for a total of 3 tablespoons of chopped pecans, and end the meal with an additional ½ cup of berries for a total of 1½ cups of berries.

. . . .

Fish and Greens

1,500-CALORIE PLAN:

Preheat oven to 425°F. Meanwhile, in a small bowl, mix together:

2	teaspoons **mayonnaise**
1	teaspoon **mustard** (preferably no more than 50 mg sodium/teaspoon, such as Gulden's)
½	teaspoon **horseradish**
1	tablespoon chopped **dill**

Rub a 5-ounce farm-raised trout fillet with a teaspoon of olive oil and place, skin-side down, in small pan sprayed with vegetable oil.

Top with the mayonnaise mixture. Cook for 8 to 12 minutes, to desired doneness.

While the fish is cooking, heat a 10-inch skillet. Spray with vegetable oil cooking spray, and add:

½ teaspoon **olive oil**

½ teaspoon **dark sesame seed oil**

Add a teaspoon of finely chopped ginger and ⅛ teaspoon of chopped garlic to the oil. Cook for 20 seconds, then add:

6 cups washed cooking **greens**, such as **spinach**, **chard**, **kale**—chopped if necessary

Stir-fry on medium-high heat for 40 seconds to 2 minutes—until just wilted. Sprinkle with a dash of salt and serve with the fish.

Serve with:

80-calorie slice of **whole-grain bread**

- - - - - - - -

1,800- and 2,100-calorie plans: Same as above, but add 1½ teaspoons of olive oil to dip bread with, and end the meal with a kiwi or another small fruit.

- - - - - - - -

2,500-calorie plan: Same as the 1,800 and 2,100 plan, but add another slice of bread, and add ½ teaspoon of olive oil for a total of 2 teaspoons of olive oil for dipping.

- - - - - - - -

· · · ·

Whole-Grain Pasta Baked with White Beans, Spinach, and Walnut Sauce

1,500-CALORIE PLAN:

Whole-Grain Pasta Baked with White Beans, Spinach, and Walnut Sauce, 1 serving (page 212)

- - - - - - - -

1,800- and 2,100-calorie plans: Same as above, but have a cup of grapes for dessert.

- - - - - - - -

2,500-calorie plan: Same as the 1,800 and 2,100 plan, plus:

Have with:

1 medium **tomato**, sliced

Dress with:

> 2 teaspoons **olive oil**
> ½ teaspoon **sherry vinegar** or **other vinegar**
> Pinch of **salt**
> Freshly ground **black pepper**

. . . .

Cod, Cauliflower, and Pea Curry with Mango and Brown Rice

1,500-CALORIE PLAN:

Cod, Cauliflower, and Pea Curry, 1 serving (page 220) with seasoned rice

Mix together:

> ½ cup cooked **brown rice**
> 2 teaspoons **olive oil**
> Dash of **salt**
> **Black pepper**

Serve with:

> ½ cup chopped **mango** as a relish for the curry

1,800- and 2,100-calorie plans: Same as above, but add ¼ cup of brown rice to the seasoned rice mixture for a total of ¾ cup of cooked brown rice. Also:

Mix together:

> ⅓ cup **nonfat plain yogurt**
> ½ cup chopped **cucumber**

Serve with the rice and curry.

2,500-calorie plan: Same as the 1,800 and 2,100 plan, but add an additional ¾ cup of chopped mango for a total of 1¼ cups of chopped mango as a relish for the curry.

. . . .

Seafood Stew and Broccoli Salad with Berries

1,500-CALORIE PLAN:

> Seafood Stew, 1 serving (page 237) and Broccoli Salad, 1 serving (page 168)
>
> **End the meal with:**

$\frac{1}{2}$ cup **berries**

1,800- and 2,100-calorie plans: Same as above, but serve with one slice of 100% whole-grain bread dipped in a half teaspoon of olive oil.

2,500-calorie plan: Same as the 1,800 and 2,100 plan, but use an additional $\frac{1}{2}$ teaspoon of olive oil for a total of one teaspoon of olive oil. End the meal with an additional $\frac{3}{4}$ cup of berries for a total of $1\frac{1}{4}$ cups of berries.

. . . .

One-Dish Lentil Soup

1,500-CALORIE PLAN:

> **In a medium pan, heat together:**

1 can **Amy's Light in Sodium Lentil Soup** (or **other bean soup** with no more than 300 mg sodium per cup)

2 tablespoons dry, **whole-wheat couscous**

1$\frac{1}{2}$ cups chopped **kale**

1 cup **water**

> Let it come to a simmer, cover, and let simmer for 5 minutes, or until couscous is cooked.

1,800- and 2,100-calorie plans: Same as above, but add an apple.

2,500-calorie plan: Same as the 1,800 and 2,100 plan, but dip the apple in $\frac{1}{3}$ cup of plain nonfat Greek yogurt mixed with one tablespoon of honey and a dash of cinnamon.

. . . .

Shrimp Grilled with Barbecue Peach Chutney with Corn Salad and Watermelon

1,500-CALORIE PLAN:

> Shrimp Grilled with Barbecue Peach Chutney, 1 serving (page 239)
> with Corn Salad, 1 serving (page 186)
>
> End meal with:

3 cups diced **watermelon** or other **fruit** of your choice

---

1,800- and 2,100-calorie plans: Same as above, but serve with a salad of:

---

2 cups shredded **cabbage** dressed with

2 teaspoons **olive oil**

1/4 teaspoon **cider vinegar**

Pinch of **sugar**

Dash of **salt**

Freshly ground **black pepper**

2,500-calorie plan: To the 1,800 and 2,100 plan, add 2 tablespoons of chopped pecans to the cabbage salad.

. . . .

Salad with Avocado and Hardboiled Eggs

NOTE: Whole eggs should be eaten in moderation because they are high in cholesterol. See note on page 56 for the full explanation of how to fit eggs and other high-cholesterol foods into your diet.

1,500-CALORIE PLAN:

Combine:

4 cups **mixed greens**

1/2 **Hass avocado**, sliced

2 tablespoons chopped **dill** (or other **herb**)

1/2 cup **garbanzo beans** (no salt added or low sodium)

Whisk in small bowl:

> ½   teaspoon **lemon juice**
>
> ½   teaspoon **balsamic vinegar**
>
> ½   teaspoon **mustard** (preferably no more than 50 mg sodium/teaspoon, such as Gulden's)
>
> 1 ½   teaspoons **olive oil**

Toss salad dressing with the greens. Top with:

> 1   **hardboiled egg**, cut in half and sprinkled with pepper and a dash of salt

Serve with:

> 1   slice **whole-wheat bread** (70–80 calories)

1,800- and 2,100-calorie plans: Same as above, but add another egg for a total of two eggs and use an additional 2 tablespoons of garbanzo beans for a total of ½ cup plus 2 tablespoons of garbanzo beans.

2,500-calorie plan: To the 1,800- and 2,100 plan, add 1 tablespoon of crumbled feta, and end the meal with ¾ cup of grapes.

. . . .

Haddock Tacos with Sliced Tomato

1,500-CALORIE PLAN:

Haddock Tacos, 1 serving or 2 tacos (page 223)

Serve with:

> 1   medium **tomato**, sliced, dressed with:
>
> 2   teaspoons **olive oil**
>
> ¼   teaspoon **lime juice**

End the meal with:

> ½   cup **berries**

1,800- and 2,100-calorie plans: Same as above, but add ½ cup of berries for a total of one cup of berries topped with 1 tablespoon of chopped pecans.

2,500-calorie plan: Same as the 1,800 and 2,100 plan, but top the berries with an additional 1½ tablespoons of chopped pecans for a total of 2½ tablespoons of chopped pecans.

. . . .

Eggplant Stuffed with Lentils with Tomato Salad

1,500-CALORIE PLAN:

Eggplant Stuffed with Lentils, 1 serving (page 201)

Serve with a tomato salad; toss together:

1	medium **tomato**, diced
1½	teaspoons **olive oil**
¼	teaspoon **sherry vinegar** or ½ teaspoon **other vinegar** of your choice
	Black pepper
⅛	teaspoon **salt**

1,800- and 2,100-calorie plan: Same as above, but have one slice of whole-wheat bread with a teaspoon of olive oil for dipping.

2,500-calorie plan: Same as the 1,800- and 2,100 plan, but end the meal with 1 ¼ cups of berries.

. . . .

Clams with Tomatoes, Garlic on Whole-Grain Pasta with Wilted Spinach

1,500-CALORIE PLAN:

Clams with Tomatoes and Garlic on Whole-Grain Pasta, 1 serving (page 217)

Top with:

3	tablespoons grated **Parmesan cheese**

Serve with:

4	cups **spinach**

Tossed with:

2	teaspoons **olive oil**

Wilt in 350°F oven for 3 minutes.

Top spinach with:

Dash of **salt**

Freshly ground **black pepper**

1,800- and 2,100-calorie plans: Same as above, but end the meal with 1¼ cups of berries.

2,500-calorie plan: Same as the 1,800 and 2,100 plan, but top the berries with two tablespoons of chopped pecans.

. . . .

Curried Tuna Garbanzo Apricot (makes 2 servings)

1,500-CALORIE PLAN:

Combine in a medium bowl:

1   15-ounce can **garbanzo beans**, drained (preferably no salt added)

1   6-ounce can of water-packed **"skipjack"** or **"chunk light" tuna** (preferably low sodium)

⅓   cup chopped **dried apricots** (preferably Turkish)

½   cup of chopped **cilantro**

¼   cup roasted unsalted **almonds** (whole or roughly chopped)

In a small bowl, whisk together:

2   tablespoons **plain nonfat yogurt**

2   teaspoons **olive oil**

½   teaspoon **curry powder**

⅛   teaspoon of **salt** (skip it if the beans and tuna are not low-sodium)

Toss dressing with the bean mixture, divide in half.

Serve with:

One large stalk of **celery** per serving

NOTE: You can sub in a cup of halved grapes or chopped apples for the apricots.

1,800- and 2,100-calorie plan: Same as above, but use an additional ¼ cup of almonds for a total of ½ cup of almonds for the entire recipe (2 servings).

2,500-calorie plan: To the 1,800 and 2,100 plan, add 100 calories of a whole-grain cracker per serving.

EXTRA 150-CALORIE SNACKS

(2,500-calorie plan only)

Extra snack stats: 150 calories, no more than 175 mg sodium.
NOTE: If you're on the 2,500-calorie plan, you get three snacks: two 150-calorie snacks and one fruit/vegetable snack (200 calories). For the two 150-cal snacks, you can either have 2 calcium snacks (list begins on page 292) or have one calcium snack and one of the snacks below. For guidance on how to create your own using food groups, see page 98 in Chapter 8. The ratio of omega-6 to omega-3 fats is, on average, 1 to 1.

Black Bean Roll Up Wrapped in Romaine (page 249)

Chickpeas Roasted with Oregano (page 250)

Yogurt Avocado Dip (page 253)

3 tablespoons nuts or seeds of your choice

Whole grain cracker (60 calories) spread with a tablespoon of nut butter

TREATS

Treat stats: A 100-calorie treat every other day on the 1,500-calorie plan; a daily 150-calorie treat on the 1,800-calorie plan; a daily 200-calorie treat on the 2,100-calorie plan, and a daily 250-calorie treat on the 2,500-calorie plan.

* * * *

Grape Granita (page 262)

1,500-calorie plan: 1 serving (every other day)
1,800-calorie plan: 1½ servings

2,100-calorie plan: 1½ servings topped with 1 tablespoon
   crushed almonds

2,500-calorie plan: 1½ servings topped with 3 tablespoons
   crushed almonds

. . . .

Dark Chocolate

1,500-calorie plan: ¾ ounce (every other day)

1,800-calorie plan: 1 ounce

2,100-calorie plan: 1⅓ ounces

2,500-calorie plan: 1¾ ounces

. . . .

Melon with Lemon Sauce (page 263)

1,500-calorie plan: 1 serving (every other day)

1,800-calorie plan: 1½ servings

2,100-calorie plan: 1½ servings plus ½ cup blueberries

2,500-calorie plan: 2 servings plus ½ cup blueberries

. . . .

Air-Popped Popcorn (unsalted) with Parmesan Cheese

1,500-calorie plan: 3 cups sprinkled with 2 teaspoons grated
   Parmesan cheese and a dash of salt (every other day)

1,800-calorie plan: 4½ cups sprinkled with 2 teaspoons grated
   Parmesan cheese and a dash of salt

2,100-calorie plan: 6 cups sprinkled with 1 tablespoon grated Parmesan cheese and a dash of salt

2,500-calorie plan: 6 cups sprinkled with 1 tablespoon grated Parmesan cheese, 1 tablespoon unsalted pumpkin seeds, and a
   dash of salt

. . . .

Pears Baked with Rosemary and Walnuts (page 265)

1,500-calorie plan: ½ serving (every other day)

1,800-calorie plan: ½ serving with an extra tablespoon of walnuts

2,100-calorie plan: 1 serving

2,500-calorie plan: 1½ servings

....

Ice Cream with Berries

1,500-calorie plan: ½ cup reduced-fat ice cream, with no artificial sweeteners, containing about 100 calories per half cup (such as some sorbets, and some of the Breyers, Edy's or Dreyer's offerings) topped with 2 tablespoons blueberries or other fruit (every other day)

1,800-calorie plan: ¾ cup ice cream (same type as above) with berries

2,100-calorie plan: ¾ cup ice cream (same type as above) with berries and 1 teaspoon crushed nuts

2,500-calorie plan: 1 cup ice cream (same type as above) with berries and 1 teaspoon crushed nuts

....

Flavored Yogurt

1,500-calorie plan: 100–110 calories of vanilla, fruit, or other flavored yogurt of your choice that doesn't contain artificial sweeteners (every other day)

1,800-calorie plan: Have 140 to 160 calories, such as a 6-ounce Dannon Fruit on the Bottom

2,100-calorie plan: Have 140–160 calories, but add 1 tablespoon nuts

2,500-calorie plan: Have 140–160 calories, but have a total of 2 tablespoons nuts

....

Cookies and Tea

1,500-calorie plan: 100–115 calories of cookies of your choice, such as a Sesame Coconut cookie (page 266), or 4 Mi-Del Ginger Snaps or Chocolate Snaps, with a cup of tea (every other day)

1,800-calorie plan: 140–150 calories of cookies, with a cup of tea

2,100-calorie plan: 140–150 calories of cookies and a tablespoon of almonds with a cup of tea

2,500-calorie plan: 140–150 calories of cookies and 2 tablespoons of almonds with a cup of tea

. . . .

Chocolate Cupcake with Mint Glaze (page 260)

1,500-calorie plan: 1 cupcake (Save up! This is 3 days worth of treat calories)

1,800-calorie plan: 1 cupcake (but have one less fat serving on this day!)

2,100-calorie plan: 1 cupcake

2,500-calorie plan: 1 cupcake and a cup of nonfat milk

. . . .

Sorbet

1,500-calorie plan: 100–110 calories of sorbet (half a cup for most brands) (every other day)

1,800-calorie plan: 150–160 calories of sorbet (¾ cup for most brands)

2,100-calorie plan: 200–210 calories of sorbet (1 cup for most brands)

2,500-calorie plan: 200–210 calories of sorbet (1 cup for most brands) with a cup blueberries

. . . .

Chips and Salsa

1,500-calorie plan: 100 calories of tortilla chips (preferably whole-grain) with 1–2 tablespoons salsa (every other day)

1,800-calorie plan: 150 calories of tortilla chips (preferably whole-grain) with 2–3 tablespoons salsa

2,100-calorie plan: 200 calories of tortilla chips (preferably whole-grain) with 3–4 tablespoons salsa

2,500-calorie plan: 200 calories of tortilla chips (preferably whole-grain) with 3–4 tablespoons salsa and ¼ avocado, sliced

. . . .

Chips and Guacamole

1,500-calorie plan: 50 calories of tortilla chips (preferably whole-grain) with 2 tablespoons guacamole (every other day)

1,800-calorie plan: 100 calories of tortilla chips (preferably whole-grain) with 3 tablespoons guacamole

2,100-calorie plan: 100 calories of tortilla chips (preferably whole-grain) with 4 tablespoons guacamole

2,500-calorie plan: 150 calories of tortilla chips (preferably whole-grain) with 5 tablespoons guacamole

. . . .

Glass of Red Wine (with a meal)

1,500-calorie plan: 4-ounce glass of wine (every other day)

1,800-calorie plan: *Women:* 4-ounce glass of wine with 1 tablespoon peanuts

Men: 6-ounce glass of wine (no nuts)

2,100-calorie plan: *Women:* 4-ounce glass of wine with 2 tablespoons peanuts

Men: 6-ounce glass of wine with a tablespoon peanuts

2,500-calorie plan: *Women:* 4-ounce glass of wine with 3 tablespoons peanuts

Men: 6-ounce glass of wine with 2 tablespoons peanuts

. . . .

Blueberries Baked with Sweet Corn Cake (page 259)

1,500-calorie plan: ½ serving (every other day)

1,800-calorie plan: ¾ serving

2,100-calorie plan: 1 serving

2,500-calorie plan: 1¼ servings

NOTES

～～～

Introduction

x   **"The Island Where People Forget to Die"**   D. Buettner, "The Island Where People Forget to Die," *New York Times*, Oct. 24, 2012.

x   **Men here are four times as likely**   D. B. Panagiotakos et al., "Sociodemographic and Lifestyle Statistics of Oldest Old People (>80 Years) Living in Ikaria island: The Ikaria Study," *Cardiology Research and Practice* 2011, Article 679187.

x   **It's the traditional Mediterranean diet**   W. C. Willett et al., "Mediterranean Diet Pyramid: A Cultural Model for Healthy Eating," *American Journal of Clinical Nutrition* 1995, no. 61 (Supp.): 1402S–1406S.

Part One: Your Body on Pescetarianism

1   **80 percent of heart disease cases**   H. S. Buttar et al., "Prevention of Cardiovascular Diseases: Role of Exercise, Dietary Interventions, Obesity, and Smoking Cessation," *Experimental and Clinical Cardiology* 10, no. 4 (2005): 229–249. See also M. de Lorgeril et al., "Mediterranean Alpha-Linolenic Acid-Rich Diet in Secondary Prevention of Coronary Heart Disease," *Lancet* 343, no. 8911 (1994): 1454–1459.

1   **70 percent of cancer cases**   P. Anand et al., "Cancer Is a Preventable Disease That Requires Major Lifestyle Changes," *Pharmaceutical Research* 25, no. 9 (September 2008): 2097–2116. See also R. U. Newton and D. A. Galvão, "Exercise in Prevention and Management of Cancer," *Current Treatment Options in Oncology* 9, nos. 2–3 (June 2008): 135–146.

1   **90 percent of cases of type 2**   D. Mozaffarian et al., "Lifestyle Risk Factors and New-Onset Diabetes Mellitus in Older Adults: The Cardiovascular Health Study," *Archives of Internal Medicine* 169, no. 8 (2009): 798–807.

2   **Obesity alone is responsible**   S. D. Hurstings and S. M. Dunlap, "Obesity, Metabolic Dysregulation, and Cancer: A Growing Concern and an Inflammatory (and Microenvironmental) Issue," *Annals of the New York Academy of Sciences* 1271 (2012): 82–87.

Chapter 1: Your Fabulous Pescetarian Figure

4   **Pescetarians are, on average, about 20 pounds lighter**   G. E. Fraser, "Vegetarian Diets: What Do We Know of Their Effects on Common Chronic Diseases?" *American Journal of Clinical Nutrition* 2009, no. 89 (Supp.): 1607S–1612S.

4   **A Spanish study tracking university students**   J. J. Beunza et al., "Adherence to the Mediterranean Diet, Long-Term Weight Change, and Incident Overweight or Obesity: The Seguimiento Universidad de Navarra (SUN) Cohort," *American Journal of Clinical Nutrition* 2010, no. 92: 1484–1493.

5   **Check out these results** C. M. Shay et al., "Food and Nutrient Intakes and Their Associations with Lower BMI in Middle-Aged U.S. Adults: The International Study of Macro-/Micronutrients and Blood Pressure (INTERMAP)," *American Journal of Clinical Nutrition* 2012, no. 96: 483–491.

6   **The National Weight Control Registry** H. R. Wyatt et al., "Lessons from Patients Who Have Successfully Maintained Weight Loss," *Obesity Management* 1 (Apr. 2005): 56–61.

7   **research from the Boston Children's Hospital** C. B. Ebbeling et al., "Effects of Dietary Composition on Energy Expenditure During Weight Loss Maintenance," *Journal of the American Medical Association* 307, no. 24 (2012): 2627–2634.

7   **Genetics are thought to account for** J. R. Fernandez et al., "Genetic Influences in Childhood Obesity: Recent Progress and Recommendations for Experimental Designs," *International Journal of Obesity* (2011): 1–6.

8   **It's even worse for some people** J. M. McCaffery et al., "Obesity Susceptibility Loci and Dietary Intake in the Look AHEAD Trial," *American Journal of Clinical Nutrition* 2012, no. 95: 1477–1486.

8   **brain chemical imbalance that leaves them unsatisfied** A. N. Gearhardt et al., "Neural Correlates of Food Addiction," *Archives of General Psychiatry* 68, no. 8 (Aug. 2011).

8   **Some people are genetically programmed** A. A. Bremer et al., "Toward a Unifying Hypothesis of Metabolic Syndrome," *Pediatrics* 129, no. 3 (2012): 557–570.

9   **Your genes drive you to eat frequently** McCaffery et al., "Obesity Susceptibility Loci."

9   **It takes a lot of food to feel full** S. Fulton, "Appetite and Reward," *Frontiers in Neuroendocrinology* 31 (2010): 85–103.

10 **Typical American fare seems to encourage** K. Harris et al., "Is the Gut Microbiota a New Factor Contributing to Obesity and Its Metabolic Disorders?" *Journal of Obesity* 2012, Article 879151.

10 **Researchers at the University College in Cork** M. J. Claesson et al., "Gut Microbiota Composition Correlates with Diet and Health in the Elderly," *Nature* 488 (Aug. 2012): 178–184. For more on this, see "Eldermet" at eldermet.ucc.ie.

11 **A National Institute on Aging study** A. Koster et al., "Waist Circumference and Mortality," *American Journal of Epidemiology* 167, no. 12 (2008): 1465–1475.

12 **whole grains are rich in magnesium** N. M. McKeown et al., "Whole- and Refined-Grain Intakes Are Differentially Associated with Abdominal Visceral and Subcutaneous Adiposity in Healthy Adults: The Framingham Heart Study," *American Journal of Clinical Nutrition* 92, no. 5 (Nov. 2010): 1165–1171.

12 **Calcium. Eating calcium-rich foods is linked** M. B. Zemel et al., "Dairy augmentation of total and central fat loss in obese subjects," *International Journal of Obesity* 29(4) (April 2005); 391–7.

13 **The higher the intake** J. Halkjær et al., "Intake of Macronutrients as Predictors of 5-Y Changes in Waist Circumference," *American Journal of Clinical Nutrition* 84, no. 4 (2006): 789–797.

Chapter 2: Age-Proofing Your Body

14 **And it shortens your telomeres** M. Lee et al., "Inverse Association Between Adiposity and Telomere Length: The Fels Longitudinal Study," *American Journal of Human Biology* 23, no. 1 (2011): 100–106.

16 **A recent study found that Italians** E. Azzini et al., "Mediterranean Diet Effect: An Italian Picture," *Nutrition Journal* 10 (2011): 125.

17 **There's a condition that ignites** L. G. Gilstrap et al., "Community-Based Primary Prevention Programs Decrease the Rate of Metabolic Syndrome Among Socioeconomically Disadvantaged Women," *Journal of Women's Health* 22, no. 4 (Apr. 2013): 322–329.

17 **It strikes over a third of American adults** R. B. Ervin, "Prevalence of Metabolic Syndrome Among Adults 20 Years of Age and Over, by Sex, Age, Race, and Ethnicity, and Body Mass Index: United States, 2003–2006," *National Health Statistics Report* no. 13, May 5, 2009.

17 **It's "metabolic syndrome,"** "About metabolic syndrome," American Heart Association website, updated August 16, 2012, available at www.heart.org /HEARTORG/Conditions/More/MetabolicSyndrome/About-Metabolic-Syndrome _UCM_301920_Article.jsp, accessed September 25, 2013.

18 **The good news is that 90 percent** A. A. Bremer et al., "Toward a Unifying Hypothesis of Metabolic Syndrome," *Pediatrics* 129, no. 3 (March 2012): 557–570.

18 **University of Laval, Canada, study** C. Richard et al., "Effect of the Mediterranean Diet with and without Weight Loss on Markers of Inflammation in Men with Metabolic Syndrome," *Obesity* 21, no. 1 (2013): 51–57.

18 **Erectile dysfunction (ED)** B. G. Schwartz and R. A. Kloner, "Cardiovascular Implications of Erectile Dysfunction," *Circulation* 123 (2011): e609–e611.

18 **study from the University of Naples** F. Giugliano et al., "Adherence to Mediterranean Diet and Erectile Dysfunction in Men with Type 2 Diabetes," *Journal of Sexual Medicine* 7, no. 5 (2010): 1911–1917.

18 **Research is still sparse on this** F. Giugliano et al., "Adherence to Mediterranean Diet and Sexual Function in Women with Type 2 Diabetes," *Journal of Sexual Medicine* 7, no. 5 (2010): 1883–1890.

19 **Now consider this: Nearly 40 percent** V. L. Roger et al., "Heart Disease and Stroke Statistics—2011 Update: A Report from the American Heart Association," *Circulation* 123: (2011): e18–e209.

19 **A diet like the Pescetarian Plan cuts** H.S. Buttar et al., "Prevention of Cardiovascular Diseases: Role of Exercise, Dietary Interventions, Obesity, and Smoking Cessation," *Experimental and Clinical Cardiology* 10, no. 4 (2005): 229–249. See also de Lorgeril et al., "Mediterranean Alpha-Linolenic Acid-Rich Diet."

19 **People who ate a diet highest in omega-3** D. Mozaffarian et al., "Plasma Phospholipid Long-Chain ω-3 Fatty Acids and Total and Cause-Specific Mortality in Older Adults," *Annals of Internal Medicine* 158, no. 7 (2013).

19 **People at risk for heart disease** R. Estruch et al., "Primary Prevention of Cardiovascular Disease with a Mediterranean Diet," *New England Journal of Medicine* 368, no. 14 (2013): 1279–1290.

20 **Eating fish just one to two times** B. London et al., "Omega-3 Fatty Acids and Cardiac Arrhythmias: Prior Studies and Recommendations for Future Research: A Report from the National Heart, Lung, and Blood Institute and Office of Dietary Supplements Omega-3 Fatty Acids and Their Role in Cardiac Arrhythmogenesis Workshop," *Circulation* 116 (2007): e320–e335.

20 **A diet like the one in this book** De Lorgeril et al., "Mediterranean Alpha-Linolenic Acid-Rich Diet." (Page 317 for complete reference)

20 **More than a quarter of Americans** Y. F. Li et al., "Awareness of Prediabetes— United States, 2005–2010," *Morbidity and Mortality Weekly Report* 62, no. 11 (2013).

20 **And of the 8.3 percent** "Diabetes Statistics," American Diabetes Association website, available at www.diabetes.org/diabetes-basics/diabetes-statistics/, accessed September 25, 2013.

20 **In fact, cases are rising so fast** J. Boyle et al., "Projection of the Year 2050 Burden of Diabetes in the U.S. Adult Population: Dynamic Modeling of Incidence, Mortality, and Prediabetes Prevalence," *Population Health Metrics* 8, no. 29 (2010).

20 **Too much body fat is the cause** "Do You Know the Health Risks of Being Overweight? Type 2 Diabetes," Weight Control Information Network (WIN), National Institute of Diabetes and Digestive and Kidney Diseases (NIDDK) website, available at win.niddk.nih.gov/publications/health_risks.htm#b, accessed September 25, 2013.

20 **If you're overweight, losing about 7 percent** W. C. Knowler et al., "Reduction in the Incidence of Type 2 Diabetes with Lifestyle Intervention or Metformin," *New England Journal of Medicine* 346, no. 6 (2002): 393–403.

21 **In a study of men and women living in Spain** J. Salas-Salvadó et al., "Reduction in the Incidence of Type 2 Diabetes with the Mediterranean Diet: Results of the PREDIMED-Reus Nutrition Intervention Randomized Trial," *Diabetes Care* 34, no. 1 (2011): 14–19.

21 **The Look AHEAD Trial found** E. W. Gregg et al., "Association of an Intensive Lifestyle Intervention with Remission of Type 2 Diabetes," *Journal of the American Medical Association* 308, no. 23 (2012): 2489–2496.

21 **In an Italian study, only 44 percent** K. Esposito et al., "Effects of a Mediterranean-Style Diet on the Need for Antihyperglycemic Drug Therapy in Patients With Newly Diagnosed Type 2 Diabetes: A Randomized Trial," *Annals of Internal Medicine* 151, no. 5 (2009): 306–314.

22 **People of various ethnicities** M. Purba et al., "Skin Wrinkling: Can Food Make a Difference?" *Journal of the American College of Nutrition* 20, no. 1 (2001): 71–80.

22 **People living along the Mediterranean Sea** C. Fortes, "A Protective Effect of the Mediterranean Diet for Cutaneous Melanoma," *International Journal of Epidemiology* 37, no. 5 (Oct. 2008): 1018–1029.

23 **That means that 90 to 95 percent** Anand et al., "Cancer Is a Preventable Disease."

23 **Diet can prevent up to 35 percent** Anand et al., "Cancer Is a Preventable Disease."

23 **exercise up to 40 percent** R. U. Newton and D. A. Galvão, "Exercise in Prevention and Management of Cancer," *Current Treatment Options in Oncology* 9, no. 2–3 (Jun. 2008): 135–146.

23 **avid extra-virgin olive oil** Psaltopoulou et al., "Olive Oil Intake Is Inversely Related to Cancer Prevalence: A Systematic Review and a Meta-Analysis of 13800 Patients and 23340 Controls in 19 Observational Studies," *Lipids in Health and Disease* 10, no. 127 (2011).

23 **thirty-plus phenolic compounds in extra-virgin olive oil** A. Bendini et al., "Phenolic Molecules in Virgin Olive Oils: A Survey of Their Sensory Properties, Health Effects, Antioxidant Activity, and Analytical Methods. An Overview of the Last Decade," *Molecules* 12 (2007): 1679–1719.

23 **The appetite-suppressing foods** "Obesity and Cancer Risk," National Cancer Institute fact sheet, available at www.cancer.gov/cancertopics/factsheet/Risk/obesity, accessed September 25, 2013.

23 **I do want to point out results** E. H. J. Kim et al., "Diet Quality Indices and Postmenopausal Breast Cancer Survival," *Nutrition and Cancer* 63, no. 3 (Apr. 2011): 381–388.

Chapter 3: This Is Your Brain on Fish

26 **Americans' omega-6 to omega-3** A. McManus et al., "Omega-3 Fatty Acids: What Consumers Need to Know," *Appetite* 57 (2011): 80–83.

26 **The Pescetarian Plan has a 1-to-1** Karr et al., "Omega-3 Polyunsaturated Fatty Acids and Cognition Throughout the Lifespan: A Review," *Nutritional Neuroscience* 14, no. 5 (2011): 216–225.

27 **Depression rates are up to 65 times higher** J. R. Hibbeln, "Fish Consumption and Major Depression," *Lancet* 351, no. 9110 (1998): 1213.

27 **Young women who switched to a Mediterranean-style diet** L. McMillan et al., "Behavioural Effects of a 10-day Mediterranean Diet: Results from a Pilot Study Evaluating Mood and Cognitive Performance," *Appetite* 56, no. 1 (Feb. 2011): 143–147.

27 **Those who ate the most fish** C. Chrysohoou et al., "Fish Consumption Moderates Depressive Symptomatology in Elderly Men and Women from the IKARIA Study," *Cardiology Research and Practice* 2011, Article 219578.

27 **Eating fatty fish may lower the risk** A. A. Colangelo et al., "Long-Chain Omega-3 Polyunsaturated Fatty Acids Are Inversely Associated with Depressive Symptoms in Women," *Nutrition* 25, no. 10 (Oct. 2009): 1011–1019.

27 **Depressed people averaged 27 percent less DHA** J. Assies et al., "Plasma and Erythrocyte Fatty Acid Patterns in Patients with Recurrent Depression: A Matched Case-Control Study," *PLoS ONE* 5(5): e10635 (2010).

27 **In countries where women eat** J. R. Hibbeln, "Seafood Consumption, the DHA Content of Mothers' Milk and Prevalence Rates of Postpartum Depression: A Cross-National, Ecological Analysis," *Journal of Affective Disorders* 69 (2002): 15–29.

28 **Exercise triggers the formation of** A. C. Pereira, et al., "An In Vivo Correlate of Exercise-Induced Neurogenesis in the Adult Dentate Gyrus," *PNAS* Vol 104, no. 3 (March 27, 2007): 5638–5643.

28 **Exercise plays an enormous role.** J. A. Blumenthal et al. "Effects of Exercise Training on Older Patients with Major Depression," *Archives of Internal Medicine* 159 (1999): 2349–2356. See also B. M. Hoffman et al., "Exercise and Pharmacotherapy in Patients with Major Depression: One-Year Follow-Up of the SMILE Study," *Psychosomatic Medicine* 73 (2011): 127–133.

28 **The research linking omega-3 intake** B. Koletzko et al., "Dietary Fat Intakes for Pregnant and Lactating Women," *British Journal of Nutrition* 98, no. 5 (Nov. 2007): 873–877.

29 **Women who ate at least 12 ounces** J. R. Hibbeln et al., "Maternal Seafood Consumption in Pregnancy and Neurodevelopmental Outcomes in Childhood (ALSPAC study): An Observational Cohort Study," *Lancet* 369, no. 9561 (Feb. 2007): 578–585.

29 **Boys who regularly ate fish at age 15** Aberg et al., "Fish Intake of Swedish Male Adolescents Is a Predictor of Cognitive Performance," *Acta Paediatrica* 98, no. 3 (Mar. 2009): 555–560.

29 **The more fatty fish people ate** S. Kalmijn et al., "Dietary Intake of Fatty Acids and Fish in Relation to Cognitive Performance at Middle Age," *Neurology* 62 (2004): 275–280.

29 **Chicagoans aged 65 to 94** M. C. Morris et al., "Consumption of Fish and N-3 Fatty Acids and Risk of Incident Alzheimer's Disease," *Archives of Neurology* 60 (2003): 940–946.

29 **Elderly men who ate little** B. M. van Gelder et al., "Fish Consumption, N-3 Fatty Acids, and Subsequent 5-Y Cognitive Decline in Elderly Men: The Zutphen Elderly Study," *American Journal of Clinical Nutrition* 85 (2007): 1142–1147.

30 **Seniors with mild cognitive impairment** N. Scarmeas et al., "Mediterranean Diet and Mild Cognitive Impairment," *Archives of Neurology* 66, no. 2 (Feb. 2009): 216–225.

30 **After examining the diets** Y. Gu et al., "Nutrient Intake and Plasma β-Amyloid," *Neurology* 78 (2012): 1832–1840.

30 **Other research has found that people** S. A. Cosentino et al., "Plasma β-Amyloid and Cognitive Decline," *Archives of Neurology* 67, no. 12 (2010): 1485–1490. See also N. Schupf et al., "Peripheral Aβ Subspecies as Risk Biomarkers of Alzheimer's Disease," *Proceedings of the National Academy of Sciences* 105, no. 37 (2008): 14052–14057.

Chapter 4: Pescetarian Ultra-Nutrition

32 **Americans are big on protein** S. A. Bowman et al., "Retail Food Commodity Intakes: Mean Amounts of Retail Commodities per Individual, 2007–08," U.S. Department of Agriculture, Agricultural Research Service, Beltsville, Maryland, and U.S. Department of Agriculture, Economic Research Service, Washington, D.C., 2013, available at www.ars.usda.gov/SP2UserFiles/Place/12355000/pdf/ficrcd /FICRCD_Intake_Tables_2007_08.pdf, accessed September 25, 2013.

32 **People who eat more fish live** Mozaffarian et al., "Plasma Phospholipid Long-Chain ω-3 Fatty Acids." (See page 317 for complete reference.)

32 **A Norwegian study found** H. Strøm, "Fish, N-3 Fatty Acids, and Cardiovascular Diseases in Women of Reproductive Age: A Prospective Study in a Large National Cohort," *Hypertension* 59, no. 1 (Jan. 2012): 36–43.

32 **Dutch men and women eating the most fish** J. de Goede et al., "Marine (N-3) Fatty Acids, Fish Consumption, and the 10-Year Risk of Fatal and Nonfatal Coronary Heart Disease in a Large Population of Dutch Adults with Low Fish Intake," *Journal of Nutrition* 140, no. 5 (May 2010): 1023–1028.

32 **Fish eaters have a 12 percent** S. Wu et al., "Fish Consumption and Colorectal Cancer Risk in Humans: A Systematic Review and Meta-Analysis," *American Journal of Medicine* 125, no. 6 (June 2012): 551–559.e5.

32 **Also, you make more molecules** P. C. Calder, "Omega-3 Fatty Acids and Inflammatory Processes," *Nutrients* 2, no. 3 (2010): 355–374.

32 **international Cardiovascular Disease and Alimentary Comparison (or CARDIAC) study** Y. Yamori et al., "Low Cardiovascular Risks in the Middle Aged Males and Females Excreting Greater 24-Hour Urinary Taurine and Magnesium in 41 WHO-CARDIAC Study Populations in the World," *Journal of Biomedical Science* 17 (Supp. 1) (2010): S21.

33 **People who ate the most meat** R. Sinha et al., "Meat Intake and Mortality," *Archives of Internal Medicine* 169, no. 6 (2009): 562–571.

33 **Every daily serving of red meat** A. Pan et al., "Red Meat Consumption and Mortality," *Archives of Intern Medicine* 172, no. 7 (2012): 555–563.

34 **Eating little to no meat for twenty** P. N. Singh et al., "Does Low Meat Consumption Increase Life Expectancy in Humans?" *American Journal of Clinical Nutrition* 78 (Supp.) (2003): 526S–532S.

34 **A study led by researchers** R. A. Koeth et al., "Intestinal Microbiota Metabolism of L-Carnitine, a Nutrient in Red Meat, Promotes Atherosclerosis," *Nature Medicine* 19, no. 5 (May 2013): 576–585.

37 **We were designed for** A. McManus et al., "Omega-3 Fatty Acids: What Consumers Need to Know," *Appetite* 57 (2011): 80–83.

38 **a recent paper by Remko Kuipers** R. S. Kuipers et al., "Saturated Fat, Carbohydrates, and Cardiovascular Disease," *Netherlands Journal of Medicine* 60, no. 9 (September 2011): 372–378.

40 **Some act as antioxidants** J. A. Menendez et al., "Xenohormetic and Anti-Aging Activity of Secoiridoid Polyphenols Present in Extra Virgin Olive Oil: A New Family of Gerosuppressant Agents," *Cell Cycle* 12, no. 4 (2013): 555–578.

40 **One analysis of the major research** T. Psaltopoulou et al., "Olive Oil Intake Is In-versely Related to Cancer Prevalence: A Systematic Review and a Meta-Analysis of 13800 Patients and 23340 Controls in 19 Observational Studies," *Lipids in Health and Disease* 10, no. 127 (2011).

41 **University of Vermont College of Medicine** C. L. Kien et al., "Substituting Dietary Monounsaturated Fat for Saturated Fat Is Associated with Increased Daily Physi-cal Activity and Resting Energy Expenditure and with Changes in Mood," *American Journal of Clinical Nutrition* 97, no. 4 (Apr. 2013): 689–697.

43 **Numerous studies show** M. V. L. da Silva and C. G. Alfenas, "Effect of the Glycemic Index on Lipid Oxidation and Body Composition," *Nutrición Hospitalaria* 26, no. 1 (2011): 48–55.

43 **Legumes and whole grains** J. P. Karl and E. Saltzman. "The Role of Whole Grains in Body Weight Regulation," *Advances in Nutrition* 3, no. 5 (Sept. 2012): 697–707. See also C. P. Marinangeli and P. J. Jones, "Pulse Grain Consumption and Obesity: Effects on Energy Expenditure, Substrate Oxidation, Body Composition, Fat Depo-sition, and Satiety," *British Journal of Nutrition* 108 (Supp. 1) (Aug. 2012): S46–S51.

44 **Consider this: Soft drinks** G. Singh et al., "Mortality Due to Sugar Sweetened Beverage Consumption: A Global, Regional, and National Comparative Risk Assess-ment," *Circulation* 127 (2013).

44 **But new research is indicating** Kuipers et al., "Saturated Fat, Carbohydrates, and Cardiovascular Disease." (See page 322 for complete reference.)

44 **These sugar-based compounds trigger** H. Vlassara and G. E. Striker, "AGE Restric-tion in Diabetes Mellitus: A Paradigm Shift," *Nature Reviews Endocrinology* 7, no. 9 (2011): 526–539.

45 **I recommend that you stick to** World Health Organization, "Diet, Nutrition, and the Prevention of Chronic Diseases," *WHO Technical Report Series* no. 916 (TRS 916), ch. 4.2, available at www.who.int/dietphysicalactivity/publications/trs916 /download/en/index.html, accessed September 25, 2013.

47 **While it's true that cheese** M. Chen et al., "Effects of Dairy Intake on Body Weight and Fat: A Meta-Analysis of Randomized Controlled Trials," *American Journal of Clinical Nutrition* 96 (2012): 735–747.

47 **research shows that dairy eaters** P. Elwood et al., "The Consumption of Milk and Dairy Foods and the Incidence of Vascular Disease and Diabetes: An Overview of the Evidence," *Lipids* 45 (2010): 925–939.

47 **Low-fat dairy (nonfat and 1-percent milk and yogurt)** L. Wang et al., "Dietary In-take of Dairy Products, Calcium, and Vitamin D and the Risk of Hypertension in Middle-Aged and Older Women," *Hypertension* 51 (2008): 1073–1079.

47 **Some studies show that men** J. W. Lampe, "Dairy Products and Cancer," *Journal of the American College of Nutrition* 30 (5 Supp. 1) (Oct. 2011): 464S–470S.

47 **One study showed an increased risk** J. M. Genkinger et al., "Dairy Products and Ovarian Cancer: A Pooled Analysis of 12 Cohort Studies," *Cancer Epidemiology, Bio-markers, and Prevention* 15, no. 2 (Feb. 2006): 364–372.

47 **dairy reduces the risk of this cancer** M. A. Merritt et al., "Dairy Foods and Nutri-ents in Relation to Risk of Ovarian Cancer and Major Histological Subtypes," *Inter-national Journal of Cancer* 132, no. 5 (Mar. 2013): 1114–1124.

47 **Meanwhile, people consuming more milk** Lampe, "Dairy Products and Cancer." (See above for complete reference.)

48 **Studies indicate that yogurt fans** S. N. Meydani and H. Woel-Kyu, "Immunologic Effects of Yogurt," *American Journal of Clinical Nutrition* 71 (2000): 861–872.

48 **study in Australia linked yogurt** K. L. Ivey et al., "Association Between Yogurt,

Milk, and Cheese Consumption and Common Carotid Artery Intima-Media Thickness and Cardiovascular Disease Risk Factors in Elderly Women," *American Journal of Clinical Nutrition* 94 (2011): 234–239.

48 **They also reduce the risk of blood clots** J. C. Ruf, "Wine and Polyphenols Related to Platelet Aggregation and Atherothrombosis," *Drugs Under Experimental and Clinical Research* 25, no. 2–3 (1999): 125–131.

48 **Red wine has about ten times** S. Arranz et al., "Wine, Beer, Alcohol, and Polyphenols on Cardiovascular Disease and Cancer," *Nutrients* 4 (2012): 759–781.

49 **For example, a National Cancer Institute** C. A. McCarty et al., "Alcohol, Genetics, and Risk of Breast Cancer in the Prostate, Lung, Colorectal, and Ovarian (PLCO) Cancer Screening Trial," *Breast Cancer Research and Treatment* 133, no. 2 (June 2012): 785–792.

Chapter 5: The Seven Pescetarian Principles

59 **Some studies show organic produce** C. Smith-Spangler et al., "Are Organic Foods Safer or Healthier Than Conventional Alternatives? A Systematic Review," *Annals of Internal Medicine* 157, no. 5 (2012): 348–366.

59 **These lists are courtesy of** The Environmental Working Group's website is www.ewg.org.

67 **A number of studies show** E. Ros, "Health Benefits of Nut Consumption," *Nutrients* 2 (2010): 652–682.

71 **Water drinkers average 9 percent fewer calories** B. M. Popkin et al., "Water and Food Consumption Patterns of U.S. Adults from 1999 to 2001," *Obesity Research* 13, no. 2 (2005): 2146–2152.

71 **People who drank two cups** E. A. Dennis et al., "Water Consumption Increases Weight Loss During a Hypocaloric Diet Intervention in Middle-Aged and Older Adults," *Obesity* 18, no. 2 (Feb. 2010): 300–307.

Chapter 7: Upgrade Your Diet and Maintain Your Weight

83 **What makes it so super** Unless specifically noted in references that follow, much of the information in the Standout Superfoods chart can be found in the following sources: M. Russo et al., "Phytochemicals in Cancer Prevention and Therapy: Truth or Dare?" *Toxins* 2 (2010): 517–551. See also R. J. Nijveldt et al., "Flavonoids: A Review of Probable Mechanisms of Action and Potential Applications," *American Journal of Clinical Nutrition* 74 (2001): 418–425; and A. V. Rao and L. G. Rao, "Carotenoids and Human Health," *Pharmacological Research* 55 (2007): 207–216.

83 **These four berry types** J. Joseph et al., "Grape Juice, Berries, and Walnuts Affect Brain Aging and Behavior," *Journal of Nutrition* 139 (2009): 1813S–1817S.

83 **Scientists keep finding new benefits** Allen, E. N. et al., "Reversal of Age-Related Motor Deficits Following Stilbene Dietary Supplementation," 244th National Meeting & Exposition of the American Chemical Society (2012).

85 **Plus, they can help you lose weight** B. W. Bolling et al., "Tree Nut Phytochemicals: Composition, Antioxidant Capacity, Bioactivity, Impact Factors: A Systematic Review of Almonds, Brazils, Cashews, Hazelnuts, Macadamias, Pecans, Pine Nuts, Pistachios, and Walnuts," *Nutrition Research Reviews* 24 (2011): 244–275.

85 **SUPER HERBS AND SPICES** P. K. Lai and J. Roy, "Antimicrobial and Chemopreventive Properties of Herbs and Spices," *Current Medicinal Chemistry* 11, no.11 (2004): 1451–1460.

87   **A 2013 study of nearly 18,000**   V. L. Folgoni III et al., "Avocado Consumption Is Associated with Better Diet Quality and Nutrient Intake and Lower Metabolic Syndrome Risk in U.S. Adults: Results from the National Health and Nutrition Examination Survey (NHANES) 2001–2008," *Nutrition Journal* 12, no. 1 (2013).

88   **Studies show that if you cook**   G. K. Beauchamp et al., "Failure to Compensate Decreased Dietary Sodium with Increased Table Salt Usage," *Journal of the American Medical Association* 258 (1987): 3275–3278.

93   **Penn State University study**   C. N. Sciamanna et al., "Practices Associated with Weight Loss versus Weight-Loss Maintenance Results of a National Survey," *American Journal of Preventive Medicine* 41, no. 2 (2011): 159–166.

93   **In addition, here are tips**   J. G. Thomas and R. R. Wing, "Maintenance of Long-Term Weight Loss," *Medicine and Health* 92, no. 2 (Feb. 2009).

93   **The NWCR participants who**   R. R. Wing and S. Phelan, "Long-Term Weight Loss Maintenance," *American Journal of Clinical Nutrition* 82, no. 1 (July 2005): 222S–225S.

Chapter 9: Exercise, Sleep, Love

106   **A fifteen-minute walk**   C. P. Wen et al., "Minimum Amount of Physical Activity for Reduced Mortality and Extended Life Expectancy: A Prospective Cohort," *Lancet* 378, no. 9798 (2011): 1244–1253.

106   **For a sample exercise program**   "Adding Physical Activity to Your Life," Centers for Disease Control website, available at www.cdc.gov/physicalactivity/everyone /getactive/index.html, accessed September 25, 2013.

107   **Here's what the American College of Sports Medicine**   C. E. Garber, "Quantity and Quality of Exercise for Developing and Maintaining Cardiorespiratory, Musculoskeletal, and Neuromotor Fitness in Apparently Healthy Adults: Guidance for Prescribing Exercise," *Medicine and Science in Sports and Exercise* 43, no. 7 (July 2011): 1334–1359.

107   **If you need to lose weight**   J. E. Donnelly, "Appropriate Physical Activity Intervention Strategies for Weight Loss and Prevention of Weight Regain for Adults," *Medicine and Science in Sports and Exercise* 41, no. 2 (Feb. 2009): 459–471.

109   **Another good resource**   "Growing Stronger—Strength Training for Older Adults," Centers for Disease Control website, available at www.cdc.gov/physicalactivity/ growingstronger/index.html, accessed September 25, 2013.

109   **Experts say we need seven**   "2013 Exercise and Sleep," National Sleep Foundation 2013 poll, March 4, 2013, available at www.sleepfoundation.org/2013poll, accessed September 25, 2013.

110   **Getting six hours or less**   C. S. Möller-Levet et al., "Effects of Insufficient Sleep on Circadian Rhythmicity and Expression Amplitude of the Human Blood Transcriptome," *Proceedings of the National Academy of Sciences* 110, no. 12 (2013): E1132–E1141.

Chapter 10: Catches to Reel In, Catches to Toss Back

116   **Safety standards in these countries**   "Seafood Buying Guide 2008," Food & Water Watch, available at http://documents.foodandwaterwatch.org/doc/Seafood BuyingGuide2.pdf, accessed September 25, 2013.

116   **high levels of persistent organic pollutants**   D. Hayward et al., "Polybrominated Diphenyl Ethers and Polychlorinated Biphenyls in Commercially Wild Caught and

Farm-Raised Fish Fillets in the United States," *Environmental Research* 103, no. 1 (Jan. 2007): 46–54.

117 **I was surprised to find out** "Mercury in the Aquatic Environment: Sources, Releases, Transport and Monitoring," United Nations Environment Programme, November 2011, available at www.unep.org/hazardoussubstances/Portals/9 /Mercury/Documents/coal/Microsoft%20Word%20-%20Final%20Merged %20report.pdf, accessed September 25, 2013.

118 **But here's the surprise twist** P. W. Davidson et al., "Fish Consumption and Prenatal Methylmercury Exposure: Cognitive and Behavioral Outcomes in the Main Cohort at 17 Years from the Seychelles Child Development Study," *Neurotoxicology* 32, no. 6 (Dec. 2011): 711–717.

118 **In fact, experts recommend** B. Koletzko et al., "Dietary Fat Intakes for Pregnant and Lactating Women," *British Journal of Nutrition* 98, no. 5 (Nov. 2007): 873–877.

119 **That means they're still polluting** "Polychlorinated Biphenyls (PCBs), TEACH Chemical Summary," Environmental Protection Agency, 2009, available at www .epa.gov/teach/chem_summ/PCB_summary100809.pdf, accessed September 25, 2013.

119 **cuts POPs by up to 94 percent** M. Sprague et al., "Effects of Decontaminated Fish Oil or a Fish and Vegetable Oil Blend on Persistent Organic Pollutant and Fatty Acid Compositions in Diet and Flesh of Atlantic Salmon (Salmo Salar)," *British Journal of Nutrition* 103, no. 10 (May 2010): 1442–1451.

120 **The cut-off points** "Mercury Contamination in Fish: A Guide to Staying Healthy and Fighting Back," Natural Resources Defense Council website, available at www .nrdc.org/health/effects/mercury/guide.asp, accessed September 25, 2013.

129 **The Centers for Disease Control and Prevention (CDC)** J. A. Painter et al., "Attribution of Foodborne Illnesses, Hospitalizations, and Deaths to Food Commodities by Using Outbreak Data, United States, 1998–2008," *Emerging Infectious Diseases* 19, no. 3 (2013): 407–415.

130 **But raw seafood is riskier** A. Butt et al., "Infections Related to the Ingestion of Seafood. Part I: Viral and Bacterial Infections," *Lancet Infectious Diseases* 4 (2004): 201–212.

Chapter 11: Environmentally Friendly Pescetarianism

134 **85 percent of the world's fisheries** "Wild Seafood Issue: Overfishing: Are We Too Good at Catching Fish?" Monterey Bay Aquarium Seafood Watch, available at www.montereybayaquarium.org/cr/cr_seafoodwatch/issues/wildseafood _overfishing.aspx, accessed September 25, 2013.

134 **In 1930 alone, 70 to 90** "Brief History of the Groundfishing Industry of New England," Northeast Fisheries Science Center, National Oceanic and Atmospheric Agency, available at www.nefsc.noaa.gov/history/stories/groundfish/grndfsh1 .html, accessed September 25, 2013.

138 **For instance, in the United States and Canada** Author interview with Michael Rust, PhD, science coordinator for office of aquaculture, National Oceanic and Atmospheric Administration (NOAA).

138 **Fewer fish are escaping** Ø. Jensen et al., "Escapes of Fishes from Norwegian Sea-Cage Aquaculture: Causes, Consequences, and Prevention," *Aquaculture Environment Interactions* 1 (2010): 71–83. See also "Atlantic Salmon and Rainbow Trout," Directorate of Fisheries, Norway, available at www.fiskeridir.no/english/statistics

/norwegian-aquaculture/aquaculture-statistics/atlantic-salmon-and-rainbow
-trout, accessed September 25, 2013.

Appendix C

285 **You must grind flaxseeds** D. C. Nieman et al., "Chia Seed Supplementation and Disease Risk Factors in Overweight Women: A Metabolomics Investigation," *Journal of Alternative and Complementary Medicine* 18, no. 7 (2012): 700–708.

INDEX

A

Abdominal (visceral) fat, 2, 8, 11–12, 15, 44

Addictive eating, 60, 111

Advanced glycation end-products (AGEs), 17, 44–45, 85, 149

Aerobic exercise, 92, 104, 107–8, 281

AGEs (advanced glycation end-products), 17, 44–45, 85, 149

ALA (alpha linoleic acid), 36, 37, 285

Alcohol consumption. *See also* Red wine
  and cancer risk, 23
  health benefits of, 48–49, 83, 87
  moderate, 61–62, 72
  and sleep problems, 110

Almond Butter, 68
  English Muffin, and Pear, 288–89

Almond milk, 66

Almonds
  in Black Rice Pudding, 155
  Chia Pudding with Berries and, 158, 286
  Flounder Baked with Grapes and, 222
  as healthy fat source, 68
  Latte and, 293
  monounsaturated fat in, 35
  on-the-run, 290, 298
  as superfood, 85

Alpha linoleic acid (ALA), 36, 37, 285

Alzheimer's disease, 15, 29, 30, 91

Amaranth, 64

American College of Sports Medicine, 106, 107

American diet, health drawbacks of, vii, xii, 16, 31, 35

American Heart Association, 20

Amino acids, 84

Anthocyanins, 46, 49, 83, 84, 87, 155

Antioxidants
  and brain function, 25
  and cancer prevention, 23, 83
  in red wine, 48, 87
  and skin health, 22

Appetite quelling foods, 9, 15, 57, 85, 281

Apple(s)
  Oatmeal, 289
  Peanut Butter and, Open-Faced, 300
  pesticide levels, 60
  with Spiced Sesame, 255, 302

Apricot Tuna Garbanzo, Curried, 311

Aquaculture (fish farming)
  contaminants in, 116, 119
  eco-seals in, 139
  environmental threats from, 138, 139

Aquaculture Stewardship Council, 139

Arctic Char
  safety/sustainability, 56, 121
  Seafood Stew, 237–38

Arctic Char (*cont'd*):
  servings, 56
  as superfood, 86
Arnold, Jeff, xii
Arugula
  with Roasted Garlic Fig Dressing, 164
  Sardines, Broiled, with Green Onion
    on, 232–33
  Shrimp Salad, Black Rice with, 297
Asparagus, 60
Attention deficit hyperactivity disorder
    (ADHD), 26
Avocado
  Cucumber, and Mango Kebab, 257,
    302
  Dressing, Creamy, Cucumber and
    Fennel with, 172
  Dressing, Thick, 274
  fat serving, 68
  guacamole and chips treat, 315–16
  in Haddock Tacos, 223–24
  as healthy fat source, 68
  monounsaturated fat in, 35
  Mozzarella, and Tomato Sandwich,
    294–95
  nutrients in, 87
  pesticide level, 60
  Salad with Hardboiled Eggs and,
    308–9
  serving size/calorie level, 79
  in Shrimp Taco Salad, 240
  as a superfood, 87
  Yogurt Dip, 253

B
Bacteria
  in fish, 130–31, 132
  intestinal, 10, 34, 42, 44
  in shellfish, 131
Balsamic Vinegar, Beets with Onions,
  Rosemary and, 166

Banana(s)
  in Black Rice Pudding, 155
  Frozen with Cocoa and Peanuts,
    256, 302
  in Green Shake, 160
  on-the-run, 290, 297–98
  with Pancakes, Whole-Grain, 162, 289
  Sliced, with Chia Pudding with
    Berries and Almonds, 286
  Yogurt, Peanut Butter Pop, 254, 292
Barbecuing, and cancer risk, 149
Barley
  in Black-Eyed Pea Stew, 197–98
  fiber in, 42
  as superfood, 84
  as whole grain, 64
Basil
  Potato and Celery Root Mashed
    with, 189
  Summer Squash Salad with Lemon
    and, 181
  as superfood, 85
  Tomato, and Peach Salad, 182
  Trout in Paper with Summer
    Squash, Green Onions and,
    245–46
Bass, safety/sustainability, 126
Bay scallops, 124
Bean(s). *See also* Black Bean(s);
    Garbanzo Bean(s)
  Black-Eyed Pea Stew, 197–98
  Cannellini Bean Spread on Toast,
    300–1
  dried, cooking, 268
  fresh shell, cooking, 268–69
  Green, in Sardine Niçoise, 234–35,
    297
  Pasta, Whole-Grain, Baked with
    White Beans, Spinach, and Walnut
    Sauce, 212–13, 305–6
  as protein source, 56–57

in Sloppy Joe, Tofu, 205–6
in Veggie Burger, 207
Beck, Judith, 112
Beck Diet Solution, The, 112
Beef, calories/fats in, 33
Beer
  health benefits of, 49, 87
  moderate consumption of, 61
Beet(s)
  with Onions, Balsamic Vinegar, and
    Rosemary, 166
  Slaw, 165
Bell Pepper(s)
  pesticide level, 60
  Red, Garbanzo Bean, Pumpkin
    Seed, and Olive Salad, 298–99
  Sweet Red, Seared Salmon with
    Fennel, Mushroom and, 228–29
Belly fat, 2, 8, 11–12, 15, 44, 106
Berries
  Chia Pudding with Almonds and,
    158, 286
  French Toast with, 290–91
  Ice Cream with, 314
  pesticide levels, 60
  as superfood, 83
*Best Life Diet and Total Body
  Makeover, The* (Greene), 104
Beta-amyloid, 30
Beta-carotene, 24, 83, 84
Betaglucan, 84
Beverages. *See also* Alcohol
    consumption; Coffee; Tea
  cocoa, 87
  Green Shake, 160, 288
  in meal plan, 97
  Peach Cinnamon Smoothie, 251, 292
  Strawberry Milk, 232
  sugary, 44, 70–71, 72
  tracking consumption, 281
  water, 70–72

Bifidobacteria, 48
Biodiversity, and aquaculture, 138
Bipolar disorder, 91
Black bass, safety/sustainability, 126
Black Bean(s)
  Roll Up Wrapped in Romaine, 249
  Salsa, and Eggs, 286–87
  in Shrimp Taco Salad, 240
  Tilapia with Green Onions, Garlic,
    Ginger and, 243–44
Blackberries, 83
Black-Eyed Pea Stew, 197–98
Black Rice, 270
  with Arugula Shrimp Salad, 297
  Pudding, 155, 287
  with Sesame and Green Onions,
    185
  as superfood, 84
  in Veggie Burger, 207
  as whole grain, 64
Bladder cancer, 47
Blood pressure, 19, 32, 83, 85, 88
Blood sugar, 9, 17, 21, 41, 42, 43, 44,
    83, 86
Blueberries
  Baked with Sweet Corn Cake, 259,
    316
  French Toast with Berries, 290–91
  pesticide level, 60
  as superfood, 83
Bluefish, 120, 128
Body Mass Index (BMI), 11
Body weight
  healthy, 2, 11, 23
  and inflammation, 15
  and microbiota, 10
  recording, 74, 83–84, 92, 283–84
  and waistline measurement, 11–12
Bowman, Sheila, 134
Brain chemicals (neurotransmitters),
    25–26

Bread, Whole-Wheat, with Seeds and Nuts, 194–95

Breakfast, 155–62
Black Rice Pudding, 155
Carrot Muffins, 156–57
Chia Pudding with Berries and Almonds, 158, 286
English Muffin, Almond Butter, and Pear, 288–89
French Toast with Berries, 290–91
Granola, 159
Granola, Crunchy, with Soy Milk, 288
Green Shake, 160, 288
meal plans, xiii, 99, 102, 285–91
on-the-run, 290
Pancakes, Whole-Grain, with Banana, 162, 289
protein sources for, 66–67
Trout and Scrambled Egg, 161, 287
Yogurt, Fruit, and Chia, 287–88

Breast cancer, 23, 47, 49, 86

Broccoli
Quick Roasted with Cilantro, Ginger, and Garlic, 167
Salad, 168, 307

Brown Rice, 64
Cod, Cauliflower and Pea Curry with Mango and, 306
in Eggplant Stuffed with Lentils, 201

Brown Rice Noodles, Shiitake Quick Broth with Edamame and, 203–4, 296

Brussels Sprouts
Marinated with Sesame and Rice Vinegar, 169
Pan-Roasted, 170

Buckwheat, 64

Bulgur. See Cracked Wheat

Bulgur wheat, 42, 85

Burger(s)
Cod, 218–19, 295
Sloppy Joe, Tofu, 205–6, 304
Veggie, 207

Butter, 69

C

Cabbage
in Haddock Tacos, 223–24
pesticide level, 60
Slaw, Beet, 165
Stuffed with Tofu, Walnuts, Cracked Wheat, and Raisins in a Sweet and Sour Tomato Sauce, 199–200

Cake
Chocolate Cupcake with Mint Glaze, 260–61, 315
Sweet Corn, Blueberries Baked with, 259, 316

Calcium
and "belly fat," 12–13
and blood pressure, 47
and body weight, 47
food sources of, 12–13, 47, 66, 90
high-calcium snacks, 292–93
supplements, 65, 89–90

Calorie levels, daily. See also Serving size/calorie level
in-between level, 79–80
meal plans, 78, 95, 101–2, 285–316
selecting, 75
men, 76–77
women, 76
and weight maintenance, 92

Calories
from fat, 8, 35, 36
from fish, 33
on packaged foods, 75
and pescetarian diet, 8, 9, 35, 54
from sugar, 44, 45
for treats, 60, 61, 75, 282

Cancer, 1, 2
  and alcohol consumption, 49
  and barbecuing, 149
  and body fat, 8, 11
  and dairy consumption, 47
  dietary prevention of, 23–24, 40, 46,
    83, 84, 86
  and inflammation, 15, 17
  and meat consumption, 33–34
  skin, 22
  and sugar consumption, 44
Cannellini Bean Spread on Toast,
  300–1
Canola oil, 68
Cantaloupe
  pesticide level, 60
  Trout and Scrambled Egg with
    Almond Milk and, 287
Carbohydrates
  dairy products, 46–48
  fruits and vegetables, 45–46
  and glycemic index (GI), 9, 41,
    42–43
  starches, 41, 43–44
  sugar, 44–45
  types of, 41–42
Cardiovascular Disease and
  Alimentary Comparison
  (CARDIAC) study, 32–33
Carrot(s)
  and Cashew Soup, 171
  Greek Yogurt Dip, 293
  Muffins, 156–57, 290
  on-the-run, 298
  in Veggie Burger, 207
  in Veggie Meatballs over Whole-
    Grain Spaghetti, 208–9
  Yogurt Avocado Dip, 253
Cashew(s)
  and Carrot Soup, 171
  as healthy fat source, 68

Cashew butter, 68
Cast iron searing, 150
Catalan Institute of Oncology, 40
"Catches to Reel in, Catches to Toss
  Back" chart, 121–29, 140
Catfish
  Cornmeal Crusted, with Cucumbers,
    215–16
  safety/sustainability, 120, 122
Cauliflower, Cod and Pea Curry,
  220–21, 306
Celery, 60
Celery Root and Potato Mashed with
  Basil, 189
Centers for Disease Control and
  Prevention (CDC), 109, 129
Cereal
  Fruit, and Milk, 286
  Granola, 159
  Granola, Crunchy, with Soy Milk,
    288
  Oatmeal, Apple, 289
  serving/calorie level, 62, 63
Cheddar, Pear, and Walnuts, 293
Cheerios, 42, 44
Cheese
  protein from, 65
  serving size, 55, 56, 79
Chia (seeds)
  grinding, 285
  as healthy fat source, 36, 68
  Pudding with Berries and Almonds,
    158, 286
  as superfood, 85
  Yogurt, Fruit and, 287–88
Chickpeas. See Garbanzo Beans
Chilean sea bass, 128
Chips
  and guacamole, 315–16
  and salsa, 315
Chives, 86

Chocolate
Banana Frozen with Cocoa and
Peanuts, 256, 302
Cupcake with Mint Glaze, 260–61,
315
dark, as treat, 313
saturated fat in, 36
Cholesterol
HDL, 17, 21
high-cholesterol proteins, 56
LDL, 21, 32, 38, 48, 83, 87
in meat, 34
reduction of, 84, 85, 86
Chowder, Scallop Corn, with Leeks,
236
Chutney, Barbecue Peach, Shrimp
Grilled with, 239, 308
Cilantro
Broccoli, Quick Roasted with
Ginger, Garlic and, 167
in Haddock Tacos, 223–24
Red Lentils with Lime and, 191, 296
in Shiitake Quick Broth with
Edamame and Brown Rice
Noodles, 203–4
as superfood, 85
in Tuna Garbanzo Apricot, Curried,
311
Cinnamon
Peach Smoothie, 251, 292
as superfood, 86
Citrus fruit, 60
Clams
bacteria in, 131
farming, 138
nutrients in, 86
safety/sustainability, 122
steaming, 148–49
with Tomatoes and Garlic on Whole-
Grain Pasta, 217, 310–11
Cleveland Clinic, 34

Cocoa
Banana Frozen with Peanuts and,
256, 302
as superfood, 87
Coconut
fat serving, 68
in Granola, 159
Sesame Cookies, 266
Coconut milk, 66
Coconut oil, 69
Cod
Burger, 218–19, 295
Cauliflower and Pea Curry, 220–21,
306
overfishing of, 134
safety/sustainability, 122
Coffee
cafe au lait, 289
health benefits of, 87
latte and almonds, 293
latte, on the run, 290
servings, 72
Cognition, and omega-3 intake, 29–30
Collard Greens
Mackerel with Sweet Potatoes, Okra
and, 225–26
pesticide level, 60
Colon cancer, 47, 49, 86
Colorectal cancer, 23, 47
Columbia University, 30
Contaminants in seafood
locally caught, 120
mercury, 116, 117–18, 128–29
persistent organic pollutants (POPs),
116, 118–20
raw, 129–32
and safety standards (U.S., Canada,
Europe), 116
and selection guidelines, 115–17,
120–29
and size of fish (wild), 115, 116

Cookies
  Sesame Coconut, 266
  and Tea, 314
Cooking seafood
  cast iron searing, 150
  grilling, 147
  high-temperature methods, 149
  oven-roasting, 146–47
  pan-roasting, 144–45
  poaching, 149–50
  steaming, 148–49
Coriander, 86
Corn
  Chowder, Scallop, with Leeks, 236
  pesticide level, 60
  Salad, 186, 308
  in Veggie Burger, 207
Cornmeal, 63, 64
  Corn Cake, Sweet, Blueberries
    Baked with, 259, 316
  Crusted Catfish with Cucumbers,
    215–16
Corn syrup, 45
Couscous
  in Lentil Soup, One-Dish, 307
  Whole-Wheat, with Rice Vinegar
    and Herbs, 193, 295–96
  Whole-Wheat, with Root Vegetables
    and Garbanzo Beans, 210–11
Crabs
  safety/sustainability, 122
  steaming, 148
Cracked Wheat (bulgur)
  Cabbage Stuffed with Tofu, Walnuts,
    Raisins and, in a Sweet and Sour
    Tomato Sauce, 199–200
  in Cod Burger, 218–19
  in Eggplant Stuffed with Lentils, 201
  glycemic index, 42, 44
  with Golden Raisins and Pistachios,
    187

as superfood, 85
as whole grain, 64
C-reactive protein, 18
Cream, 69
Cream cheese, 69
Cruciferous vegetables, 46, 83
Cucumber(s)
  with Catfish, Cornmeal Crusted,
    215–16
  with Fennel and Creamy Avocado
    Dressing, 172
  Mango, and Avocado Kebab, 257,
    302
  pesticide level, 60
  Seaweed Salad with Peanut Butter
    and, 178
  Yogurt, 292
Cumin, 86
Cupcake, Chocolate, with Mint Glaze,
  260–61, 315
Curry(ied)
  Cod, Cauliflower and Pea, 220–21,
    306
  Tuna Garbanzo Apricot, 311

D
Dairy allergy, and pescetarian meal
  plan, 97
Dairy foods
  as calcium source, 47, 90
  and food poisoning, 129–30
  low-fat/nonfat, 65–67
  pros and cons of, 46–48
  serving size/calorie level, 79
Defenders of Wildlife, 137
Depression, 27–28, 91
Desserts, 259–66
  Blueberries Baked with Sweet Corn
    Cake, 259, 316
  Chocolate Cupcakes with Mint
    Glaze, 260–61, 315

Desserts (cont'd):
  Cookies, Sesame Coconut, 266
  Cookies and Tea, 314
  Granita, Grape, 262
  Ice Cream with Berries, 314
  Melon with Lemon Sauce, 263
  Oranges and Pomegranate with
    Candied Pistachio, 264
  Pears Baked with Rosemary and
    Walnuts, 265, 313
  Sorbet, 315
DHA (docosahexaenoic acid), 25, 26,
  27, 28, 29, 37, 91, 118
Diabetes, 1, 2, 8
  dietary prevention/reversal of, 4,
    20–21, 83, 86
  and erectile dysfunction, 18
  and inflammation, 15, 17
  pre-diabetes, 11, 20
  and raw seafood risk, 132
  and saturated fat, 39
  and sugar consumption, 44
Dietary Guidelines, 39
Dinner meal plans, xiii, 99–100, 102,
  303–11
Dips and spreads
  Cannellini Bean Spread on Toast,
    300–1
  Greek Yogurt Dip, 293
  guacamole and chips, 315–16
  salsa and chips, 315
  Yogurt Avocado Dip, 253
Disease risk
  and body fat, 2, 8, 11–12, 20
  and chronic inflammation,
    14–19
  and dairy consumption, 46–47
  lifestyle factors, 23
  and meat consumption, 33–34
  and overweight, 20
  and sugar consumption, 44–45

Docosahexaenoic acid (DHA), 25, 26,
  27, 28, 29, 37, 118
Docosapentaenoic acid (DPA), 36
DPA (docosapentaenoic acid), 36
Dredging, 137

E
Eating habits
  addictive, 60, 111
  emotional triggers, 103, 111–12,
    281–82
  food cravings, 8
  tracking, 92, 280–81
Eco-labels, 139, 140
E. coli, 129
Edamame
  servings/calorie level, 55
  Shiitake Quick Broth with Brown
    Rice Noodles and, 203–4, 296
Egg(s)
  Black Beans, Salsa and, 286–87
  French Toast with Berries, 290–91
  Hardboiled, Salad with Avocado and,
    308–9
  in Sardine Niçoise, 234–35, 297
  Scrambled, Trout and, 161, 287
  servings of, 55
Eggplant
  pesticide level, 60
  Stuffed with Lentils, 201–2, 310
Eicosapentaenoic acid (EPA), 36, 37, 91
Emotional eating, 103, 111–12, 281–82
Energy
  achieving on Pescetarian Plan, 103
  and caffeine, 72
  and exercise, 106
  and Pescetarian Tracker, 280, 281
  and water, 71
Endometrial cancer, 23
English Muffin, 63
  Almond Butter, and Pear, 288–89

Environmental defense, 137
Environmental problems. *See* Pollution
Environmental Protection Agency (EPA), 116
EPA (eicosapentaenoic acid), 36, 37, 91
Erectile dysfunction, 18
European Union, 118
Exercise
    aerobic, 92, 104, 107–8, 281
    and "belly fat," 12
    energy for, 5
    excuses for not exercising, 104–5
    flexibility training (stretching), 109
    health benefits of, 1, 12, 17, 18, 19, 21, 23, 28, 106
    at middle level of fitness, 104
    and mood, 7, 28
    as Pescetarian principle, 72
    prescription, 106–9
    recording weekly minutes, 281
    and sleep, 111
    strength training, 109
    and weight maintenance, 13, 72, 92, 103, 106, 107

F
Fairburn, Christopher, 112
Farmed fish. *See* Aquaculture
Fat, body
    and diabetes risk, 20
    and genetics, 8
    visceral (abdominal), 8, 11–12, 15, 44
Fat, dietary. *See also* Oils; Omega-3 fats; Omega-6 fats; Saturated fat
    balance in, 39–40, 68–69
    calories from, 8, 35, 36
    imbalance in, 37
    and inflammation, 16
    monounsaturated, 16, 35, 36, 40, 41
    polyunsaturated, 35–36
    serving size/calorie level, 67–68, 79, 80
    and skin health, 22
    trans fat, 39, 69
Fennel
    in Beet Slaw, 165
    with Cucumber and Creamy Avocado Dressing, 172
    Salmon, Seared, with Mushroom, Sweet Red Pepper and, 228–29
    in Seafood Stew, 237–38
Fetal brain development, 28–29
Fiber, dietary, 12, 42
Fig Dressing, Roasted Garlic, Arugula with, 164
Fish. *See also* Pescetarian diet
    bacteria in, 130–31, 132
    contaminants in. *See* Contaminants in seafood
    cooking. *See* Cooking seafood
    fatty, 55, 56, 79, 118
    has healthy fat source, 70
    nutrients in, 32–33, 86
    as protein source, 3–4
    raw, 129–32
    safety/sustainability guidelines, 115–17, 120–29
    shopping for. *See* Shopping for seafood
    storage of, 143–44
    white-fleshed, 55
Fish dishes
    Catfish, Cornmeal Crusted, with Cucumbers, 215–16
    Cod Burger, 218–19, 295
    Cod, Cauliflower and Pea Curry, 220–21, 306
    Fish and Greens, 304–5
    Flounder Baked with Grapes and Almonds, 222

Fish dishes (*cont'd*):
  Haddock Tacos, 223–24, 309
  Mackerel with Sweet Potatoes,
    Collard Greens, and Okra, 225–26
  Salmon Salad, 227, 299
  Salmon, Seared, with Fennel,
    Mushroom, and Sweet Red
    Pepper, 228–29
  Salmon with Tahini and Toasted
    Nuts, 230–31, 303–4
  Sardine Niçoise, 234–35, 297
  Sardines, Broiled with Green Onion
    on Arugula, 232–33
  Sardines and Greens, 295–96
  Sardines on Toast, 294
  Seafood Stew, 237–38, 307
  Tilapia with Black Beans, Green
    Onions, Garlic, and Ginger,
    243–44
  Tilapia Fish Sticks, 241–42
  Trout in Paper with Summer
    Squash, Green Onions, and Basil,
    245–46
  Trout and Scrambled Egg, 161, 297
  Trout, Whole with Thyme and
    Preserved Lemon, 247
  Tuna Garbanzo Apricot, Curried, 311
  Tuna Salad Sandwich, 298
Fisheries
  destroying/harming of, 136–37
  fishing sustainably, 135–36
  overfishing, 133–35
  and pollution problems, 137
Fish farms. *See* Aquaculture
Fish oil
  compared to plant-based omega-3,
    36–37
  DHA, 25, 26, 27, 28, 29, 37, 91, 118
  EPA, 36, 37, 91
  in farmed fish, 119
  supplementing with, 91

Flatfish, safety/sustainability, 122
Flaxseed oil, 68
Flaxseeds
  grinding, 285
  as healthy fat source, 36, 68
  as superfood, 85
Flexibility training (stretching), 109
Flounder
  Baked with Grapes and Almonds,
    222
  safety/sustainability, 116, 122
Flour
  refined, 16, 38, 42, 44, 63, 64
  whole-grain, 42, 63, 64, 65
Food addiction, 60, 111
Food and Agriculture Organization
    (FAO), 29, 135
Food allergies, xv, 46, 47, 97
Food cravings, 8
Food and Drug Administration (FDA),
    39, 116, 128
Food poisoning, 129
Food and Water Watch, 137
Forman, Sidra, xii, 144, 152–53
French Toast with Berries, 290–91
Freshness, selecting seafood for, xvi,
    141–43
Friends of the Sea, 139
Frozen food, 82
Frozen seafood
  selecting, 143
  thawing, 144
Fructose, 41, 44, 45
Fruit. *See also* Berries; *specific fruits*
  and body fat, 13
  Cereal, and Milk, 286
  fiber in, 42
  freshness of, 59
  frozen, 82
  Green Shake, 160
  increasing consumption of, 57–58

nutrients in, 45–46
organic *vs.* conventional, 59
pesticide levels, 60
serving size/calorie level, 58, 79, 80
snacks, 100, 102, 302
in starch dishes, 63–64
superfoods, 83
Yogurt, and Chia, 287–88
"Full" signal, 9, 15

G
Garbanzo Bean(s) (chickpeas)
Couscous, Whole-Wheat, with Root
Vegetables and, 210–11
Red Pepper, Pumpkin Seed, and
Olive Salad, 298–99
Roasted with Oregano, 250
Tuna Garbanzo Apricot, Curried, 311
Garlic
Broccoli, Quick Roasted with
Cilantro, Ginger and, 167
Clams with Tomatoes and, on
Whole-Grain Pasta, 210–11, 217
health benefits of, 86
Roasted, 271
Roasted, Fig Dressing, Arugula with,
164
Roasted, Kale with, 173
Tilapia with Black Beans, Green
Onions, Ginger and, 243–44
Tomatoes with, Roasted, 183
Genetics
and cancer risk, 49
and weight loss, 7–10, 111
Gillnetting, 136
Ginger
Broccoli, Quick Roasted with
Cilantro, Garlic and, 167
as superfood, 86
Tilapia with Black Beans, Green
Onions, Garlic and, 243–44

Glucose, 41
Gluten allergy, and pescetarian meal
plan, 97
Gluten-Free Chocolate Cupcake with
Mint Glaze, 260–61
Gluten-free whole grains, 63
Glycemic index (GI), 9, 41, 42
Grains. *See also* Whole-Grain(s);
specific grains
fiber in, 42
glycemic index, 42–43, 44, 85
health benefits of, 84, 85
servings/calorie level, 62, 63, 78,
79
Granita, Grape, 262, 312
Granola, 159
Crunchy, with Soy Milk, 288
Grape(s)
Flounder Baked with Almonds and,
222
Granita, 262, 312
pesticide level, 60
as superfood, 83
Grapefruit, 60, 83
Gratin, Sweet Potato, 192
Gray snapper, safety/sustainability of,
127
Greek Yogurt Dip, 293
Green Beans, 60
in Sardine Niçoise, 234–35, 297
Greene, Bob, xii, 91, 104, 105, 109,
112
Green Onion(s)
Black Rice with Sesame and, 185
Mushrooms, Oven Roasted with
Thyme and, 177
with Sardines, Broiled, on Arugula,
232–33
in Shiitake Quick Broth with
Edamame and Brown Rice
Noodles, 203–4

Green Onion(s) (*cont'd*):
  Tilapia with Black Beans, Garlic,
    Ginger and, 243–44
  Trout in Paper with Summer
    Squash, Basil and, 245–46
Greenpeace, 147
Greens. *See also specific greens*
  and Fish, 304–5
  and Sardines, 295–96
  as superfood, 84, 288
Green Shake, 160
Grilling seafood, 147
Groats, 64
Grouper, safety/sustainability, 128
Guacamole and chips treat, 315–16

H
Haddock
  overfishing of, 134
  safety/sustainability, 122
  Tacos, 223–24, 309
Halibut, safety/sustainability, 126
Harpooning, 135
Harvard Health Professionals
    Follow-Up Study, 33–34
Harvard Nurse's Health Study, 23, 34,
    47
HCAs (heterocyclic amines), 149
HDL cholesterol, 17, 21
Health benefits of pescetarian diet,
    ix–x, xii, xiii, 1–2
  anti-inflammatory, 15–17
  belly fat reduction, 12–13
  brain function, 25–27
  cancer prevention, 23–24
  dementia prevention, 29–30
  diabetes prevention, 20–21
  diabetes reversal, 21
  fetal brain development, 28–29
  heart disease prevention, 19–20
  psychological, 2, 27–28

red wine and beer, 48–49, 83, 87
  sexual function, 18
  skin protection, 22
  of superfoods, 83–87
Heart disease, 1, 2
  and body fat, 8, 11
  and cholesterol level, 38
  dietary prevention of, 19–20, 33, 86,
    87
  and erectile dysfunction, 18
  and fish oil, 91
  and inflammation, 15, 17
  and meat consumption, 33, 34
  and saturated fat, 34, 35, 37–38
  and sugar consumption, 44
Hemochomatosis, 132
Hemp milk, 66
Heptopancreas, 116
Herbs, superfoods, 85
Herring, safety/sustainability, 123
Heterocyclic amines (HCAs), 34,
    149
Hibbeln, Joseph, 27
Hicks, Doris T., 130
High blood pressure, 4, 17, 83
Hunger scale, in Pescetarian Tracker,
    280–81
Hungry, 4, 13, 54, 76, 77, 79, 97, 280,
    281

I
Ice Cream
  with Berries, 314
  saturated fat in, 70
Ikaria (Greece), viii, 27, 89
Immune system, and raw seafood
    risk, 132
Inflammation
  acute, 15
  anti-inflammatory agents, 16, 32,
    38–39

in brain, 26
chronic, 14–19
and saturated fat, 38, 44
and sugar consumption, 45
Insulin resistance, 17, 86
Intelligence (children's), and
    omega-3 intake during pregnancy,
    28–29
INTERMAP, 5–6
Intestinal bacteria, 10, 34, 42, 44

J
Japanese diet, ix, 32–33
Jibrin, Sami and Najla, xiii

K
Kale
    in Black-Eyed Pea Stew, 197–98
    with Garlic, Roasted, 175
    Green Shake, 160
    in Lentil Soup, One-Dish, 307
    pesticide level, 60
    Salad with Sesame Dressing, 173
    Soup, Creamy and Quick, 174,
        294–95
Kearney-Cooke, Ann, 91, 112
Kebab, Cucumber, Mango, and
    Avocado, 257, 302
Kefir, 47–48
Kidney Beans, in Tofu Sloppy Joe,
    205–6
Kiwi, 60, 83
Kuipers, Remko, 38

L
Lactation, and low-mercury fish
    consumption, 118
Lactobacillus adiophilus, 48
Lactobacillus casei, 48
Lactose, 41
Lactose intolerance, 46, 47, 48

Latte
    and Almonds, 293
    on-the-run, 290
L-carnitine, 34
LDL cholesterol, 21, 32, 38, 48, 83, 86,
    87
Leeks
    Scallop Corn Chowder with, 236
    as superfood, 86
Legumes. See also Bean(s); Lentil(s)
    fiber in, 12, 42
    health benefits of, 43–44, 84
    as protein source, 4, 56–57
    servings/calorie level, 63
Lemon(s)
    Preserved, 272
    Preserved, Spinach with Olives and,
        180
    Preserved, Trout Whole with Thyme
        and, 247
    Quinoa with Olive Oil, Pomegranate
        and, 190, 303–4
    Sauce, Melon with, 263, 313
    Summer Squash Salad with Basil
        and, 181
    as superfood, 83
Lentil(s)
    Eggplant Stuffed with, 201–2, 310
    Red, with Lime and Cilantro, 191,
        296
    Soup, One-Dish, 307
Lettuce, pesticide level, 60
Life You Want, The: Get Motivated,
    Lose Weight, Be Happy (Jibrin,
    Greene and Kearney-Cooke), 91,
    112
Lime
    Red Lentils with Cilantro and, 191,
        296
    as superfood, 83
Listeria monocytogenes, 132

Liver disease, and raw seafood risk, 132
Lobster, safety/sustainability, 116, 127
Longlining, 136
Look AHEAD trial, 21
Lunch meal plans, xiii, 99, 102, 294–301
Lung cancer, 49
Lutein, 84
Lycopene, 84

M
Macadamia nuts, 68
Mackerel
  king, 129
  safety/sustainability, 123
  servings of, 56
  Spanish, 128
  with Sweet Potatoes, Collard Greens, and Okra, 225–26
Macular degeneration, 84
Mahimahi, safety/sustainability, 127
Mango
  Cod, Cauliflower and Pea Curry with Brown Rice and, 306
  Cucumber, and Avocado Kebab, 257, 302
  pesticide level, 60
  as superfood, 83
Marine Stewardship Council (MSC), 134–35, 139
Mayonnaise, fat serving, 68
Meal plans, xiii, 95–102, 285–316
  and affordability, xvi, 101
  balanced, 100
  beverages in, 97
  breakfast, xiii, 99, 102, 285–91
  calorie levels in, 101–2
  designing your own, 98–100
  dinner, xiii, 99–100, 102, 303–11
  flexibility of, 96, 97, 98
  and food allergies, 97
  and food groups, 98
  lunch, xiii, 99, 102, 294–301
  selecting food items for, 95–96, 101
  snacks, 97, 99, 100, 102, 292–93
  sticking to, 96
  treats, 100, 102, 312–16
Meat
  and food poisoning, 129–30
  health drawbacks of, xv, 33–34
  saturated fat in, 70
  and skin aging, 22
  trans fat in, 39
Meatballs, Veggie, over Whole-Grain Spaghetti, 208–9
Meat substitutes, xiv–xv
Mediterranean diet
  cognitive benefits of, 30
  and diabetes prevention, 21
  and heart disease prevention, 19–20
  and mood enhancement, 27–28
  and sexual function, 18
  and skin health, 22
  traditional, ix, x–xi
  and weight loss, 24
Mediterranean Diet Score, xi
Melanoma, 22
Melon
  Cantaloupe, Trout and Scrambled Egg with Almond Milk and, 287
  with Lemon Sauce, 263, 313
Men, calorie level for weight loss/ maintenance, 76–77
Mercury contamination, 116, 117–18, 128–29
Metabolic syndrome, 17–18
Metabolism, and weight loss, 6–7
Microbiota, 10
Milk
  as calcium source, 90
  lactose intolerance, 46, 47, 48

low-fat/nonfat, 65, 66
nondairy, 66, 67
saturated fat in, 47, 70
serving size/calorie level, 79
Strawberry, 232, 292
Mint
Glaze, Chocolate Cupcake with, 260–61, 315
as superfood, 85
Monkfish, safety/sustainability, 127
Monounsaturated fat, 16, 35, 36, 40, 41, 87
Monterey Bay Aquarium, 137
Seafood Watch, 134
Mood enhancement, 27–28, 41
Mortality, and meat consumption, 33–34
Mozzarella, Tomato, and Avocado Sandwich, 294–95
Muffins, Carrot, 156–57, 290
Mullet, striped, safety/sustainability, 123
Multivitamins, 90
Mushroom(s)
Marinated, 176
Oven Roasted with Green Onion and Thyme, 177
pesticide level, 60
Salmon, Seared, with Fennel, Sweet Red Pepper and, 228–29
Shiitake Quick Broth with Edamame and Brown Rice Noodles, 203–4, 296
Mussels
farming, 138
nutrients in, 86
safety/sustainability, 116, 123
steaming, 148–49
Mustard
Grainy, 273
Vinaigrette, 275

N
National Cancer Institute, 33, 49
National Institute on Aging, 11
National Weight Control Registry (NWCR), 6, 93–94
Natural Resources Defense Council, 120, 128–29
Nectarines, 60
Neurotransmitters, 25–26
Noodles, Brown Rice, Shiitake Quick Broth with Edamame and, 203–4, 296
Nut(s). *See also specific nuts*
allergy, xiii, 67, 97
fat serving, 67, 68
health benefits of, 15, 85
healthy fats in, 67
monounsaturated fat in, 35
serving size/calorie level, 68, 78, 79
as superfoods, 85
Toasted, Salmon with Tahini and, 230–31, 303–4
Whole-Wheat Bread with Seeds and, 194–95
Nut allergy, and pescetarian meal plan, 97
Nut Butter
Dressing, 276
fat serving, 68
Nutrition. *See also* Pescetarian principles
and alcohol consumption, 48–49
carbohydrates, 41–48
fats, 35–41
macronutrients, 31
protein, 31, 32–33
and sodium reduction, 87–89
superfoods, 81–87
vitamin and mineral supplements, 89–91
Nutrition labels, 39

O

Oat flour, 64

Oatmeal
  Apple, 289
  glycemic index, 42
  Onion Cake, 188
  in Pears Baked with Rosemary and
    Walnuts, 265
  as whole grain, 64

Oats
  fiber in, 42
  in Granola, 159
  servings/calorie level, 63
  as superfood, 84
  as whole grain, 64

Obesity, 2, 6, 10
  and Body Mass Index, 11
  and cancer risk, 23
  and chronic inflammation, 15
  and diabetes risk, 20

Oceana, 137

Ocean Conservancy, 137

Oceans, pollution of, 137

Oceans Futures Society, 137

Octopus, 116, 147

Oils. See also Fish oil; Olive oil
  fat serving, 68
  healthy, 68
  partially hydrogenated, 39
  serving size/calorie level, 79

Oil spills, 137

Okra, Mackerel with Sweet Potatoes,
  Collard Greens and, 225–26

Olive(s)
  fat serving, 68
  Garbanzo Bean, Red Pepper, and
    Pumpkin Seed Salad, 298–99
  Spinach with Preserved Lemons
    and, 180

Olive oil
  health benefits of, 23, 40, 87
  as healthy fat source, 35, 67, 68,
    70

Omega-3 fats
  and Alzheimer's disease, 30
  as anti-inflammatory agent, 16,
    32
  average amount on Pescetarian
    Plan, 40, 68
  and brain-boosting powers of, 25,
    26, 118
  cognitive benefits of, 29–30
  and disease prevention, 19, 36
  and fetal brain development, 28–29
  in fish, 32–33, 86
  food sources of, 68, 85
  and heart disease, 19, 91
  and mood enhancement, 27, 41
  and omega-6 ratio, 16, 26, 37, 40
  plant vs. fish, 36–37
  and skin health, 22
  supplements, 89, 91

Omega-6 fats
  food sources of, 69
  and omega-3 ratio, 16, 26, 37, 40
  polyunsaturated, 35–36

Onions. See also Green Onion(s)
  Oatmeal Onion Cake, 188
  pesticide level, 60
  as superfood, 86

On-the-run meals, 290, 297–98

Opiates, 26

Oranges
  and Pomegranate with Candied
    Pistachio, 264
  Spinach Salad with Poppy Seeds
    and, 179
  as superfood, 83

Oregano
  Chickpeas Roasted with, 250
  as superfood, 85

Organic produce, 59–60

Ornish, Dean, 14–15
Osteoarthritis, 91
Ovarian cancer, 47
Oven-roasting seafood, 146–47
Overcoming Binge Eating (Fairburn), 112
Overfishing, 133–35
Overweight
  Body Mass Index (BMI), 11
  and chronic inflammation, 15
  and diabetes risk, 20–21
  visceral (abdominal) fat, 2, 8, 11–12,
    15, 44
Oysters
  bacteria in, 131
  farming, 138
  nutrients in, 86
  post-harvest processed, 131
  safety/sustainability, 116, 123
  steaming, 148–49
Oz, Mehmet, xii

P
Packaged foods, calories on, 75
PAHs (Polycyclic aromatic
    hydrocarbons), 149
Pancakes, Whole-Grain, with Banana,
    162, 289
Pancreatic cancer, 23, 86
Pan-roasting seafood, 144–45
Papaya, 83
Parmesan Cheese, with Air-Popped
    Popcorn (unsalted), 313
Parsley, 85
Partially hydrogenated oil, 39
Pasta
  servings/calorie level, 63
  Spaghetti, Whole-Grain, Veggie
    Meatballs over, 208–9
  Whole-Grain, Baked with White
    Beans, Spinach, and Walnut
    Sauce, 212–13, 305–6

Whole-Grain, Clams with
    Tomatoes and Garlic on, 217,
    310–11
Pea(s)
  Cod, and Cauliflower Curry,
    220–21, 306
  pesticide level, 60
  servings/calorie level, 63
Peach(es)
  Chutney, Barbecue, Shrimp Grilled
    with, 239, 308
  Cinnamon Smoothie, 251, 292
  pesticide level, 60
  Tomato, and Basil Salad, 182
Peanut Butter
  and Apple, Open-Faced, 300
  Dressing, Nut Butter, 276
  fat serving, 68
  as healthy fat source, 68
  Seaweed Salad with Cucumber and,
    178
  Yogurt, Banana Pop, 254, 292
Peanut oil, 68
Peanuts
  Banana Frozen with Cocoa and, 256,
    302
  as healthy fat source, 68
Pear(s)
  Baked with Rosemary and Walnuts,
    265, 313
  Cheddar, and Walnuts, 293
  English Muffin, and Almond Butter,
    288–89
  Yogurt, and Pistachio, 292
Pecans, 68
Pepper(s). *See* Bell Pepper(s)
Persistent organic pollutants (POPs),
    116, 118–20
Pescetarian diet. *See also* Meal plans;
    Nutrition; Weight loss; Weight
    maintenance

Pescetarian diet (cont'd):
  common questions about, xiv–xvi
  defined, ix
  health benefits of. See Health
    benefits of Pescetarian diet
  Mediterranean foods in. See
    Mediterranean diet
  nutrients in, 2
Pescetarian principles, xv, 53–72
  dairy foods, low-fat/nonfat/nondairy,
    65–67
  produce servings, increasing, 57–60
  protein sources, nonmeat, 55–57
  put into action, 73–80
  starchy foods, portioning, 62–65
  treats/alcohol consumption, limits
    on, 60–62
  water consumption, 70–72
Pescetarian Tracker, 73, 92, 279–82
Pesticides, on fruit and vegetables, 59,
  60
Pew Institute for Ocean Science, 137
Phytonutrients, 2, 16, 46, 82, 83
Phytoplankton, 137
Pineapple, 60
Pistachio(s)
  Candied, Oranges and Pomegranate
    with, 264
  Cracked Wheat with Golden Raisins
    and, 187
  as healthy fat source, 68
  Yogurt, and Pear, 292
Plums, 83
Poaching seafood, 149–50
Polenta, 63
Poll fishing, 135
Pollock, safety/sustainability, 123
Pollution
  and cancer risk, 22, 23
  and fish farming, 138, 139
  sources of, 137

Polycyclic aromatic hydrocarbons
  (PAHs), 149
Polyphenols, 40
Polyunsaturated fat, 35–36. See also
  Omega-3 fats; Omega-6 fats
Pomegranate
  in Eggplant Stuffed with Lentils, 201
  and Oranges with Candied
    Pistachio, 264
  Quinoa with Lemon, Olive Oil and,
    190, 303–4
  as superfood, 83
Pop, Yogurt, Banana, Peanut Butter,
  254, 292
Popcorn, 64
  Air-Popped (unsalted), with
    Parmesan Cheese, 313
Poppy Seed(s)
  Dressing, 277
  Spinach Salad with Oranges and, 179
Portfolio Diet, 85
Portion size. See Serving size; Serving
  size/calorie level
Postpartum depression, 27–28
Potato(es)
  and Celery Root Mashed with Basil,
    189
  pesticide level, 60
  in Sardine Niçoise, 234–35, 297
  servings/calorie level, 63
  in Trout and Scrambled Egg, 161
Poultry
  and food poisoning, 129–30
  health drawbacks of, xv
  saturated fat in, 70
Prawns, safety/sustainability, 116, 125
Pregnancy
  depression during, 28
  fatty fish consumption during, 118
  fetal brain development during,
    28–29

low-mercury fish consumption
during, 118, 128
and raw/smoked fish risk, 132
Preserved Lemon(s), 272
Spinach with Olives and, 180
Trout Whole with Thyme and, 247
Probiotic supplements, 10
Prostate cancer, 23, 47, 49, 83, 86
Protein
and body fat, 13
from fish, 3–4, 32–33
from legumes, 56–57
serving size/calorie level, 55–56, 79,
80
Prunes, 83
Psychological benefits of pescetarian
diet, 2, 27–28
Pudding(s)
Black Rice, 155, 287
Chia with Berries and Almonds,
158, 286
Pumpkin Seed, Garbanzo Bean, Red
Pepper, and Olive Salad, 298–99
Purse seining, 136

Q
Quinoa
in Granola, 159
with Lemon, Olive Oil, and
Pomegranate, 190, 303–4
as superfood, 84

R
Rainbow trout, safety/sustainability,
125
Raisins
Cabbage Stuffed with Tofu, Walnuts,
Cracked Wheat and, in a Sweet
and Sour Tomato Sauce, 199–200
Golden, Cracked Wheat with
Pistachios and, 187

Raspberries, 83
Raw seafood, 130–32
Red Lentils with Lime and Cilantro,
191, 296
Red Pepper
Garbanzo Bean, Pumpkin Seed, and
Olive Salad, 298–99
Sweet, Seared Salmon with Fennel,
Mushroom and, 228–29
Red snapper, safety/sustainability,
127
Red wine
health benefits of, 48–49, 83, 87
recommended amounts, 61
as treat, 316
Resveratrol, 87
Rice, 64. *See also* Black Rice; Brown
Rice
Rice milk, 66
Rice Vinegar, Whole-Wheat Couscous
with Herbs and, 193
Rice Vinegar, Brussels Sprouts
Marinated with Sesame and, 169
Rockfish, safety/sustainability, 127
Romaine, Black Bean Roll Up
Wrapped in, 249
Rosemary
Beets with Onions, Balsamic
Vinegar and, 166
Pears Baked with Walnuts and, 265,
313
as superfood, 85
Runoff, rainwater, 137
Rush Institute for Healthy Aging, 29
Rye, 65
Rye berries, 64

S
Sablefish, safety/sustainability, 127
Safety guidelines, for seafood
selection, 115–17, 120–29

Safety standards, 116
Salad(s)
    Arugula with Roasted Garlic Fig
        Dressing, 164
    Arugula Shrimp, Black Rice with,
        297
    with Avocado and Hardboiled Eggs,
        308–9
    Beet Slaw, 165
    Broccoli, 168, 307
    Corn, 186, 308
    Cucumber with Fennel and Creamy
        Avocado Dressing, 172
    Garbanzo Bean, Red Pepper,
        Pumpkin Seed, and Olive Salad,
        298–99
    Greens and Sardines, 295–96
    Kale, with Sesame Dressing,
        173
    Salmon, 227, 299
    Sardine Niçoise, 234–35, 297
    Seaweed, with Cucumber and
        Peanut Butter, 178
    Shrimp Taco, 240, 303
    Spinach, with Poppy Seeds and
        Oranges, 179
    Tomato, 310
    Tomato, Peach, and Basil, 182
    Tuna Garbanzo Apricot, Curried,
        311
    Walnut, 295
Salad Dressing
    Avocado, Creamy, Cucumber and
        Fennel with, 172
    Avocado Thick, 274
    Garlic, Roasted, Fig, Arugula with,
        164
    Nut Butter, 276
    Poppy Seed, 277
    Sesame, Kale Salad with, 173
    Vinaigrette, Mustard, 275

Salmon
    farm-raised, safety/sustainability of,
        116, 119, 127
    fats in, 33
    Salad, 227, 299
    Seared, with Fennel, Mushroom,
        and Sweet Red Pepper, 228–29
    servings of, 56, 86
    skin removal, 120
    with Tahini and Toasted Nuts,
        230–31, 303–4
    wild, safety/sustainability of, 116,
        119, 124
    wild, as superfood, 86
Salmonella, 129
Salmon roe, 124
Salsa
    Black Beans, and Eggs, 286–87
    and chips, 315
    Fresh, Shrimp Taco Salad with, 303
Salt
    craving, 8
    reduction of, 87–89
    snacks, 5, 60
Salt shaker, 88
Sandwich(es). See also Burger(s)
    Mozzarella, Tomato, and Avocado,
        294–95
    Peanut Butter and Apple, Open-
        Faced, 300
    Sardines on Toast, 294
    Tuna Salad, 298
Sardine(s)
    Broiled with Green Onion on
        Arugula, 232–33
    Greens and, 295–96
    Niçoise, 234–35, 297
    safety/sustainability, 118, 119, 124
    servings of, 56
    as superfood, 86
    on Toast, 294

Saturated fat
  in chocolate, 36
  in dairy products, 47
  in fish *vs.* beef, 33
  food sources of, 35, 70
  and heart disease, 34, 35, 37–38
  limit on, 40
  substitutes for, 70
  types of, 69
Sauce(s)
  Lemon, Melon with, 263, 313
  Tomato, Sweet and Sour, Cabbage
    Stuffed with Tofu, Walnuts,
    Cracked Wheat, and Raisins in a,
    199–200
  Walnut, Whole-Grain Pasta Baked
    with White Beans, Spinach and,
    212–13, 305–6
Scallions. *See also* Green Onion(s)
  as superfood, 86
Scallop(s)
  cast iron searing, 150
  Corn Chowder with Leeks,
    236
  oven-roasting, 146
  pan-roasting, 145
  safety/sustainability, 116, 124
  Seafood Stew, 237–38
  steaming, 148
Scarmeas, Nikolaos, 30
Seafood. *See* Fish; Fish dishes;
    Pescetarian diet; Shellfish;
    Shellfish dishes
Seafood Stew, 237–38, 307
Sea lice, 138
Searing, cast iron, 150
Sea scallops, 124
Seaweed Salad with Cucumber and
    Peanut Butter, 178
Sedentary lifestyle, and cancer risk, 22,
    23

Seed butter
  fat serving, 68
  health benefits of, 85
Seeds. *See also specific seeds*
  fat serving, 67, 68
  in Granola, 159
  healthy fats in, 67
  serving size/calorie level, 79
  Whole-Wheat Bread with Nuts and,
    194–95
Semolina, 64, 65
Serotonin, 26
Serving size
  in meal plan, 99–100
  measuring/gauging, 73–74, 78–79,
    282
  recording/logging, 73–74
Serving size/calorie level, 54
  alcoholic beverages, 61–62, 78
  dairy, low-fat/nonfat/nondairy,
    65–66
  drinking water, 71–72
  fats, healthy, 67–68, 78
  food group chart, 78
  fruits, 57–58, 78
  protein, 56–57, 78
  starches, 62–65
  treats, 60, 61, 78
  vegetables, 58–59, 78
Sesame
  Black Rice with Green Onions and, 185
  Brussels Sprouts Marinated with
    Rice Vinegar and, 169
  Coconut Cookies, 266
  Dressing, Kale Salad with, 173
  in Shiitake Quick Broth with
    Edamame and Brown Rice
    Noodles, 203–4
  Spiced, Apple with, 255
Seventh-day Adventists, weight loss
    study of, 4

Sexual dysfunction, 18
Shad, safety/sustainability, 124
Shake, Green, 160, 288
Sharecare.com, xii
Shark, safety/sustainability, 116
Shellfish. *See also* Pescetarian diet
  bacteria in, 131
  contaminants in. *See* Contaminants in seafood
  cooking. *See* Cooking seafood
  nutrients in, 86
  as protein source, 3–4
  raw, 129–32
  safety/sustainability guidelines, 115–17, 120–32
  serving size/calorie level, 55
  shopping for. *See* Shopping for seafood
  storage of, 143–44
Shellfish dishes
  Clams with Tomatoes and Garlic on Whole-Grain Pasta, 217
  Scallop Corn Chowder with Leeks, 236
  Seafood Stew, 237–38, 307
  Shrimp Arugula Salad, Black Rice with, 297
  Shrimp Grilled with Barbecue Peach Chutney, 239, 308
  Shrimp Taco Salad, 240, 303
Shiitake Quick Broth with Edamame and Brown Rice Noodles, 203–4, 296
Shopping for seafood
  "Catches to Reel in, Catches to Toss Back" chart, 121–29, 140
  and eco-labels, 139, 140
  freshness tips, xvi, 141–43
  frozen seafood, 143
  guidelines for, 115–17
  live seafood, 142
  raw oysters, 131

Shrimp
  Arugula Salad, Black Rice with, 297
  Grilled with Barbecue Peach Chutney, 239, 308
  grilling, 147
  oven-roasting, 146
  pan-roasting, 145
  safety/sustainability, 116, 125
  Seafood Stew, 237–38
  steaming, 148
  Taco Salad, 240, 303
Sierra Club, 137
Skin cancer, 22, 49
Skin protection
  and Mediterranean diet, 22
  and vitamin D supplements, 89
Slaw, Beet, 165
Sleep, 5
  good sleep hygiene, 110–11
  lack of, 103, 109–10
  tracking/recording, 280
Sloppy Joe, Tofu, 205–6, 304
Smoking, and cancer risk, 23, 24
Smoothie, Peach Cinnamon, 251, 292
Snacks, xiii, 240–57. *See also* Dips and spreads
  Apple with Spiced Sesame, 255
  Banana Frozen with Cocoa and Peanuts, 256
  Black Bean Roll Up Wrapped in Romaine, 249
  Cheddar, Pear, and Walnuts, 293
  Chickpeas Roasted with Oregano, 250
  Cucumber, Mango, and Avocado Kebab, 257
  Cucumber Yogurt, 292
  extra (2,500-calorie plan), 312
  fruit and vegetable, 100, 102, 302
  high-calcium, 292–93
  latte and almonds, 293

meal plans, 97, 99, 100, 102, 292–93
Popcorn, Air-Popped (unsalted), with Parmesan Cheese, 313
salty, 5, 60
Smoothie, Peach Cinnamon, 251, 292
Strawberry Milk, 252, 292
Yogurt, Banana, Peanut Butter Pop, 254
Yogurt, Pistachios, and Pear, 292
Snapper, safety/sustainability, 127
Sodium. See also Salt
and blood pressure, 19
reduction of, 87–89
Sorbet treat, 315
Sorghum, 64
Soup(s)
Carrot and Cashew, 171
Corn Chowder, Scallop, with Leeks, 236
Kale, Creamy and Quick, 174, 294–95
Lentil, One-Dish, 307
Shiitake Quick Broth with Edamame and Brown Rice Noodles, 203–4, 296
Sour cream, 69
Soy milk, 66
Soy yogurt, 66
Spaghetti, Whole-Grain, Veggie Meatballs over, 208–9
Spanish mackerel, 128
Spelt, 65
Spices, superfoods, 86
Spinach
with Olives and Preserved Lemons, 180
Pasta, Whole-Grain, Baked with White Beans, Walnut Sauce and, 212–13, 305–6
pesticide level, 60

Salad with Poppy Seeds and Oranges, 179
in Trout and Scrambled Egg, 161
Wilted, Clams with Tomatoes and Garlic on Whole-Grain Pasta with, 310–11
Squash, Summer. See Summer Squash
Squid
grilling, 147
safety/sustainability, 116, 125
Starches
defined, 41
health benefits of, 43–44
servings/calorie level, 62–65, 78
Starchy vegetables, 62, 78, 79, 80
Steaming seafood, 148–49
Stearic acid, 36
Stew(s)
Black-Eyed Pea, 197–98
Seafood, 237–38, 307
Stivers, Tori, 131
Storage of seafood, 143–44
Strawberry(ies)
Milk, 232
pesticide level, 60
as superfood, 83
Strength training, 109
Stress
and cancer risk, 22, 23
and overeating, 103, 281
Stretching (flexibility training), 109
Striped bass, safety/sustainability, 126
Sucrose, 41
Sugar
added, 16, 45
in beverages, 70–71, 72
calories from, 44, 45
cravings, 5, 8
and inflammation, 16, 44–45
milk (lactose), 46

Sugar (cont'd):
  on Pescetarian Plan, xv, 45
  types of, 41
Sugar alcohols, 41
Sulforaphane, 46
Summer Squash
  Salad with Lemon and Basil, 181
  Trout in Paper with Green Onions,
    Basil and, 245–46
Sun exposure, and cancer risk, 22, 23, 89
Sunflower Seeds, in Whole-Wheat
  Bread with Seeds and Nuts,
  194–95
Superfoods, 81–87
Sushi, 129, 130, 131–32
Sustainable fishing methods,
  135–36
Sustainable seafood
  "Catches to Reel in, Catches to Toss
    Back" chart, 121–29
  certification for, 134–35, 139
  eco-labels, 139
Sweeteners, 9, 16, 45. See also Sugar
  artificial, 72
Sweet Potato(es)
  Gratin, 192
  Mackerel with Collard Greens, Okra
    and, 225–26
  nutrients in, 84
  pesticide level, 60
  serving size/calorie level, 63
Sweet and Sour Tomato Sauce,
  Cabbage Stuffed with Tofu,
  Walnuts, Cracked Wheat, and
  Raisins in a, 199–200
Swordfish, 115, 116, 118
Synaptic cleft, 25–26

T
Tacos, Haddock, 223–24, 309
Taco Salad, Shrimp, 240, 303

Tahini
  Salmon with Toasted Nuts and,
    230–31, 303–4
  Sesame Coconut Cookies, 266
  in Sesame Dressing, Kale Salad
    with, 173
  in Sesame, Spiced, Apple with,
    255
Tangerines, 83
Taurine, 32–33
Tea
  cookies and, 314
  servings of, 72
  as superfood, 87
Telomeres, 14
TheBestLife.com, xii
Thyme
  Mushrooms, Oven Roasted with
    Green Onion and, 177
  as superfood, 85
  Trout, Whole with Preserved Lemon
    and, 247
Tilapia
  with Black Beans, Green Onions,
    Garlic, and Ginger, 243–44
  fats in, 33
  Fish Sticks, 241–42
  safety/sustainability, 120, 125
Tilefish, safety/sustainability, 116
TMAO, 34
Tofu
  Cabbage Stuffed with Walnuts,
    Cracked Wheat, Raisins and, in a
    Sweet and Sour Tomato Sauce,
    199–200
  in Corn Cake, Sweet, Blueberries
    Baked with, 259
  in Melon with Lemon Sauce, 263
  in Muffins, Carrot, 156
  servings of, 55
  Sloppy Joe, 205–6, 304

Veggie Meatballs over Whole-Grain Spaghetti, 208–9

Tomato(es)

Clams with Garlic and, on Whole-Grain Pasta, 217, 310–11

health benefits of, 84

Mozzarella, and Avocado Sandwich, 294–95

Roasted, with Garlic, 183

Salad, 310

Salad, Peach, Basil and, 182

Salsa, Fresh, Shrimp Taco Salad with, 303

Sauce, Sweet and Sour, Cabbage Stuffed with Tofu, Walnuts, Cracked Wheat, and Raisins in a, 199–200

in Spaghetti, Whole-Grain, Veggie Meatballs over, 208–9

Total Body Makeover (Greene), 109

Trans fats, 39, 69

Traps and pots, 135–36

Trawling, 136–37

Treats. *See also* Desserts

calorie counting, 60, 61, 75, 282

in meal plans, 100, 102, 312–16

Trigger foods, 60

Triglycerides, 17, 32

Triticale, 65

Trolling, 135

Trout

farm-raised, 119, 120, 125

locally caught, 120

in Paper with Summer Squash, Green Onions, and Basil, 245–46

safety/sustainability, 116, 119, 120, 125

and Scrambled Egg, 161, 287

servings of, 56, 86

skin removal, 120

Whole with Thyme and Preserved Lemon, 247

Tuna

albacore, 128

bigeye, 116

Garbanzo Apricot, Curried, 311

safety/sustainability, 127, 128

Salad Sandwich, 298

servings of, 56

yellowfin, 128

Turmeric, 86

U

Ulcerative colitis, 15

V

Vegetable oil

partially hydrogenated, 39

pesticide level, 60

Vegetables. *See also specific vegetables*

and body fat, 13

cruciferous, 83

fiber in, 42

and food poisoning, 129

freshness of, 59

frozen, 82

increasing consumption of, 57–58

nutrients in, 45–46

organic *vs.* conventional, 59

Root, Whole-Wheat Couscous with Garbanzo Beans and, 210–11

seasonal, 153

serving size/calorie level, 58–59, 79, 80

starchy vegetables, 62, 78, 79, 80

snacks, 100, 102, 302

in starch dishes, 63–64

superfoods, 83–84

Veggie Burger, 207

Veggie Meatballs over Whole-Grain Spaghetti, 208–9

Vegetarian/vegan diet, protein sources in, 3–4

Veggie Burger, 207

Veggie Meatballs over Whole-Grain
Spaghetti, 208–9

Vibrio infection, 131

Villalon, Jose R., 139

Vinaigrette, Mustard, 275

Visceral (abdominal) fat, 2, 8, 11–12,
15, 44

Vitamin A, 84

Vitamin B12, 90

Vitamin C, 83

Vitamin D, 89, 90

Vitamin and mineral supplements, 24,
89–91

W

Waistline measurement, 11–12, 17, 74,
283–84

Wakame

Seaweed Salad with Cucumber and
Peanut Butter, 178

in Shiitake Quick Broth with
Edamame and Brown Rice
Noodles, 203–4

Walnut(s)

Cabbage Stuffed with Tofu,
Cracked Wheat, Raisins and, in a
Sweet and Sour Tomato Sauce,
199–200

Cheddar, and Pear, 293

in Granola, 159

as healthy fat source, 36, 68

Pears Baked with Rosemary and,
265, 313

Salad, 295

Sauce, Whole-Grain Pasta Baked
with White Beans, Spinach and,
212–13, 305–6

as superfood, 85

in Veggie Meatballs over Whole-
Grain Spaghetti, 208–9

Whole-Wheat Bread with Seeds and
Nuts, 194–95

Water consumption, 70–72

Watermelon, 60

Water pollution. *See* Pollution

Weight. *See* Body weight

Weight loss, xiv, 54. *See also*
Pescetarian principles

appetite quelling foods in, 9, 15, 57,
85, 281

belly fat, 11–13

biological/psychological factors in,
4–5

and calorie level, 76–77

and dairy products, 47

and genetics, 7–9, 111

gradual, 13

INTERMAP study, 5–6

and legumes, 57

and Mediterranean foods, 4

on the Pescetarian Plan, 3–5

seafood as protein source in, 3–4

and water consumption, 71

Weight maintenance

and addictive eating, 111

and calorie level, 76, 77

and emotional eating, 111–12

and exercise, 13, 72, 92, 103, 106,
107

guidelines for, 91–94

and Pescetarian Plan, 6–7

successful losers, 91, 93–94

Whale and Dolphin Conservation
Society, 137

Wheat Berries

as superfood, 85

as whole grain, 65

in Whole-Wheat Bread with Seeds
and Nuts, 194–95

White Beans

in Veggie Burger, 207

Whole-Grain Pasta Baked with
Spinach, Walnut Sauce and,
212–13, 305–6
White fish, safety/sustainability, 126
Whiting, safety/sustainability, 126
Whole Grain(s)
and abdominal fat reduction, 12
Couscous with Rice Vinegar and
Herbs, 193, 295–96
definition of, 64
glycemic index, 42, 44
nutrients in, 44
vs. refined grains, 64–65
Pancakes with Banana, 162, 289
Pasta Baked with White Beans,
Spinach, and Walnut Sauce,
212–13, 305–6
Pasta, Clams with Tomatoes and
Garlic on, 217, 310–11
serving/calorie level, 63
Spaghetti, Veggie Meatballs over,
208–9
types of, 64–65
Whole-Wheat
Bread with Seeds and Nuts, 194–95
Couscous with Root Vegetables and
Garbanzo Beans, 210–11
Whole-wheat flour, 65
Wildlife Conservation Society, 137
Wild rice, 65
Wine. *See also* Red wine
health benefits of, 48–49
recommended amounts, 61–62
Women, calorie level for weight loss/
maintenance, 76

World Health Organization, 45, 86
World Wildlife Fund, 137, 139

Y
Yellow Squash, Summer Squash Salad
with Lemon and Basil, 181
Yogurt
Avocado Dip, 253
Banana, Peanut Butter Pop, 254,
292
Cucumber, 292
in Eggplant Stuffed with Lentils,
201
flavored, as treat, 314
Fruit, and Chia, 287–88
Greek Yogurt Dip, 293
health benefits of, 46, 47–48
nonfat/low-fat, 66
on-the-run, 297–98
in Pancakes, Whole-Grain, with
Banana, 102
Pistachio, and Pear, 292
plain, 66
serving size/calorie level, 79
in Tuna Garbanzo Apricot, Curried,
311

Z
Zinc, 86
Zucchini
Summer Squash Salad with Lemon
and Basil, 181
Trout in Paper with Summer
Squash, Green Onions, and Basil,
245–46

JANIS JIBRIN, M.S., R.D., is contributing nutrition editor at *SELF* magazine and the lead nutritionist for Best Life (a weight loss and wellness company), writing weekly blogs for TheBestLife.com. She has written hundreds of articles for *Family Circle, Good Housekeeping, More, Men's Health, SELF, Prevention,* and other popular publications. She is the co-author (with Best Life founder, Bob Greene) of *The Life You Want* and *The Best Life Guide to Managing Diabetes and Pre-Diabetes,* and she also wrote *The Supermarket Diet* series, all of which have been *New York Times* bestsellers.

SIDRA FORMAN is a chef, florist, urban farmer, and recipe contributor to Janis Jibrin and Bob Greene's books who lives in Washington, D.C. Her philosophy of cooking, whether for her family, friends, or clients, is that the best-tasting and best-for-you foods should be one and the same.

ThePescetarianPlan.com

ABOUT THE TYPE

This book was set in Scala, a typeface designed by Martin Majoor in 1991. It was originally designed for a music company in the Netherlands and then was published by the international type house FSI FontShop. Its distinctive extended serifs add to the articulation of the letterforms to make it a very readable typeface.